A Century of Service

Mark Loughrey trained as a general nurse at St Vincent's Hospital, Dublin, before specialising in intensive-care nursing. In addition to his postgraduate qualifications in intensive-care nursing from UCD and master's degree in nursing from UCC, he was awarded a PhD in history from UCD in 2015. He currently works as a research nurse.

A Century of Service

A History of the Irish Nurses' and Midwives' Organisation, 1919–2019

Mark Loughrey

Foreword by Liam Doran

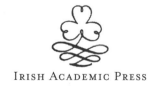

IRISH ACADEMIC PRESS

First published in 2019 by
Irish Academic Press
10 George's Street
Newbridge
Co. Kildare
Ireland
www.iap.ie

© Mark Loughrey, 2019

9781788550628 (Cloth)
9781788550635 (Kindle)
9781788550642 (Epub)
9781788550659 (PDF)

British Library Cataloguing in Publication Data
An entry can be found on request

Library of Congress Cataloging in Publication Data
An entry can be found on request

Typeset in Minion Pro 11/14 pt

Jacket front: 'Charlie's Angels': nurses protest in Dublin in 1978.
Courtesy Derek Speirs.
Jacket back: INMO Whitworth building.
Courtesy Lisa Moyles.

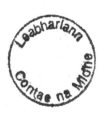

INMO
Irish **Nurses** and **Midwives** Organisation
Working Together

Contents

Author's Note

The views expressed in this book are those of the author and various commentators who took part in oral history interviews or supplied testimonies. They do not necessarily reflect the official position of the Irish Nurses' and Midwives' Organisation. The author apologises for any and all errors and omissions; these are honest and unintentional. All reasonable efforts have been made to contact the owners, or descendants of owners, of copyrighted images/ text reproduced herein; no copyright infringement is intended.

Acknowledgements

This book would not have been possible were it not for the help I received from a number of people and organisations. First and foremost, I would like to thank the Irish Nurses' and Midwives' Organisation (INMO) for facilitating me in accessing their archives and for welcoming me each time I visited their headquarters and attended their Executive Council meetings and annual delegate conferences. In particular, I would like to thank Liam Doran, Martina Harkin-Kelly, Dave Hughes, Phil Ní Sheaghdha, Clare Treacy, Elizabeth Adams, Cathriona Lacey, Marion Behan, Olympic gold medallist Lorcan Byrne, Albert Murphy, Dr Edward Mathews, Muriel Haire and the organisation's Executive Council, past and present. I would also like to thank P.J. Madden, Noreen Muldoon and Lenore Mrkwicka, all former staff of the organisation.

Some individuals went over and beyond the call of duty in assisting me and deserve a special mention. At the INMO they include Lisa Moyles, Freda Hughes, Oona Sugrue, Annette Kennedy, Sheila Dickson, Claire Mahon, Michaela Ruane and the excellent staff at the INMO's library, namely Niamh Adams, Aileen Rohan, Rhona Ledwidge and Edel Reynolds. At the School of Nursing, Midwifery and Health Systems at University College Dublin (UCD) they include Dr Martin McNamara and Professor Gerard Fealy – gentlemen and scholars alike. A big thank you too to Dr Una Molloy for sharing a desk (and a few coffees and laughs) with me while we completed our PhDs at UCD. (We finally made it, Una!) A very big thank you also goes to all those who took part in oral history interviews and contributed testimonies – this book wouldn't have been the same without you. A special mention must go to the INMO's Editorial Committee for their many suggestions and for keeping me on the straight and narrow, especially Kay Craughwell for her mind, memory and meticulous attention to detail. Sincere gratitude also to Conor Graham, Fiona Dunne and the team at Irish Academic Press/Merrion Press for taking on this project and bringing it to fruition.

A number of other individuals and organisations were also of assistance. They include MedMedia, Dublin; Dr Odette Best, Queensland University of Technology; Noelle Dowling, Dublin Diocesan Archives; Francis Devine; the Irish Association of Directors of Nursing and Midwifery; John Kane, Medical Laboratory Scientists' Association; Séamas Sheils, Irish Bank Officials'

Association; the Irish Municipal Public and Civil Trade Union; the Services
Industrial Professional and Technical Union; the Teachers' Union of Ireland;
the Association of Secondary Teachers, Ireland; Professor Adrian Frazier,
NUI, Galway; the National Archives, Ireland, in particular, Brian O'Donnell;
Fiona Bourne, Royal College of Nursing Archives; Dr John Sweeney,
University College Cork; Martina Kearns; Liz Gillis; Derek Speirs; Press 22;
Lensmen; Mark Stedman; Áine Duggan; Photocall Ireland; the Nursing
and Midwifery Board of Ireland, in particular, Catherine Rooney; Professor
Richard English, University of St Andrews; Dr Emmet O'Connor, University
of Ulster; the International Labour Organisation; the International Council
of Nurses; Debbie Emerson; Warren Hawkes, Michael D'Amario and Helen
Anotoniak, New York State Nurses' Association; Christen Tracey, Australian
Nurses' Federation; Victoria Branch; Rita Martin, New South Wales Nurses'
Association; UCD Archives; Phillip Martin, Irish Newspaper Archives; the
Irish Press; the *Irish Independent*; Irish Labour History Society Archives; the
National Archives, Kew, England; James Hardiman Library Archives, NUI,
Galway; Cork City and County Archives; Therese Bradley; Ruth Geraghty;
Dr Mary Bell; Dr Seán Lucey; Eamon Devoy, the Technical Engineering and
Electrical Union; the administrative staff at Mount Jerome Cemetery, Dublin;
the greatly missed Margaret Ó hÓgartaigh; the Military Archives, Dublin; the
Catholic Nurses Guild of Ireland; the National Library of Ireland; Proinnsíos Ó
Duigneáin; John Vanek; Tony Cotton; Carl Mortished; Anne MacLellan; Eric
Wilkinson; Siobhan Horgan Ryan; Mary Hawkins; the Irish History Students'
Association; Desmond Bates; Elizabeth Anne McMahon; Ida Milne; Rosemary
Cullen Owens; Christiaan Corlett; Sandra Lefroy; Pearse Street Library, Dublin;
Trinity College Library, Dublin; NUI, Maynooth Library; UCC Library and
Audrey Drohan and staff at UCD Library.

   Finally, a really, really special word of thanks to my good friend, comrade
and mentor Dr Joan McCarthy at the School of Nursing and Midwifery at
University College Cork, for giving me a start.

No Pressure – No Progress

I wish to begin by saying what a privilege it is to be asked to write the foreword to this book celebrating the first one hundred years of this great, vibrant and growing organisation. I wish to thank the President of the Irish Nurses' and Midwives' Organisation's (INMO), Martina Harkin-Kelly, the organisation's Executive Council, the book's publishers, Irish Academic Press, and, most of all, the book's author, Mark Loughrey, for inviting me to give my reflections. I have had the great privilege of working for this organisation, in various capacities, for almost thirty-five years. In that time, I have seen it become the most visible, vocal, dynamic and active professional trade union in Ireland, and I am sure the best is yet to come.

The story told in this book and the journey travelled in the past century confirms that, in relation to nursing and midwifery, there has never been any progress without the INMO applying pressure for change and improvements in the interests of nurses, midwives, patients and other service users. I cannot remember one situation over the past one hundred years when employers have been willing to recognise, respect and pay nurses/midwives for the role they play and the work they do in the provision of health care. In fact, both the government's and management's approach over the decades has been to consistently exclude nurses and midwives from policy-making decisions and from the management of services. The years are filled with warm words, which proved nothing more than empty rhetoric from ministers and senior management. The time was never right to recognise the contribution of nurses and midwives, so the INMO had to work harder, much harder than others to ensure any degree of recognition.

The Early Years

I have often wondered what the atmosphere was like, and what was actually said, when that small group of nurses and midwives gathered in South Anne Street in 1919 and agreed to formally establish the Irish Nurses' Union (INU). These were women who had undoubtedly seen and worked through appalling working conditions and had come to the realisation that collective action was necessary to improve their situation. On that evening in February 1919, the struggle to establish a national union must have seemed daunting, but their courage overcame their concerns. Therefore, as we celebrate one hundred years, I wish to begin this foreword by saying I stand in awe of these women who started the journey that now sees the INMO represent almost 41,000 members across all health services in this country while also enjoying global recognition. The courage of that small group of women who gathered on that cold February evening in 1919 must never be forgotten and always recognised and respected.

As the early decades of this organisation's growth and development tell us, those first years saw it grow as it fostered relationships with other bodies, i.e., the Irish Women Workers' Union (IWWU) and also international bodies such as the International Council of Nurses (ICN). It can also be seen that the organisation, while constantly seeking improvements in pay and conditions, had a social side, i.e., the 'Nurses' Dance', which was also vibrant – we might smile now, but at the time this was an integral part of the organisation and what it did.

It is said history repeats itself, and I was so pleased to see the INMO purchase, redevelop and open the Richmond Hospital as our national Education and Event Centre in 2018. I also note that the first programmes for members took place in February 2018, some eighty years to the week when the Irish Nurses' Organisation (INO, as we were then known) held its first professional development programmes in the Richmond. This reaffirms the twin objectives of meeting both the socio-economic and the educational and professional development needs of members, which has always been the hallmark of this great organisation. It should also be noted that within the first fifty years, the organisation was instrumental in the commencement of programmes leading to registered qualifications in general, psychiatric, intellectual disability nursing and midwifery, together with specialist programmes in such areas as theatre and intensive/coronary care. The commencement of all of these programmes, leading to formal recognition and ultimately additional pay for certain qualifications or for those working in certain areas, only happened because the INMO applied pressure leading to progress. No pressure – no progress without the INMO.

The 1970s: Significant Change Begins

I think it is fair to say, based upon Mark's excellent work reflected in this book, that the winds of real change, leading to greater visibility, assertiveness and militancy, began in the early to mid-1970s. In the early 1970s, the public service marriage ban was lifted. In 1973, Ireland joined the European Common Market (now the European Union). Both of these events changed the face of every workplace and injected new energy into the INO.

In the context of the organisation's growth and development, perhaps the most significant event of the 1970s was the decision, taken at the Annual Conference in 1978, for the organisation to seek affiliation to the Irish Trade Union Congress (ICTU). This was a watershed moment in the history of the organisation. It was, without doubt, an expression of frustration at the treatment of nurses and midwives at the hands of government and management. It demonstrated a willingness to be more militant, assertive and demanding in the interests of members. Irreversible change had begun and continues to this day. The debate, chaired by the then President, Carmel Taaffe, was determined, eloquent, inclusive and ultimately decisive. The INO was to write to the ICTU to seek affiliation. At this point, I think it is only appropriate that I would recognise the leadership role played by Ms Taaffe, who, as a Director of Nursing, was not expected to lead the INO into a more militant 'trade union' stance. I clearly remember, as I was beginning my third year as a student intellectual disabilities nurse in St Mary's, Drumcar, Co. Louth, the vital role played by this great president as she realised the organisation must join with the wider union movement in pursuance of the interests of its members. She was a great leader.

The changes and events of the mid to late 1970s reflected the growing militancy and changing dynamic of the nursing and midwifery workforce. They also confirmed the beginning of radical change and transformation in the thinking, strategies and actions of the INO. This would gather further pace in the 1980s.

The 1980s

Just before 9:30 a.m. on Monday, 13 June 1983, I, as the INO's first Student Officer, entered 20 Lower Leeson Street to start my first day in a new job. I had qualified as an intellectual disabilities nurse and as a general nurse at St Mary's, Drumcar, Co. Louth, and at Our Lady of Lourdes Hospital, Drogheda, respectively, and had worked as a staff nurse in both services since first commencing my student nurse education on 16 November 1976. On that day, I was informed by Kevin Downey (Membership Officer), who retired only recently and was a tremendous servant to the organisation, that membership numbers were 9,200, with only 400 of these (approximately) being students. My job was to recruit all student nurses and to develop services for our student nurse members which would, following qualification, lead them to become members of the organisation. Ireland at that time was facing high levels of unemployment and mass emigration. Nurses and midwives were emigrating following qualification as there was simply no work in Ireland. The work that was available was only temporary, with payment on the minimum of the scale, no incremental credit, no holidays and no respect.

If I am honest, it is something of a mystery to me as to how the organisation, with its conservative stance on many issues in the workplace, continued to survive in the face of massive efforts to recruit nurses by the Irish Transport and General Workers' Union (ITGWU) and Psychiatric Nurses' Association (PNA). It became very obvious that unless we changed rapidly we would no longer be fit for purpose; we could no longer expect to make progress on our agenda, and ultimately, we would no longer remain relevant to nurses and midwives.

In 1985, following the retirement of the legendary Ena Meehan, the organisation appointed a new General Secretary, John Pepper, who remained in the post for approximately two years. I remember during his tenure that the organisation became actively involved in a dispute about the cost of accommodation for student nurses in hospitals across the country. This gave the organisation visibility on national television and radio. However, in 1987, following the departure of John Pepper, the organisation appointed P.J. Madden, who had been the General Secretary of the PNA. The organisation would never be the same again.

The health service continued to be seriously underfunded, leading to cutbacks in services, with all areas suffering from severe staff shortages. The then Minister for Health, Dr Rory O'Hanlon TD, when responding to a Dáil question, said nursing was a highly mobile, international, marketable commodity, and we would always see Irish-educated nurses and midwives emigrating, but they would come back. This flawed thinking continues to the present day and reflects again the lack of respect toward nurses and midwives shown by ministers and management. Against this background, the new General Secretary and Executive Council held a nationwide ballot in protest at the working conditions of members. This ballot, which provided for industrial action up to and including the withdrawal of labour, showed a two to one vote in favour of taking action in the absence of concrete measures to address the problem of staff shortages and poor pay.

In tandem with this industrial strategy, the organisation, again through the determination of the presidents of the time, Biddy Butler and Ita O'Dwyer, coupled with the energy of P.J., redoubled its efforts to affiliate to the ICTU.

The efforts to affiliate had made little progress due to such issues as spheres of influence (the name given to inter-union arrangements about membership) and the INO's possible approach, if affiliated, to an ICTU call for an all-out strike.

The INO finally affiliated in the early 1990s. This was a momentous development that brought the organisation into mainstream trade union activity. It also meant involvement in the periodic negotiations leading to social partnership agreements. These agreements not only covered pay, but increasingly agreements with regard to wider policy issues, thus affording the organisation input into these discussions on an ongoing basis. As a result of these developments, the late 1980s/early 1990s, were a time of great change for the INO. These changes sowed the seeds for the more visible, vocal, demanding and aggressive professional trade union for nurses and midwives that we have today.

1992–2008

It is my honest view that the period of 1992–2008 was when the organisation came of age. The INO was now getting into its stride. However, it was clear that improving the relative position of nursing/midwifery in terms of pay and conditions was not resting easily with either government or sister trade unions. I have to place on record that it is my absolute conviction that the INO, by applying pressure, initiated, led, shaped and delivered all of the changes in the area of pay, conditions, professional development, educational pathways, staffing levels and structures that took place during this time.

It is a constant source of frustration to me that academics, other stakeholders and the media have failed to recognise and acknowledge the role that the INO has played in the massive changes that took place over these sixteen years. I have had many discussions with academics, people from state agencies, senior people from international nursing bodies and the media. All of them, when commenting upon the changes and the events over this period, have completely underestimated the influence of, and the central role played by, the INO. That is why, in this book, I wish to state quite clearly that if you want to know why nursing and midwifery in Ireland was the subject of massive change and progress over this period, then look no further than the INO, because this great organisation made it all happen. Here is the timeframe:

1992

The INO opened its Professional Development Centre and Library for members, in its then headquarters in Fitzwilliam Place. This was a tangible demonstration of the organisation's commitment to the entire spectrum of services required by the student and qualified member. Twenty-six years later, we opened the Richmond as our state-of-the-art Education and Event Centre – real progress.

1994: Galway Diploma

Following months of discussions with senior officials in the Department of Health, the 'Galway Diploma' commenced in 1994. This saw the nursing programme in University College Hospital Galway linked with a diploma awarded by University College Galway, and was the first significant step of linking nurse education to the third level sector. The programme was so successful that in 1996, the model was adopted across the country, with partnerships being formed between all major hospitals and their local university/third level institution. This reflected the efforts of the INO, as directed by numerous motions adopted at annual conferences, to seek the introduction of an undergraduate degree programme leading to registration as a nurse in this country.

1996

In tandem with the beginnings of this revolution in undergraduate nurse education, the INO was also actively engaged in discussions at national level with health employers with regard to the pay, grading and conditions of employment applicable to all grades of nurse and midwife. These discussions culminated in what became known as the Blue Book Agreement. However, this did not resolve the level of dissatisfaction felt by members in all workplaces with regard to their pay, hours of work and staffing levels. That is why, in early 1997, the organisation obtained a mandate, following a national ballot, for the commencement of nationwide industrial action in pursuance of improvements in pay and conditions. At the last moment, and again following direct discussions, the then Minister for Health, Michael Noonan, in tandem with implementing certain pay and other revised grading structures, agreed to establish a Commission on Nursing. The commission was to be chaired by a High Court Judge. It would undertake a review of the professions and make recommendations as to how they should be reshaped and revitalised to meet the expectations of nurses, midwives and the needs of patients within a changing health service.

1997

The commission, which was chaired by High Court Judge, Justice Mella Carroll (her niece Jean still works for the INMO), was established in 1997, with the organisation represented by Eilish Hardiman (now Chief Executive Officer of the National Children's Hospital) and our then General Secretary, P.J. Madden. The commission carried out an exhaustive examination of nursing and midwifery, making some national and international comparisons, and in September 1998 it produced its final report with over 200 recommendations.

1998

As coincidence would have it, the commission reported immediately following my appointment as General Secretary. The commission's report was launched in Dublin Castle and was the subject of much media attention. It was recognised that its recommendations would decide whether the dissatisfaction of nurses and midwives would be allayed or if the potential for nationwide industrial action remained. I can vividly recall the evening of the launch of the report when the then Minister for Health, Brian Cowen said effectively that the government accepted the 197 non-pay-related recommendations. However, in relation to the three pay-related recommendations, these would have to be considered in the context of any future national or public service pay agreement.

That evening, the INO, through a press statement, indicated that if the government failed to implement all of the recommendations with timelines for full implementation, it would hold a national ballot of all members seeking a mandate for nationwide industrial action involving the withdrawal of labour. The government, supported by other public service unions, refused to agree to implement the pay-related recommendations; the ballot commenced and an overwhelming mandate was given.

1999

In the weeks and months leading up to 19 October 1999 (when the nine-day national nurses' all-out strike began), there were numerous efforts and offers made and rejected to avert the action. However, all of the offers made were in the context of existing public service pay policy and did not provide for the required uplift in the relative pay of nurses and midwives. Internally, in preparation for the nationwide action, the organisation, both through debates at annual conference and decisions of the Executive Council, decided that if the action was to go ahead it would be nationwide, involve all services, and all members with emergency care being provided, unpaid, by members working to an INO Strike Committee in every workplace. This approach to industrial action, the first of its kind to be taken by the organisation, was the subject of much heated debate. However, it was felt that for the action to be effective and to be accepted by all members, it had to be universal, inclusive and absolute. In these weeks and months, the INO became a union in every workplace, and we have never looked back.

19 October 1999

I will always remember waking up at 6:00 a.m. on Tuesday 19 October and listening to the news confirming that at 8:00 a.m., the first ever national nurses' and midwives' strike would commence. The country would only have emergency level health services in operation, with all routine work cancelled. I spent that day attending numerous picket lines. We were dealing with massive media interest, both national and international, making constant efforts to reaffirm the legitimate claims behind the dispute and confirm that the action would not endanger the health of any patient or service user. My last media engagement was on the *Vincent Browne Show* at 10:00 p.m. that night. The first question I was asked was 'Liam Doran, what gives nurses the right to let people die as a result of their strike action?' I did my best, over a very difficult forty-minute interview, to explain that all emergency cover was being provided, and while people died every day in the country's hospitals, they would not die that day, or any other day, because of any industrial action being taken by INO members.

Over the following nine days, INO members in every area of our health service were brilliant and showed remarkable dedication to each other in terms of trade union solidarity and also to their patients. Over those nine days, on a 24/7 basis, Strike Committees (all of whom were absolute heroes) organised shifts which involved the provision of an emergency level of cover (without pay) and rostering for picket duties.

Despite the best efforts of a small section of health management and the media, throughout those nine days no adverse incident leading to a negative outcome for any patient or client could be found. Our members, even in the heat of industrial action, were excellent, committed and dedicated professionals. While it was unbelievably challenging those nine days during October 1999 are something that I am immensely proud of as I was privileged to work with, and for, such people of pure class, professionalism, dignity and determination.

21 October 1999

On this day, over 10,000 members marched down O'Connell Street, and we held a mass rally outside the General Post Office. It was a tremendous show of solidarity as members from every corner of the country came together to demand fair pay. At 10:00 p.m. that evening, talks to resolve the dispute began in Government Buildings and continued until early in the morning of Monday 25 October. Outstanding issues were then referred to the Labour Court, which convened a hearing involving all parties at 2:30 p.m. that Monday afternoon. Throughout this period, the strike committees continued to manage the provision of services and organise pickets.

27 October 1999

After nine days of industrial action and six days of negotiations involving independently chaired engagement and a Labour Court hearing, a set of proposals emerged at 4:00 p.m. on Wednesday 27 October. The INO's Executive Council met immediately and decided that the court's recommendations should be recommended for acceptance by the membership. The nationwide action would be suspended to allow for information meetings and balloting, with effect from 8:00 p.m. that Wednesday night, with all normal services resuming.

For obvious reasons, the Executive Council felt it was necessary to commence information meetings with members immediately. The first was arranged for St James' Hospital, Dublin, that Wednesday evening at 8:30 p.m. I have no doubt, having attended literally hundreds of meetings, that the atmosphere at that meeting was unique. There was standing room only, and members were literally leaning in the windows demanding access to information and answers to questions. Feelings were, for legitimate reasons, running very high, and the situation was very tense, with much initial anger. Over the following ten days we held many such meetings. On the Thursday morning of 28 October 1999 at 7:30 a.m., I met with over 400 members in Beaumont Hospital, Dublin. During this meeting I had to do an interview on *Morning Ireland*, in the course of which I was asked if I would resign if the members rejected the Labour Court recommendation. This period was, without doubt, very challenging for me both personally and professionally, but through great teamwork and togetherness, led by Anne Cody, another great INO President, we survived. It also marked the INO literally coming of age as a trade union.

In the end, the Labour Court Recommendation was accepted by a vote of 63 per cent in favour and 37 per cent against. The organisation moved immediately to demand full implementation of all the recommendations.

2000: Post-Mortem and Delivering

In the immediate aftermath of the strike and the decision of members to accept the recommendations, a meeting took place with the Minister for Health, Brian Cowen, his two junior ministers and all of the senior officials in the Department of Health. This was the first time that all three ministers in the department had met with the organisation. It was obvious that in addition to securing the proposals from the Labour Court following industrial action, the INO was now on the political radar screen and was recognised as being the voice of nurses and midwives. Critically, it was now a trade union with whom the government of the day would have to be prepared to do business.

It is my view that this level of political recognition and visibility in the eyes of the public which emerged from the nine-day national strike was as important as the tangible measures, and they were significant, gained as a result of the strike settlement. I am adamant that the centrality of the organisation from that November 1999 period to the present day is measurably different to anything that existed before and is still producing benefits to INMO members.

Following the settlement of the strike, the organisation, once again showing its maturity and integrity, immediately commenced two processes:

- Implementing the strike settlement and the Commission on Nursing recommendations; and
- Initiating nationwide consultation, with members, to carry out a post-strike evaluation of what had been done, what had worked, what had not worked and what lessons must be learned for any future industrial action campaigns.

In this context, the period 1999–2001 was challenging, dynamic and exciting. It was a period when the organisation showed tremendous resilience as we engaged internally and externally on matters of huge significance all the while analysing, learning and changing.

2002–6

As a direct result of the Commission on Nursing, which was established to avoid industrial action threatened by the INO and following the national strike in 1999, the government funded the introduction of a four-year undergraduate nursing degree programme in general, intellectual disability and psychiatric nursing, which commenced in September 2002. Once again, I say if there had been no pressure applied by the INO through industrial action we would never have secured the four-year degree programmes, and we would still have the old 'apprenticeship' model. In 2006, this undergraduate four-year pathway was extended to midwifery, which saw, for the first time in this country, a direct entry, third-level midwifery programme being available. This development, which again was a long-term goal of the INO, had the effect of requiring the organisation, in 2010, to change its name from the Irish Nurses' Organisation to the Irish Nurses' and Midwives' Organisation. For the first time in a long time in Ireland, a member could be a midwife and not a nurse, and the name of the organisation had to reflect this reality.

2006: Working Hours

The organisation now moved to tackle the inequality in the working hours of nurses and midwives compared to other health professionals. This led, again after a sustained campaign involving six weeks of work-to-rule, to the introduction of a 37.5-hour week for nurses/midwives in July 2008. This was the first time in over forty years that a single group, grade, or category of worker in this country had secured for itself a reduction in the working week separate from any other adjustment in the working week for all workers in the state. The campaign of 2007/08 in relation to working hours and the working week was an example of the lessons learned from the 1999 dispute. This reduction in working hours was a remarkable achievement by the organisation and one for which I was very proud.

However, after this period of massive change, revolution and improvement in the relative pay of nurses and midwives from 1999–2008, all was now about to change. The period 2008–14 would, from a very different perspective, again test the organisation's resilience, infrastructure and unionateness.

2008

In late September 2008, only three months after the INO secured a 37.5-hour working week for members, the government was forced to introduce measures that would guarantee all of the country's major banks in terms of their liabilities, borrowings and deposits. This decision, taken in the early hours of a Friday morning, was eventually to cost the country over €64 billion, which the Irish taxpayer (that is, our children's children) will be paying for years into the future. This economic Armageddon was brought about by the reckless, greedy and craven behaviour of all of the banks, which saw senior management, who were earning millions per annum, act as if they were gods, as if they were untouchable and as if they could do no wrong. The reality is that over a number of years leading up to 2008, they borrowed, lent and created a market that was unsustainable and which would ultimately bring the country to its knees.

In order to honour the bank guarantee, the government was forced very quickly to enter into a financial arrangement with the IMF. This would see the country, for an extended period, effectively lose our economic independence, sovereignty and control over the provision of public services. All government spending decisions were subject to IMF approval, and we had the spectre of officials, from the IMF and associated entities, periodically visiting Dublin to oversee the government's recovery programme. I always thought it was somewhat ironic to see on the news these officials walk across from the Merrion Hotel (where rooms cost €500 per night) into the Department of Finance to ensure that the government imposed cuts on social welfare and pension recipients, who were trying to live on €200 or less per week. These people had the hardest of necks and had no understanding of the pressures facing ordinary families. The impact on families, and on the country, of having to avail of the loan from the IMF, was massive. All taxpayers, including all public servants, i.e., nurses and midwives, were faced with increased levels of taxes, the introduction of the Universal Social Charge and the introduction of various additional charges such as the Local Property Tax.

As part of this reflection, I would like to make the following observations about the decisions made during those dark and dismal years:

1. It is often forgotten that in September 2008, before the government introduced a public service recruitment embargo, the HSE introduced its own recruitment embargo. At that time, the HSE excluded doctors and allied health professionals from the recruitment ban. However, they refused to exclude nurses/midwives with the result that, very rapidly, staffing levels on the frontline were cut in a wholly unmanaged, damaging and indefensible way.

2. The decision to include nurses and midwives in the ban, while excluding other grades, is yet another example of management's inherent bias against nurses/midwives and total ignorance of the delivery of healthcare in the frontline. There is also a view, held by senior people in the civil service and periodically across government, that because we have thousands of nurses we can cut numbers without any damage being done to the health service. How wrong they were,

how wrong they are, and how many patients have suffered as a result of this flawed approach?

3. The insistence, particularly by the European Union that the government fully repay all bond holders (senior and junior) through the IMF programme, was, and is, indefensible, and caused hurt and damage to thousands of families across the country. We were effectively told that we had to reward risk-takers while ordinary citizens, on ordinary incomes, were faced with cuts which meant they could not pay bills, could not adequately feed their children, were forced to live in poverty and even forced to lose their homes. All of this was done to 'protect' the world's banking system. However, I believe all of this was done because the elite always look after their fellow elite, regardless of the impact upon ordinary people. It was simply a modern version of the famous phrase of Marie Antoinette: 'Let them eat cake'.

4. During this period there were repeated efforts, often as a result of alliances between the government and certain public sector unions, to target allowances and premium pay as part of the cutback measures. For the first time, we heard the phrase 'core pay', which effectively became code for leaving the pay of civil servants and administrators alone while cutting the pay of those who worked unsocial hours, weekends and night duty. In response to this, the INMO was instrumental in the establishment of the 24/7 Alliance. This saw the unions and organisations representing frontline staff (i.e., nurses, midwives, gardaí, prison officers and paramedics) come together and mount a campaign of resistance over any further cuts to those who worked unsocial hours. This campaign had two highlights, which I will always remember:

    •   The silent march, in uniform, down O'Connell Street, Dublin, which saw over 3,000 frontline public servants march in visible solidarity with each other; and

    •   The famous rally, at the National Basketball Arena, Tallaght, which saw over 4,500 frontline public servants come together to again show that they would not tolerate any further cuts targeted at them.

    I am proud to say that the INMO was at the forefront of organising the 24/7 Campaign. I am certain that without this mobilisation of uniformed frontline public servants, even more draconian measures would have been imposed upon us.

5. One of my proudest moments as General Secretary of this great union was when, in 2013, the INMO, together with three other unions,

walked out of talks with the government. The talks had begun on a Friday and by Sunday it was clear that the government, with the tacit agreement of a number of public service unions, were preparing to table measures that would see cuts in Sunday and night duty premiums. These cuts would only affect staff who worked on a 24/7 basis. The INMO negotiating team and I wish to acknowledge the strength and conviction of my great colleagues Phil Ní Sheaghdha, Dave Hughes and Eddie Mathews, who decided to leave the process as we could not accept the imposition of such measures, which would result in a further 11 per cent cut in the take home pay of an average nurse/midwife. I am happy to say that we were joined in our decision to leave the process by the Irish Medical Organisation, Unite and the Civil and Public Services Union. The remaining fourteen public service unions, together with the government representatives, remained in talks that Sunday evening, resulting in a draft agreement being finalised and made public on the Monday. In the following days, the INMO's decision to leave the process was publicly criticised by other trade unions and government spokespersons, and our commitment to represent our members was questioned. History will show that in the following six weeks the INMO, together with the other three unions and the PNA, undertook a nationwide campaign involving town hall meetings and press conferences. This resulted in a total of fourteen of the nineteen public service unions rejecting the proposals, as ordinary members of other public service unions saw and understood how flawed and unjust they were.

6. If those proposals had been accepted, we would have seen Sunday/ Bank Holiday and night duty premiums cut to time and one-sixth. As the cuts did not actually take place because the proposals were rejected, the reality is that members did not fully appreciate the importance and strength of the campaign put forward by the INMO and this union's commitment to protect its members' interests in the face of loud opposition from management and regrettably, from other public service unions. The reality is some of those public service unions have still not forgiven, or forgotten, the fact that the INMO understood their members more than they did.

7. I also believe that instead of building on the strength of unity arising from the rejection of the flawed Haddington Road 2 proposals, a number of unions quickly recommenced negotiations with the government on an individual basis. While the proposals that emerged from these talks,

which were done on a single union-to-government basis, were far less draconian, we should have collectively refused to negotiate, stood our ground and said that the earlier pension levy and pay cuts were more than enough of a contribution from public servants.

8. To add insult to injury, the Haddington Road proposals, which were ultimately accepted by individual unions following national ballots, also included an increase in the working week of between 1.5 to 2 hours. This resulted in the gain that we had obtained in 2008, of moving from 39 to 37.5 hours, being taken back, and nurses recommenced working a 39-hour week in 2013. This, undoubtedly, was one of my saddest days as General Secretary. However, it is also a reality that if we had not brokered a collective agreement between the INMO and the government, it would have used legislation to impose even more draconian cuts, including the lengthening of the working week. This would have been even more damaging to individual members.

9. It was in these negotiations that the government and senior management decided they could impose even deeper cuts on newly qualified nurses and midwives. The flawed, insulting, damaging and futile Graduate Scheme was part of the Haddington Road proposals. I vividly remember, at 4:00 a.m., meeting with senior management and telling them they were wrong and that newly qualified nurses/midwives would never accept the posts offering 85 per cent of salary (a total pay cut since 2009 of 39 per cent) and that they would simply emigrate. However, they would not listen, and in yet another show of disrespect, came forward with the scheme. History shows that, within one year, it was reckless, and instead of retaining newly qualified professionals, it was only speeding up their exit from the country. By 2017, we were once again recruiting, but the damage was done, and this is still being felt today.

Overall, the period of 2008–13 was undoubtedly very grim. No trade union General Secretary, particularly this trade union General Secretary, goes to work to tell their members, on three occasions, to accept cuts which would reduce their pay and terms and conditions of employment. It is a fact that we had no choice, as the only alternative was to allow the government, with the power of legislation, to impose even greater cuts. However, this does not in any way minimise the demoralising and damaging impact of these cuts upon members who, quite rightly, questioned what their trade union was doing for them.

2014: Restoration Begins

While having to accept and endure these measures, history will also show that the INMO, in 2014, began the process of restoring the cuts imposed during those dark years. Starting with the restoration of the Senior Staff Nurse scale, which had been abolished with other allowances in 2011, the organisation began to secure the restoration of allowances, grading structures and undergraduate pay. Recruitment recommenced while we participated in talks that began the process of restoring the pay that had been cut in 2009 and 2011. However, untold damage was done, and our current recruitment and retention crisis is as a direct result of management thinking that nurses/midwives will always be there. They will not!

To the Future

This process continues, with the INMO being central to all initiatives seeking to restore lost ground. I know that the INMO will not rest until all conditions that were cut, including the working week, have been restored and our pay claim of parity with other health professionals has been realised. The only question will be whether these totally legitimate goals will be achieved through process and procedure or whether they will require a national campaign of industrial action.

I retired from the position of General Secretary at the beginning of 2018, and Phil Ní Sheaghdha is now our General Secretary. Phil has taken over an organisation with almost 41,000 members, over seventy staff, the best education centre of any trade union in the country and local structures that are strong, dynamic and effective. This organisation, particularly throughout the last thirty years, has become a union for nurses and midwives recognised the world over as effective, responsive, visible and relevant. In other words, the journey is only starting, and I look forward to the many successes this organisation will secure in the coming years.

Thank you. It was a privilege.

Liam Doran

100 Years Young: 1919–2019

*'The belief that we have come from somewhere is closely linked
with the belief that we are going somewhere.'[1]*

1919 was a signature year for nursing in Ireland. Not only did it witness the passage of the *Nurses Registration (Ireland) Act,* which established professional regulation and registration for nurses, it also witnessed the establishment of Ireland's largest trade union and professional association for nurses and midwives. On the occasion of its centenary, this book tells the story of that union, known originally as the Irish Nurses' Union (INU), known since 1936 as the Irish Nurses' Organisation (INO) and known since 2010 as the Irish Nurses' and Midwives' Organisation (INMO). The organisation's original remit, which focussed almost exclusively on improving members' pay and working conditions, has expanded to encompass education; professional, regulatory and social policy issues; and patient advocacy.

Over the course of its 100-year history, the organisation has grown from just twenty members to some 40,000. This book is for them. It is for the minority of members who take an active role in the organisation, who attend meetings and who, as nurse/midwife representatives, assist their colleagues on a daily basis. The INMO would not be there without them. But it's also for the nurses and midwives who take a less active role in the organisation. If you are one such member, then you are in the majority. However, your membership is every bit as valid and valuable as that of the active members, perhaps more so because in *you* lies potential. So, come a little closer: there's lots to be done, and *you* can help.

The author of this history, as a nurse and member of the organisation, is aligned with and immersed in the subject matter. The history is also informed by the organisation's own publications and by interviews with the organisation's members, employees and leaders. This likely biases the story told, but the extent of that bias, and whether or not such bias is a bad thing, is up to the reader to decide. The recurring theme in this book, as indicated in its title, is service, and these pages explore the vast and varied service that the organisation provided to nurses and midwives through the years. The book also explores service from another vantage point. The vexed question of strikes within essential service-oriented professions such as nursing and midwifery was, and is, a central tension within the organisation and within nurse and midwife trade unionism more generally. Industrial action by nurses and midwives, up to and including strike action, raises ethical questions regarding patient welfare, and this book looks closely at how the organisation negotiated these tensions through the years.

Where possible, the book recounts the INMO's history in nurses' and midwives' own words, and the many interviews and testimonies add a personal perspective. They speak of struggles heretofore untold; they speak of the passion and poignancy that comes with nursing, midwifery and trade unionism more generally; they speak to the importance of history's oral tradition; they tell tales that otherwise would never have been told; and for all of posterity, they will say 'we were here'. The images scattered throughout the book's pages aim to lighten the reader's load along the way. More than that, you will see that they also tell a story in their own right. Although this history is a comprehensive one, it focusses mostly on the key events and campaigns. In order to show the reader some mercy, many aspects of the organisation's history, interesting as they were, had to be excluded. Hence, the INMO has many more untold stories awaiting a new generation of nursing, midwifery and labour historians to recount. So what's stopping you?

Presidents of the Irish Nurses' and Midwives' Organisation

1919–25	Louie Bennett
1925–34	Mary McCarry
1934–54	Nellie Healy
1954–7	Eileen O'Sullivan
1957–9	Mary Prunty
1959–63	Eileen O'Sullivan
1963–71	Maureen McCabe
1971–5	Maeve Keane
1975–9	Carmel Taaffe
1979–81	Maeve Keane
1981–5	Ita O'Dwyer
1985–9	Bridget Butler
1989–91	Ita O'Dwyer
1991–6	Kathleen Craughwell
1996–2000	Anne Cody
2000–3	Clare Spillane
2003–4	Eilish Corcoran (acting), then Ann Martin
2004–8	Madeline Spiers
2008–12	Sheila Dickson
2012–16	Claire Mahon
2016–present	Martina Harkin-Kelly

General Secretaries of the Irish Nurses' and Midwives' Organisation

1919–21	Marie Mortished
1921–9	Kathleen Nora Price
1929–43	Annie Smithson
1943–59	Eleanor Grogan
1960–84	Christina Meehan
1984–6	John Pepper
1986–98	P.J. Madden
1998–2018	Liam Doran
2018–present	Phil Ní Sheaghdha

Headquarters of the Irish Nurses' and Midwives' Organisation

1919–30	29 South Anne Street, Dublin
1930–6	28 Upper O'Connell Street, Dublin
1936–43	24 Nassau Street, Dublin
1943–51	Dawson House, 15 Dawson Street, Dublin
1951–87	20 Lower Leeson Street, Dublin
1987–2003	11 Fitzwilliam Place, Dublin
2003–present	The Whitworth Building, North Brunswick Street, Dublin
2018–present	The Richmond Building, North Brunswick Street, Dublin

CHAPTER 1

Setting the Scene

I. A (Very) Brief History of Trade Unionism in Ireland

From the late 1600s, 'combinations' of workmen, precursors to today's trade unions, were beginning to form in Ireland. Combinations comprised skilled craftsmen and had practical concerns; for example, the carpenters' society provided assistance to carpenters' widows, buried dead members and established an institution in which sick carpenters could receive care.[1] Workers also combined to maintain wage rates and working hours. Combinations were not welcomed by employers, who feared being unable to meet the cost of employees' increasing demands; capitalism dictated that market demand alone should determine wage rates and the price of goods. The state did not look upon combinations favourably, either, and a number of laws were passed in an attempt to quell their activity. These laws saw workers being whipped, imprisoned and pilloried for their involvement in combinations but did not succeed in suppressing the fledgling movements.[2]

Increasingly, violence and aggression began to characterise combination activity; employment was a valuable commodity, and when it or workers' wages were threatened, trouble ensued. Combination activity was decriminalised in 1824 but organising remained mainly associated with skilled craftsmen – earning the title 'craft unionism'. Craft unions were regarded as 'model' or 'responsible' unions as they tended to forego the use of striking as a weapon.[3] Protectionism, through the restriction of entry to trades, was their main strategy – a ploy that prevented craft labour surplus and ensured a constant demand for the skills of artisans. Members of craft unions were not permitted to work with non-unionised employees, were forbidden from working for less than the union-stipulated wage and had to serve a full apprenticeship before joining. These practices were vehemently adhered to, and their breach was treated most severely; twenty plasterers attacked a man for working for less than the union rate in 1824. In other incidents, a carpenter was beaten and subsequently died for not observing union rules; a blacksmith suffered a fractured skull for refusing to strike; and an employer was beaten for refusing to fire a non-unionised employee.[4]

As the 1800s drew to a close, a new type of trade unionism, referred to as 'new unionism' emerged. New unionism marked a departure from the relatively tame protective labour practices of the craft unions and involved organising unskilled workers. Its supporters were overt in their pursuit of better terms and conditions and had a marked tendency toward 'aggressive' strike action.[5] Proponents of new unionism sought to address their grievances not only at work but through political engagement.[6] The advent of new unionism in Ireland was most apparent through the efforts of James Larkin and the union he founded, the Irish Transport and General Workers' Union (ITGWU). The ITGWU soon found itself at the centre of one of the most pivotal events in European labour history: the 1913 Lockout. That year, much to the irritation of prominent businessman William Martin Murphy, Larkin sought to organise tram drivers. This precipitated the lockout of 25,000 trade union members from thirty-seven trade unions by a federation of 400 employers, all at Murphy's behest. The Lockout lasted six months and caused severe hardship for employees and their families, who turned to the soup kitchens for food. Workers returned to their jobs in February 1914, having won neither concessions nor union recognition. The Lockout was a battle waged against a bleak social and economic backdrop. Poverty, unemployment and an oversupply of unskilled labour was rampant in Dublin.[7] Over 25,000 families in the city lived in tenements, and four out of five of these lived in one-room dwellings.[8] The collapse of two tenement houses in Church Street claimed seven lives during the dispute and added to the poignancy of events. Writer George Russell boomed:

> You determined deliberately, in cold anger, to starve out one-third of the population of this city, to break the manhood of the men by the sight of the suffering of their wives and the hunger of their children … Your insolence and ignorance of the rights conceded to workers universally in the modern world were incredible, and as great as your inhumanity … You reminded labour you could always have your three square-meals a day while it went hungry.[9]

Russell's broadside suggested that the Lockout was about forcing men to capitulate and denounce trade unionism. The implication was that women were not unionised, but this was not wholly the case. Women too were organising, and a harder line was emerging among Irish female trade unionists. One commentator wrote:

> If there is any class of employers in Ireland more worthy of damnation … it is the class that builds up its wealth on the exploitation of girl and women

labour ... the wages paid [*sic*] women and girl workers are the lowest paid in any country with pretensions to civilisation ... But the real wonder is why womankind does not rise up in revolt and sweep the whole accursed order of exploiters into the hell that surely awaits them.[10]

The rise in the Irish women's labour movement was reflected in the formation of the Irish Women Workers' Union (IWWU), the founding of which broadly coincided with a strike of 3,000 women at the Jacob's Biscuit Factory in Dublin in 1911. The Women Workers' Union was rejuvenated by events at Jacob's during the 1913 Lockout when the company decided to employ strike-breakers.[11] What followed was bitter acrimony and a column in the *Irish Worker*, edited by Women Workers' Union Secretary Delia Larkin (sister of James Larkin and a nurse[12]) claimed: 'Jacob's and their scabs will doubtless wish they were not only dead, but dead and buried before this fight for freedom is finished.'[13] As of yet, nurses and midwives remained outside the trade union fray in spite of their sisters' activities in other occupations. This would soon change.

II. An Essential Dilemma

In 1919, unskilled men at the Ford car factory in County Cork earned £239 per year.[14] Women bank officials earned between £100–£190 per year.[15] In contrast, nurses at the Dublin Union Hospital earned £52–£65 per year and received an allowance of ¾ lb of butter and 1 st of potatoes per week, as well as a ½ pt of milk per day. They also worked sixty-five hours a week and were obliged to make up for any annual leave or sick leave they took by elongating their working days 'till the total is worked off'.[16] Many nurses had no pension entitlements. Their conditions reflected deeply engrained sexual inequalities in which men, not women, were regarded as the breadwinners. A comment by a nurse in the *British Journal of Nursing* in 1919, arguing that 'a society for the prevention of cruelty to nurses was badly needed', came very close to the mark.[17]

In early 1919, a small group of nurses and midwives in Ireland began to question whether their poor employment conditions might be best addressed by forming a trade union. Their plans, at least on the surface, appeared neither problematic nor unusual. Ireland had a long history of trade union activity; unions were by then a primary means of addressing workplace grievances and, following the drubbing that trade unionism suffered in the 1913 Lockout, union membership was in recovery. Trade union membership rose from 100,000 in 1916 to 225,000 in 1920.[18] But things were not quite that simple. The writer

of a commentary piece in the *Irish Times*, while readily acknowledging and
sympathising with the 'toil' and poor conditions of 'tender-handed' and 'self-
sacrificing' nurses, condemned their action in organising.[19] The commentator
took issue with the very idea of a nurses' trade union, which neither served the
'noble profession', the hospital nor the public.[20] Trade unions were incompatible
with the spirit of professional work, and the writer fretted that nurses were
about to 'cheapen the magnificent repute which the profession has won for
itself'.[21] The commentator reminded nurses that their role was not wholly
about material gain; rather it was about public service and such service was
incompatible with strikes in which nurses would be compelled to 'desert their
patients'.[22] But nurses and their supporters responded defiantly: 'That funny
paper, the "Irish Times" ... Comment would really spoil this gem ... we are
grateful to the newsboy who inadvertently slipped [it] into our letter-box: he
enabled us to face a new day joyously'.[23] In their defence, nurses asked:

> Although the public at large, whose servants they are, is quite loud in its
> praise of the courage and devotion of nurses ... when it comes to a question
> of supplying the practical needs of nurses ... there is a strange lack of
> understanding ... nurses are beginning to ask why poverty and slavery must
> be the necessary accompaniments of this virtue.[24]

The *Irish Times* endorsed nursing work as a public service. Such work carried
a service-obligation or implied understanding that the needs of the service
superseded the needs of the nurses. The resultant dilemma, particularly the view
that strike action contravened that obligation, was to bedevil nurses, midwives,
and the union they founded, for the next century. The contributor to the *Irish
Times* was by no means peculiar in their opinion. The International Council of
Nurses (ICN), in its *International Code of Nursing Ethics*, decreed that 'service
to mankind is the primary function of nurses'.[25] The spirit of the council's decree
was endorsed by many nurses themselves. Renowned Irishwoman Catherine
Black, who served as a personal nurse to King George V, remarked in her
autobiography: 'Nurses are born, not made ... [nursing] must be a vocation
first and a profession afterwards. It is the job that of all others demands the
most constant self-sacrifice, and we only get any satisfaction out of sacrificing
ourselves when we do it for love of someone or something'.[26] Some nurses even
paid to work. In Mercer's Hospital in Dublin, trainee nurses paid thirty-five
guineas (approximately £37) to train for four years, yet they received a salary
of just £10 per year for the first three years of their training and £20 for the
last year.[27] 'Good' nurses were clearly selfless and dedicated while 'bad' nurses

were out to indulge their own material needs.[28] Those pioneers who considered establishing a nurses' union challenged the old adages. They questioned why their role should be synonymous with self-sacrifice and hardship and why their own interests should be relegated in the interests of the service. Their stance was infused by more than just enlightened thinking: a range of other factors was also at play.

III. Context and Confluence

An auspicious meeting of a range of economic, labour and political factors was causing nurses to rethink their position outside the trade union fray. Chief among these was the First World War and its economic aftermath. Some 200,000 Irish men fought in the war and 50,000 died, leading some to suggest that nurses became alarmed that they might not be able to find a husband in the war's aftermath, thus prompting them to take a greater interest in becoming financially independent.[29] In addition, many Irish nurses enlisted in the war and were stationed at military hospitals in England or further afield.[30] These nurses were paid more than the nurses who remained at home working in voluntary hospitals[31] and higher expectations on their return may have motivated them to organise.

The post-war period was one of unemployment, recession and inflation; this period saw much economic hardship among the labour force who clamoured for financial redress. Workers' frustration found practical expression in an increasing number of strikes in a number of industries,[32] and the widespread industrial agitation at the time took the shape of what became known as 'the wages movement'. At the time, the manner in which disgruntled workers conducted their trade union activities was remarkable. The period 1917–23 is referred to as the syndicalist period in trade union organising history.[33] Syndicalism was a doctrine by which workers seized control of both government and economy and owned and managed industries. It encompassed a mindset through which trade unionists sought to remedy grievances.[34] In Ireland, it entailed sympathetic strike action between workers in different industries and the formation of the 'One Big Union', commonly referred to as the 'OBU', in which workers from many different trades unionised.[35] In 1919, syndicalism was to have a pronounced effect on how nurses chose to organise and on their new union's general reception.

The decision to establish the Irish Nurses' Union (INU) was also conceived amid intense political unrest. Dublin played host to a failed uprising in 1916 wherein insurgents sought to overthrow British rule and establish an Irish

Republic. The execution of the Rising's central protagonists caused increased hostility toward British rule and, in the years that followed, anti-British sentiment found expression in the continued rise of Sinn Féin. Following their success in the 1918 general election, Sinn Féin declared Irish independence and set up Dáil Éireann, the Irish parliament, in January 1919. Britain later moved to quash the Dáil, and a British military presence was deployed to quell insurgency. Tensions mounted and the War of Independence, the foundation of the Irish Free State (Saorstát na hÉireann) and the Civil War followed. Many women played prominent roles in the nationalist and republican struggles between 1916 and 1922. Some were nurses and midwives. Elizabeth O'Farrell, who later became a midwife at the National Maternity Hospital in Holles Street, Dublin,[36] at great danger to herself, delivered the notice of surrender to the commander of the British forces and to the rebel garrisons following the failed 1916 uprising. Up to 12,000 women were also members of organisations such as Cumann na mBan. This 'association of women' nursed wounded insurgents, provided them with safe houses and acted as couriers for munitions.[37] The membership of Cumann na mBan included nurses who, in keeping with nationalist sentiment, altered the red cross on their uniform to a green one.

One nurse, Bridget Dirrane, arrived in Dublin in 1919 to work at St Ultan's Hospital. While carrying out home nursing duties for a local family, Dirrane received a letter detailing the movements and activities of Republican insurgents. Shortly after the letter arrived, the home at which Dirrane was employed was raided by British troops. In order not to betray the cause in which she so firmly believed, Dirrane burned the letter – an offence for which she was imprisoned.[38] In essence, the prevailing sense of nationalism created a gap in the market: the College of Nursing, an English professional association representing nurses, found it increasingly difficult to recruit members in Ireland at the time, owing to 'intense national feeling as regards English institutions'; the college admitted defeat and ceased its efforts to recruit members in the Saorstát by 1925.[39] This facilitated the emergence and subsequent growth of an Irish nurses'/midwives' union, and it is not surprising that the union's first badge would prominently feature a shamrock.

Economic, labour and political factors coalesced with social change. A series of women's rights campaigns commenced in Ireland in the mid-1800s.[40] These crusades commenced with women's battle to own property independently of their husbands, ultimately achieved in 1907. Later, campaigning continued in an effort to repeal the *Contagious Diseases Acts*, which provided that women suspected of being prostitutes could be hospitalised if found to have venereal diseases; these acts were repealed in 1886. A successful campaign to permit

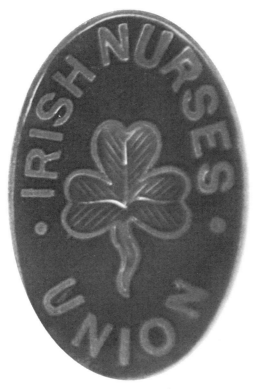

The union's first badge. The choice of a blue background, still in use today, appears to have been inspired by the blue badge of the Irish Women Workers' Union. Courtesy Lisa Moyles/INMO.

women to attend university and gain a professional qualification followed, and legislation, which permitted women entry to the professions, was enacted in 1919. These successes offered women reason for optimism, and soon attention turned to achieving suffrage. Several organisations were established to campaign for votes for women and they eventually, and fully, achieved their objective in 1922.[41] One of the central characters in the campaign for women's rights was Louie Bennett. Bennett was a middle-class Protestant, a staunch advocate of women's suffrage and founder of the Irishwomen's Reform League in 1911. She was taken aback by the suffering she had witnessed during the 1913 Lockout and began to view women's economic freedom as of equal importance to suffrage. She also increasingly viewed trade unionism as a means to achieve economic emancipation.[42] Her interest in labour issues was evident in the *Irish Citizen* newspaper. The *Citizen* began primarily as a suffrage newspaper but later expanded its remit to include labour issues.[43]

THE IRISH CITIZEN

Printed in Ireland on Irish Paper.

For Men and Women Equally
The Rights of Citizenship;
From Men and Women Equally
The Duties of Citizenship.

Monthly.
Two-Pence.
Annual Subscription
2s. 6d. post free.

Vol. 7. DUBLIN, NOVEMBER, 1919. No. 7.

CONTENTS

Current Comment

WORK FOR WOMEN.

Among other results of the coming Elections we hope to see a number of experienced and representative women placed on the committee, at present entirely male, which administer school meals; these to find out what powers are possessed by Corporations, Town Councils, Boards of Guardians, and to plan and supervise schemes for school meals, medical and dental inspection, mothers' pensions, etc. Another section might profitably deal with the problem of street trading, juvenile employment, and try to solve, possibly on American lines, the problem of the truant. We read of many complaints as to conduct of boys in streets. Cruelty to children is common. All these difficulties can only be dealt with by creating a healthy public opinion among the great mass of the people. Then common action can be agreed upon. We especially appeal to country readers to interest themselves in these reforms.

CHILD WELFARE.

The preservation and care of child life in Irish towns and in rural districts has often been put forward as the primary duty of every patriotic Irishwoman. "So much said, so little done." The society, ladies, who, a few years ago, earned a Vive-regal invitation by doing a little "health" work, are busy in other directions! But we welcome a new Children's Care Committee, with Miss D. Mellone as Hon. Secretary. St. Ultan's Children's Hospital is another splendid example of the constructive work Irishwomen are doing. But are Republican women doing all that can be done? On them will fall the main burden of planning schemes of reform, and seeing that the local authorities carry them out. As already pointed out we need a Ministry of Child Welfare. We have already Commissions of Enquiry into Irish industries, we ask for a Women's Commission on similar lines.

AUGUSTE HOLMES' IRISH C ROL.

Proud as Ireland is of the Irish nationality of the late Auguste Holmes, the greatest woman-composer and poet of the age, it may be necessary to remind some of her patriots that she wrote the "Noël d'Irlande," one of the finest Christmas carols ever published. Although born and brought up in France, Auguste Holmes knew English perfectly, but preferred to write in French, which she considered better adapted to poetical and musical purposes, nor is the fact that the "Noël d' Irlande" is composed to French words instead of English likely to render it less popular than it is in France, especially at this season. It is published by Heugel et Cie., Au Menestrel, 3 bis., Rue Vivienne, Paris.

A WOMEN'S HOSPITAL.

We have often been told that the feminist movement tends to destroy womanly modesty. For our part, we are too often horrified by the immodest practices of the most womanly of their sex. Ladies who shrink from the publicity of the polling-booth hasten to call in a man, when a doctor is needed for themselves or for their daughters. Suffragists prefer to consult women physicians. The popularity of our women doctors affords ample proof that women much prefer, in practice, to be treated by members of their own sex. As things are at present, any woman who is forced to enter a Dublin hospital has to endure treatment by men doctors, and possibly from men students. Nurses, too, have to attend to male patients, a state of affairs which "anti's" deplore without providing any remedy. Women voters must urge upon their local authorities the need for providing women's hospitals, staffed entirely by women, open to women sutdents, and training probationers to nurse women. Of course, there will be the usual outburst of opposition from the male monopolist. Truth to state, however, we like doctors as men even more than we dislike men as doctors! We can think of no more noble occupation for a man than that of nursing his own sex! We think it would be an admirable idea to send every school boy for a course of training in hygiene and nursing to the men's hospitals. A celebrated feminist has said that the ideal man of the modern feminist is a doctor. As pacificists we desire to emphasise the necessity of opposing the training of boys in scientific butchery and the lust to kill by a no less thorough inculcation of the ardent desire to preserve life and a knowledge of the principles of medicine. We understand that various women's organisations are thinking out a social reform programme for all candidates at the forthcoming elections, and we trust that the need for a women's hospital will not escape their attention. The possibility of providing public baths, creches, school meals, dental clinics, medical inspection, mothers' pensions, etc., by all local authorities throughout Ireland, not merely in the cities, will, we hope, follow as a necessary result of a vigilant and educated women's movement. The time has long gone by for Irish women of either political party to content themselves with making bandages for either Army. All women Republicans as well as loyalists, must personally enlist in the Army of Progress, and work, by every means in their power, for the Mother Country!

OUR MODEST CITY FATHERS.

A further discussion (which the "Irish Times" was apparently too modest to report) took place at a recent meeting of the Dublin Corporation on the closing up of the only Woman's Public Lavatory in this city. Had the motion not been talked out it is probable a decision to have it kept open for another three months pending the acquisition of more suitable premises, would have been arrived at. It is understood that the reason for closing the present lavatory is the fact that it has been used for other purposes that that for which it was erected; surely the police could and should have prevented such a development. Anyway, at least one decent public lavatory for women, properly fitted up and in a central part of the city is an urgent need. It is also desirable that when this want is supplied, some indication of the purpose it serves should be visible to the naked eye; numberless women must have passed the existing lavatory daily without noticing its very modest sign of identification.

WHO WILL REVOLT?

The following advertisement appeared in the "Irish Times," of the 29th October:—"Wanted, Lady Help Companion; well educated, Catholic, musical, keep accounts, knowledge shorthand, typewriting desirable; supervise servants, good knowledge cooking, needlewoman; state salary, etc." Surely the revolt of the "LadyHelp" is long overdue!

The front page of the *Irish Citizen* newspaper in 1919. Courtesy the author.

Bennett was a regular contributor and sometime editor of the newspaper and, in the wake of the 1916 Rising, was asked to assist in running the Irish Women Workers' Union. She started off a little wet behind the ears but quickly learned the ropes, mastered her brief and, by 1917, had become Secretary of the union. Bennett and the *Irish Citizen* were to play pivotal roles in the emergence of an Irish nurses' union and, amid the 'One Big Union' fervour that characterised 1919, she suggested that nurses join the Women Workers' Union as an autonomous branch. The *Irish Citizen* would become the union's primary means of communicating with prospective members and with the public until it established its own publication in 1925. The fledgling nurses' union also operated from the same Dublin address, 29 South Anne Street, as Bennett's Irishwomen's Reform League. The nurses' union utilised and benefitted from the personnel and facilities that the women's movement had established and harnessed these to its advantage.

A number of more specific influences were also at play. There was an innate solidarity between nurses and as early as the late 1800s, when some nurses were dismissed for 'levity' and 'breaches of discipline' at St Vincent's Hospital in Dublin, others resigned in sympathy.[44] In addition, midwives' enthusiasm to unionise slightly preceded that of nurses, with the latter seemingly taking their lead from the former. A letter from a disgruntled Elizabeth Moran, a midwife from Carrick-on-Shannon in County Leitrim, to the *Irish Independent* in January 1919, drew attention to the 'hardship' in midwifery that was not endured by 'any other class of nurse', and suggested organising midwives into an 'Irish Midwives' Union.'[45] The decision of the midwives to organise, marginally before the nurses did, suggests that they had a greater sense of innate unity because they were lesser in number and their roles were better circumscribed than those of nurses.[46] Moran quipped: 'Why not start at once a District Midwives' Union, and demand a living wage … Night as well as day, rain or sun, snow or frost, we must go; no car hire, or bicycle allowance, all must be taken out of the miserable salary of 10/- or 12/- per week.'[47] Moran was inundated with correspondence from midwives who felt the same way and held a midwives' meeting in Boyle, County Roscommon at which the proposed union was discussed.[48] Ultimately, in keeping with the prevalent 'One Big Union' mindset of the time, the midwives opted to affiliate to the Irish Nurses' Union at a meeting held in Dublin on 1 May 1919.[49]

The attendants and nurses employed in Ireland's 'lunatic' asylums were also displaying increasing militancy.[50] This was evident at Monaghan Asylum in January 1919, just one month before the Irish Nurses' Union came into being. Staff at the asylum, members of the Irish Asylum Workers' Union, were unhappy with their 93-hour working week and requested that it be reduced to fifty-six hours per week.[51] At a meeting of the asylum's Management Committee and the Asylum Workers' Union, the Resident Medical Superintendent outlined the working conditions of the staff: 'They work twelve hours a day for seven days, but they get off every thirteenth day, and every fourth Sunday from ten o'clock.'[52] The Chairman of the committee remarked incredulously: 'What real grievance have they[?]'[53] The employees recruited Peadar O'Donnell, an organiser for the ITGWU, to advise them. Negotiations began but when these faltered, the asylum's employees barricaded the institution's doors, mounted hoses at the windows, took the matron hostage and decided to run the asylum themselves, with O'Donnell essentially acting as governor of the embattled institution.[54]

A week-and-a-half-long standoff ensued, during which strikers and inmates entertained themselves by having dances; indeed, O'Donnell noted that inmates were 'quite enthusiastic over the prospect of having a tussle with the police', who formed a cordon around the building.[55] The employees' demands were ultimately met and, in black humour, O'Donnell wrote to the Asylum Committee, reassuring them that he would not be seeking payment for his stint as governor.[56] By occupying the asylum as opposed to withdrawing their labour, the employees, consistent with their service-obligation to patients, found a novel manner in which to take industrial action while simultaneously 'minimising the potential for accusations of neglect'.[57] Allegedly, the mortality rate at the asylum decreased during the occupation.[58]

Increasingly testing and risky clinical conditions characterised the period during which nurses and midwives sought to organise. This may have caused some to seek increased rewards for the dangers to which they were exposed at work. The spring of 1918 witnessed the beginning of the worldwide influenza epidemic, which infected up to 800,000 people in Ireland and claimed 20,000 lives.[59] The Royal City of Dublin Hospital in Baggot Street could not find sufficient beds to accommodate its high number of patients and was forced to accommodate some on the floor.[60] Half of the nurses at Dublin's Meath Hospital became ill, leaving the remainder to deal with 141 influenza cases.[61] Further evidence of the number of nurses who contracted influenza can be gleaned from the large number claiming insurance benefit at this time.[62]

Midwifery and nursing are regarded as having become professionalised with the passage of the *Midwives (Ireland) Act* of 1918 and the *Nurses Registration (Ireland) Act* of 1919, respectively.[63] These acts provided for the establishment of the Central Midwives' Board of Ireland and the General Nursing Council (Ireland) – both statutory bodies charged with the maintenance of a roll and

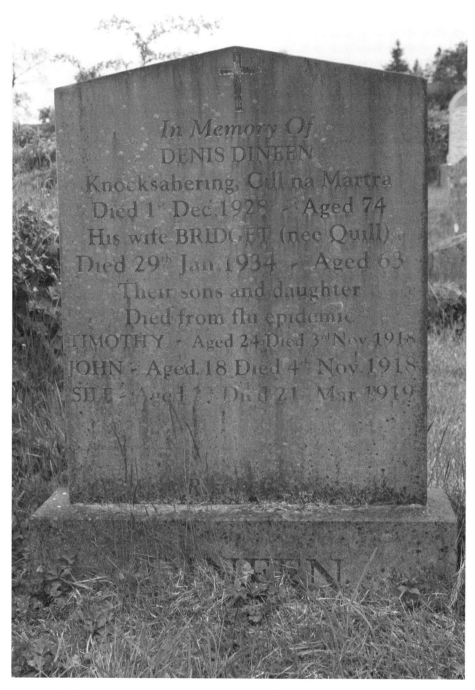

A grave in Ballyvourney, Cork, in which three siblings who succumbed to influenza were laid to rest on 3 and 4 November 1918 and 21 March 1919. Courtesy the author.

register of midwives and nurses, respectively, and with the approval of training institutions, the preparation of syllabi and the conduct of examinations. These developments increased the status of both occupations and it is likely that the nurses and midwives anticipated an increased reward for this, effectively influencing their decision to dally with trade unionism. True, some professionals, such as bank officials, in spite of their discontent with their salary, shunned trade unionism because they considered it 'beneath [their] dignity' to organise in the same manner as 'ordinary working people'.[64] Consequently, professional groups tended to organise in professional associations as opposed to trade unions. This is evident in teacher representative organisations with the Irish National Teachers' Organisation and the Association of Secondary Teachers, Ireland, founded as 'professional associations' in 1868 and 1907, respectively. Crucially, however, amid the widespread inflation that followed the First World War, these associations opted to become trade unions, the former in 1918 and the latter in 1919.[65] Economic hardship could persuade even professionals to forego their status consciousness and consider trade unionism.

The inflation that accompanied the First World War led to widespread calls by workers for financial redress. Syndicalism provided the means and manner by which workers could achieve this redress. The prevailing sense of nationalism and the support provided by the women's movement also loomed large. Added to this was the solidarity among and between nurses, the preemptive action of midwives, the industrial strife in Ireland's asylums, the clinical stresses and strains and the recent victory of registration for nurses and midwives. The drivers for the establishment of a trade union for nurses and midwives were now firmly in place.

CHAPTER 2

The Foundation of the Irish Nurses' Union

In 1919, a small second-floor room at 29 South Anne Street housed the Dublin Esperanto Club. Esperanto had gained in popularity following the Russian Revolution and was seen as a means whereby unity between the world's workers, all speaking in the same tongue, could be advanced.[1] One evening in late February that year, as the weekly Esperanto class finished and the students filed out onto the street, they passed by a group of twenty nurses and midwives who had been given permission to hold a meeting in the Esperantists' room. That night the nurses and midwives discussed their poor employment conditions and took the controversial decision to establish a trade union in response. It is fitting that from this point on the Dublin Esperanto Club, concerned with establishing unity among and between workers, would share a room with the budding INU, concerned with establishing unity among and between nurses and midwives.

I. The First Steps

The INU was declared 'the first Trade Union for Hospital Nurses in the world'.[2] Did the union have the right to lay claim to such a lofty distinction? It appears so. True, a midwives' union was operational in England in 1910 but this did not comprise nurses.[3] True too that health service staff in Russia, including nurses, had to join trade unions in the wake of the Russian Revolution,[4] but these unions were general healthcare unions that also comprised doctors and pharmacists.[5] Moreover, the other nurse representative associations that existed at the time were not trade unions per se. Rather, they were professional associations. Indeed, the second ever nurses' trade union, the Professional Union of Trained Nurses, was founded in England by nurse Maude MacCallum, who had trained at Dublin's Adelaide Hospital and seemingly took her inspiration from the establishment of the INU some months beforehand.[6]

From the outset, the INU was markedly different from other organisations representing nurses. Organisations such as the Irish Nurses' Association[7] and

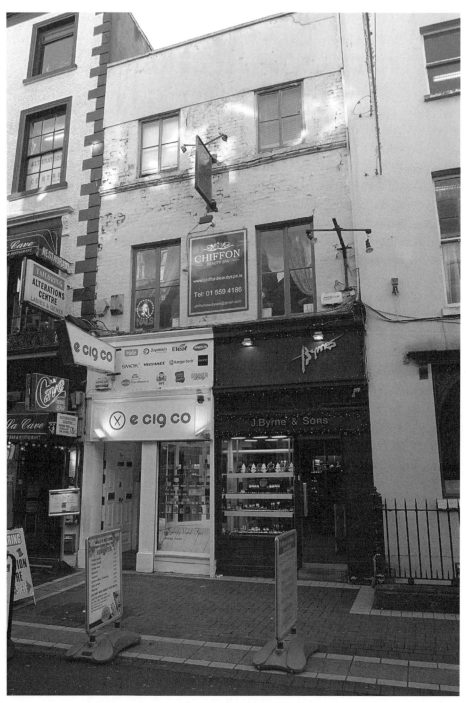

Birthplace of the Irish Nurses' Union: 29 South Anne Street, Dublin, as it appears today. The Union's office was located on the second floor of the building. Courtesy Lisa Moyles/INMO.

the Irish Matrons' Association were well established, but both were formed to campaign mainly in relation to professional issues such as nurse education and registration.[8] The INU contrasted with these associations as it was highly unionate, with a focus on achieving improved conditions of employment.[9] For the INU, any approach other than that of trade unionism would mean nurses forging alliances with associations that might not advance their cause:

> [Irish nurses should be wary of] matrons and a group of benevolent people of the middle, or even the aristocratic class, who will give balls for us, provide us with a Club perhaps, or a holiday home and invite us to tea parties in their country homes, but who, when questions of higher salaries or shorter hours are raised, gently explain to us why the present time is not a suitable one to give them to us! If nurses choose [this] method of organisation they will retain the position of heroines whose mission it is to live in poverty … so as to bring ease to the sick and help the Government and the general public to practise economy. If they choose Union organisation, they will [be] … sure of a just reward for their services, and free from any sense of obligation to benefactors, or of servitude to matrons – or employers.[10]

The impetus in forming the union was an approach made to Louie Bennett by a nurse from Dublin's Pigeon House Road Hospital. As previously mentioned, Bennett was Secretary of the IWWU by then and suggested that nurses should join the IWWU as an autonomous branch. In that way, the INU could formulate its own policy but would benefit from the guidance and administrative support of the IWWU. The IWWU had registered as a trade union in 1918 and was affiliated to the Labour Party and the Irish Trade Union Congress (ITUC), meaning that, from the outset, so too was the INU.[11] Delegates from the INU attended the annual Trade Union Congress from 1920 onwards.

Bennett's suggestion that nurses and midwives should join the IWWU was not solely an expression of her wider concern for women workers. The IWWU was founded in 1911 as a branch of the ITGWU with James Larkin as President and his sister Delia as General Secretary. Similar to the INU's relationship with the IWWU, the IWWU was once provided with financial assistance from the ITGWU, however, by 1919, the IWWU and ITGWU had parted ways; the IWWU was losing members to the ITGWU owing to concerns over the effectiveness of the former, and its financial reserves were dwindling. In response, it began to recruit members from outside of Dublin. The IWWU's situation worsened when the First World War ended and up to 150,000 soldiers returned home to displace women from their jobs and from IWWU membership. Some women also began defecting to the ITGWU because it made sense that just one union, and not many unions, would negotiate with a particular industry or employer. This trend further reduced the membership of the IWWU.[12] Nurses and midwives represented a unique opportunity for recruitment into the IWWU's dwindling fold, as almost all of them were women, few were already unionised, and the prospect of men displacing women in this sector was unlikely. Thus, the relationship between nurses/midwives and Bennett's IWWU was most likely a mutually beneficial one, and the IWWU is described as actively 'courting' them, with Bennett leaving instructions that 'the big drawing room [be] cleared up to give an air of high respectability for [the] occasion' of a meeting of the nurses.[13]

A provisional committee was established at the INU's first meeting in February 1919. Louie Bennett was nominated President and Marie Mortished was nominated Secretary. Bennett is a compelling character. She was educated in Britain but became disillusioned with British colonialism and returned to Ireland, where she was many things to many people: novelist, women's rights campaigner, trade unionist, nationalist and pacifist.[14] Far less is known about Marie Mortished and the other founders of the INU. Mortished, born Marie Shields but often referred to as Bid or Biddy, was one of eight children of Adolphus Shields and Fanny Sophie Ungerland. Money was tight for the Shields and being unable to pay their bills, they regularly moved around Dublin from one rented accommodation to the next.[15] They also had to regularly pawn their father's suit until pay day and then attempt to buy it back. The Shields' children were inculcated with a sense of defiance from an early age, as well as a love of the arts and altruism.[16] No surprise then that Marie, having helped her parents to rear her younger siblings, trained to become a nurse in England and returned to Ireland to work at the Royal City of Dublin Hospital, Baggot Street.[17]

Marie was immersed in trade unionism from an early age. Her father, Adolphus, was a compositor and prominent trade union figure; he was associated with the National Union of Gas Workers and General Labourers. He also founded the Independent Labour Party and was Secretary of the Dublin Socialist Society. Marie's husband, Ronald Mortished, was an intellectual, a member of the Socialist Party of Ireland and Assistant Secretary of the Labour Party and Trade Union Congress.[18] He became the first Chairman of the Irish Labour Court and worked for the International Labour Office (ILO) in later years. Ronald was also President of the Esperanto Association and was a friend of Louie Bennett.[19] This friendship suggests that he helped procure the office premises for the Nurses' Union, introduced Marie to Bennett and perhaps recommended her for the position of Secretary of the INU. The minutes of

Ronald Mortished and Adolphus Shields were speakers at this series of public lectures organised by the Socialist Party of Ireland. Courtesy of the James Hardiman Library Archives, NUI Galway.

IWWU meetings refer to both Marie and Ronald supervising the INU's work in its early days. This suggests that Ronald was equally as involved as Marie in the fledgling union.[20]

Notwithstanding her pivotal role in the burgeoning INU, it is largely through the notoriety of her brothers that anything has been recorded of Marie Mortished. One brother, Arthur Shields, was a rebel in the 1916 Rising. Based at the General Post Office and at Moore Street, he attempted to transmit the Proclamation by means of radio during the conflict. He was imprisoned firstly in Cheshire and subsequently at Frongoch in Wales. He was also a renowned stage and film actor.[21] Another brother, Barry Fitzgerald, was also an actor, albeit much better known – he won an Oscar for his role in the 1944 movie *Going My Way*.

The union had assembled for itself a managerial staff with talent and know-how, and Bennett and Mortished were soon joined by clerical assistant Kathleen Nora Price. The union's first democratically elected Executive Committee was formed in June 1919 when many members of the provisionally appointed committee, in place since February, were re-elected. Members of the committee consisted of nurses and midwives and had to be resident in Dublin in order to attend meetings. The union's strategies were decided at an Annual Council meeting in which delegates from the union's slowly expanding network of branches convened. Each branch was overseen by a branch secretary who had the (unenviable) task of collecting subscriptions from members and forwarding the monies to the union's headquarters in Dublin, where, between the hours of 4:30 and 6:30 each weekday evening, Mortished and Price took care of the union's day-to-day affairs.

The INU was a product of its time and its activities were in keeping with the economic and labour context in which it was founded. One feature of the syndicalist period was the formation of workers' co-operatives.[22] Co-operatives were championed by labour leaders, such as James Connolly, who implored workers to 'organise as a class to meet our masters and destroy their mastership [and to] organise to wrench from their robber clutch the land and workshops on and in which they enslave us'.[23] Nurses' homes or hostels were institutions in which nurses resided and from which they were despatched to nurse patients in the patients' own homes. In 1919, when the manager of a nurses' home in Dublin increased the fees charged to nurses for securing work for them, a number of nurses left in protest. This prompted the INU to contemplate establishing its own 'Irish Nurses' Union Co-Operative Home'.[24] The home aimed to share profits equally between the nurses employed by the co-operative and was later established at 21 Great Denmark Street in Dublin.

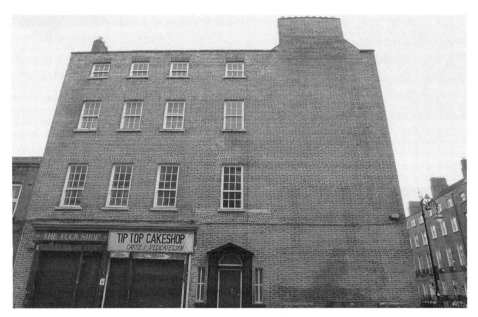

The site of the Irish Nurses' Union's ill-fated Co-operative Home at 21 Great Denmark Street, Dublin, as it appears today. Courtesy Lisa Moyles/INMO.

The home contrasted with the existing nurses' homes, which were considered 'nothing but extremely profitable commercial speculations from which doctors and matrons derive a high rate of interest' by charging high fees to the nurses who were engaged for duty through them.[25]

An article in the *Irish Citizen* boasted that the home's success would defy the 'cynics who say that Nurses [*sic*] are absolutely devoid of any business instinct, and that such a project is bound to fail'.[26] Ultimately, their words were prophetic, as by March 1920, the INU reported that the venture had failed and asked the IWWU to relinquish the £20 in shares it had contributed. The INU's foray into the co-operative home suggests the presence of a socialist consciousness among its leaders. It also indicated a sense of ambition in the union that, in the short term, was only partially realised. Owing to a range of factors from dwindling membership to matronly disapproval, the union would soon be beset by challenges.

II. Recruitment Difficulties

The union amassed an impressive 700 members in its first year. Part of the INU's success in recruitment can be attributed to the IWWU, which lent

accomplished staff, such as Helena Molony, to assist in its efforts.[27] Molony
had been involved in the 1916 Rising and was imprisoned afterwards for her
role in it. An attempt to escape prison, apparently by digging her way out with
a spoon, was unsuccessful, but she and her colleagues in the IWWU brought
that same tenacity to the INU and helped recruit nurses to the INU at the same
time as recruiting women, more generally, to the IWWU.[28] But the INU's initial
success with regard to recruitment was short-lived, and a number of factors
soon stifled its growth. The ongoing War of Independence hindered rail travel
and interrupted the postal system, making the organisation of meetings and
correspondence with members challenging; it is not clear if the INU meeting
held in Miss Ryan's sweet shop in Kilkenny in November 1919 amounted to
bribery or sheer desperation![29] The theft of a number of members' subscriptions
from the union's headquarters in the early days did not help matters. Following
the war, partition also negatively affected member numbers; delegates from
counties such as Down and Armagh are listed as attendees at the INU's first
conference in 1920 but not at subsequent conferences.

Nurses and midwives were scattered across numerous state-run and
voluntary hospitals as district nurses and midwives, which further militated
against organising. Louie Bennett sought to overcome this obstacle by replacing
the union's occasional circulars (few of which have survived) with a gazette,
which she envisaged would be the primary means of organising and which
would include, alongside INU matters, 'gossipy notes' and 'a few jokes' and be
sold nationwide, its cost defrayed by advertising.[30] Bennett's suggestion was
adopted, and the *Irish Nurses' Union Gazette* appeared triannually from 1925
onwards. In spite of these efforts, the INU's first decade was characterised by
frequent appeals for nurses to join its ranks. Membership in 1925 stood at
795 members.[31] By 1927, membership had dropped to 668.[32] Census records
indicate that there were 491 midwives and 5,341 nurses in Ireland at the
time,[33] meaning that the union's density was low, at approximately 11 per cent.
The economic boom that accompanied the First World War was followed by
recession and unemployment. This heralded a period of decline in membership
of Irish trade unions, which contrasted sharply with the acute rise in union
membership experienced during the syndicalist period. Membership of the
ITGWU fell from over 100,000 members in 1920 to just 16,000 in 1930.[34] In
short, economic prosperity facilitated trade unions in achieving improved
conditions for their members and enabled recruitment, whereas recession had
the opposite effect.

The INU's association with the IWWU may also have hampered recruitment.
The union was sometimes criticised because its association with the IWWU

meant that its managing body included people who were not nurses. Miss Carson-Rae of the rival Irish Nurses' Association asked: 'If nurses are to "control their own profession," should they not be able to control their own union?'[35] Carson-Rae got her way and Louie Bennett did not contest the INU Presidency beyond 1925 because of 'criticism about the union not being run by nurses'.[36] Some disgruntled nurses went further and reminded Bennett that nurses were 'quite capable of managing their own affairs without outside interference'.[37]

Matrons did not help matters. They were an integral aspect of hospitals' managerial structure. They had a say in hospital budgets, played a role in deciding nurses' salaries[38] and possibly feared that improvements in nurses' conditions, won by the INU, may have impacted on their hospital's finances. Their opposition to the union was made clear in a report of an INU meeting, carried in the *Evening Telegraph* in 1919:

> Matrons were preponderantly vocal at the meeting. Nurses are fairly used to the matrons doing all the talking for and at them. But the matrons did not get things quite all their own way … a very large number of the nurses present were careful to bring away their Application Forms to fill them up later … It is natural, perhaps, that some matrons should feel a little hurt, after so many years of unquestioned dictatorial authority, to find that their subordinates are determined now to have a say … nurses should be the more heartily in favour of the Irish Nurses' Union the more they find matrons denouncing it.[39]

III. Money, Men and the Middle Class: More Challenges Manifest

Nurses' demands for improved working conditions could be interpreted as having a detrimental effect on hospital services. In 1919, after improving nurses' conditions, the managers at Dublin's Adelaide Hospital published a series of front-page advertisements in the national press.[40] The hospital warned that the concessions made to nurses would cost £1,000 and that this sum would need to be recouped in voluntary donations or wards at the institution would close.[41] The subsidies of voluntary hospitals, like the Adelaide, were devalued by the inflation that followed the First World War. Adding to its financial woes, the Adelaide had a Protestant ethos and, following Irish Independence, many of its benefactors left the country. Strategies like those employed by the Adelaide had the potential to unsettle nurses, and some prospective members of the INU expressed doubts regarding whether hospitals could afford to meet the cost of the union's claims.

Another issue that beset Mortished's and Bennett's INU was the emergence, at the same time, of another identically titled union for nurses. This competitor union proved problematic, not least because it was run by a man. A letter from Mr J. Shelly, organising Secretary of the (alternative) Irish Nurses' Union, published in a national newspaper in February 1919, expressed amazement that Mortished's and Bennett's Irish Nurses' Union had been conceived. Shelly, clearly disgruntled, remarked: 'It is rather strange, when practically all the spade-work has been done, that we find people who never interested themselves in the city nurses taking a deep interest now.'[42] Shelly took a thinly veiled swipe at Bennett in stating that he believed nurses to be 'quite capable' of managing their own organisation.[43] The situation was further complicated by the fact that advertisements for both identically named unions occasionally appeared side-by-side in the press. After this, Shelly sought to differentiate both entities by reminding readers that his Irish Nurses' Union 'has no connection with any other Union'.[44] It is not clear what became of Shelly's venture, but it is clear that it had support. Men had established a track record in trade unionism. One nurse wrote to the press:

> I heard of an organisation recently founded by 'J. Shelly', whom I took to be a woman. I ignored it, because, during my course of training and since, I have listened to Matrons re the improving of our profession, both socially and financially; but it all ended simply in 'cackle.' Now that I know 'J. Shelly' is a man, I call upon every trained nurse in Ireland to rally round him, and to help him to win our cause.[45]

Men, it appears, carried more credibility; indeed, a decade earlier, John Brennan wrote a scathing article in *Bean na h-Éireann* regarding nurses' working conditions. Brennan remarked that a nurse's life was neither noble nor respectable, describing the profession as 'degrading' and likened nurses to slaves.[46] It transpired that Brennan, masquerading as a 'strong Wexford farmer', was actually Sidney Gifford, a female proponent of the women's movement who wrote under a male pseudonym in order to garner more 'respect' from readers.[47]

The social class of nurses presented more challenges. The fees for nurse training were high and deterred many young women from poorer working-class families; the yearly fees charged to trainee nurses at St Vincent's Hospital, Dublin matched the salary of a female teacher.[48] Unsurprisingly, the archives at Cork's South Infirmary show that the fathers of trainee nurses were farmers; business people, such as shopkeepers; teachers or navy officers.[49] Notwithstanding feminist concern with the validity of judging women's social class on the basis of their fathers' occupation, much of the evidence suggests that Irish nurses were from reasonably comfortable backgrounds. While the INU's founders and early members were clearly not perturbed by the associations between trade unionism and the working class, the mass of nurses appears to have questioned the appropriateness of trade union organisation. The 'grubby syndicalist look [of the Labour Party and Trade Union Congress] … did not attract the middle class'[50] and, in 1927, nurses indicated that the INU's affiliation to the Labour Party and ITUC dissuaded them from joining.[51] Some nurses also considered their professional status to be incompatible with trade union activity. The union received a letter from a disgruntled nurse in November 1920, who objected to its attempts to organise in Bray, County Wicklow:

> I must … tell you that having always looked upon my work as a profession not a trade, I can have no sympathy with any form of 'Trades Union' even though adopted by a certain class of nurses, so called. I consider the formation of any sort of Trades Union as degrading to an honourable profession … Many thoroughly trained nurses resent, as I do, this idea of Trades Unionism.[52]

A hastily scribbled note on the back of the letter, probably from Marie Mortished to Kathleen Nora Price went: 'I'm afraid I'll have to ask you to try to reply to this lady', and the union sent her some promotional literature in the unlikely hope that she might change her mind. The union learned to anticipate these sentiments and implored nurses not to think of trade unionism as 'being beneath them'.[53] Support came from Dr Tom Hennessy, the Irish Medical Secretary of the British Medical Association and later a member of Dáil Éireann. Hennessy was present at the union's inaugural public meeting and reported having been 'pestered' by nurses into helping them organise.[54] He reminded nurses that the 'dangling of a spurious respectability' was a ploy to dissuade them from joining a union and reassured them that they would not 'demean themselves by being associated with Trades Unionism or Labour'.[55] But for all the challenges that the INU faced, one was to prove the most contentious and enduring: the challenge of reconciling nurses' and midwives' service-obligation with trade unionism and, most especially, with strike action.

IV. 'My first duty is to my patient'

The inaugural meeting of the union's founders was followed by a number of public meetings. The first of these was convened in the Oak Room of Dublin's Mansion House on the afternoon of Friday 28 February 1919. The choice of

such a salubrious venue was most likely a tactic to confer some respectability on
the project. The meeting was a fractious one, with many present expressing fears
that the unionisation of nurses might precipitate a strike. There had been an
increase in strike activity in Ireland during and after the First World War. Strike
activity even spread to sectors that were not usually associated with striking,
including those of general nursing and midwifery. The Secretary of the Cork
Nurses' Association[56] wrote to the Board of the Macroom Workhouse in 1920:
workhouses effectively became hospitals in the years following the Famine and
the Secretary of the Association warned that should the board fail to grant the
workhouse nurses a 'living wage', a withdrawal of labour would ensue.[57]

The threat was successful. Two years later, a number of midwives wrote
to the same board in an individual capacity. One expressed her dissatisfaction
with her salary and warned the board that if it did not consider granting her
an adequate wage then she would 'adopt the only remedy open to a victimised
worker, namely – to go on strike'.[58] The actions of these nurses and midwives
in threatening strike action were exceptional and, back at the Mansion House,
one disgruntled nurse commented: 'My first duty is to my patient, and I shall
not allow any person to get me to decline my responsibility to my patient.'[59]
Another nurse asked if she could be compelled to strike as a member of the
INU. Louie Bennett, presiding, responded that only 'nurses themselves could
call upon her to strike'.[60] Fears of nurses being compelled to strike by other
occupational groups were associated with a number of factors. James Larkin was
a past President of the IWWU, of which the INU was a branch. Larkin, or rather
'Larkinism', had become synonymous with militancy and sympathetic striking,[61]
which constituted a large part of Larkin's understanding of syndicalism.[62] This
was unsettling for some nurses, one of whom wrote to the *Irish Independent*
concerning an upcoming INU meeting: 'I refuse to attend this meeting, which
is … organised by *Larkin's women workers* [original emphasis].'[63] Another nurse
pondered whether prospective INU members could be called on to strike in
sympathy with other members of the IWWU, such as waitresses.[64]

Concerns that the unionisation of nurses/midwives might precipitate
a strike were not well-founded. Bennett largely conducted her trade union
activity by conciliatory means. She considered a strike by INU members as
'unthinkable' and reminded nurses that they could advance their industrial
claims without resorting to strike action.[65] The INU's first Annual Conference
was held at the IWWU Hostel at Larch Hill, Rathfarnham, Dublin on the
first weekend in September 1920. The fourteen delegates in attendance were
reassured in the matter of strikes: 'There is no actual provision for a strike laid
down in our rules and should drastic action be necessary in any case, it would

be directed towards the responsible authority, and in no case would the patient be allowed to suffer.'[66]

The INU's stance regarding strikes was not entirely consistent, however, as Marie Mortished did not unequivocally rule out a strike and noted that if nurses wanted to strike, then they could do so. She did distance the union from the prospect of sympathetic strikes by adding that nurses could not be compelled to strike by the IWWU, the Executive of the INU or any other body but the members themselves.[67] Mortished also wrote to the *British Journal of Nursing* in 1920 and recounted an incident, which she described as a 'strike' of sorts and which she seemed to condone – at least subtly.[68] The incident concerned an INU member whom the union had instructed to cease carrying out what were perceived to be non-nursing duties, namely compiling lists of patients' belongings. The nurse was dismissed as a result. The INU maintained that compiling lists of patients' belongings was 'obviously not a nurse's work ... [and might] very seriously interfere with the due carrying out of the nurse's proper duties'.[69] The nurse was later reinstated following representation on her behalf by the union and Mortished concluded: 'Were it not for the "strike" [we] should not have been able to secure so speedy and satisfactory an arrangement of the matter ... [People are] inclined to attach too much blame to the nurse who is driven to strike ... and too little blame to the authorities who are responsible for driving her to this extreme.'[70]

The INU also agreed to contribute to any strike levy that the IWWU believed necessary to impose on the union as a whole,[71] suggesting that nurses and midwives did not rule out the prospect of having to draw on the fund one day themselves. Nor did the union rule out other, albeit unspecified, forms of industrial action. Union hospitals were institutions whose workers were employed directly by the state. These hospitals contrasted with voluntary hospitals, which were ostensibly independent. In 1920, trouble arose at one union hospital, the Dublin Union Hospital, where the INU complained that the hospital's board was procrastinating on its pay claim.[72] The nurses' union complained that the board was taking advantage of the fact that nurses could not take strike action but reminded the hospital's managers '[that] its hopes that no other forcible means can be found are doomed to disappointment. Sick patients must, of course, be attended to, but the Nurses can, if they decide on such a course, make themselves unpleasant to the Board in many ways.'[73]

Following friction at the maiden public meeting of the INU, the rival Irish Nurses' Association convened a meeting in March 1919. In attendance were representatives of the INU and the Nurses' Association, most notably the Nurses' Association's President, Alice Reeves, and Margaret Huxley, both prominent figures in nursing in Ireland at that time. Accounts of the meeting show that the Nurses' Association was in agreement with the INU on many of its concerns, with Reeves remarking that nurses' working conditions warranted improvement.[74] Opinions diverged with regard to how best to address these concerns. Sir Arthur Chance, surgeon, President of the Royal College of Surgeons (RCSI) (and son-in-law of William Martin Murphy), spoke at the meeting and requested that employers deal with nurses' grievances 'on lines other than those of trade unions'.[75]

Chance's sentiments mirrored those of the Irish Nurses' Association, which then formally declared its position: 'However beneficial it may be for the other bodies of Women Workers, a trades union is not the best, or only way, for nurses to remedy their grievances.'[76] The INU deployed one of its most notable protagonists in its defence: Albinia Brodrick. Brodrick was born into

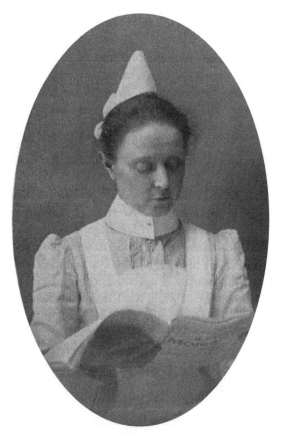

Albinia Brodrick, aka Gobnait Ní Bhruadair, in uniform in 1904. Image reproduced courtesy of the Board of Trinity College, Dublin, the University of Dublin.

an aristocratic Protestant family in Middlesex, England in 1861. In her youth, she was moved by the poverty she witnessed on a visit to Connemara, Ireland. She later became a nurse and midwife and moved to County Kerry, where she built a hospital called *Baile an Chúnaimh*, meaning the Household of Help. She was a staunch opponent of Westminster rule and described Ireland as the 'bastard product of a conquest miscalled civilising'.[77] She learned the Irish language, changed her name to Gobnait Ní Bhruadair, became a Sinn Féin councillor, joined Cumann na mBan and gave refuge to Republican insurgents. She was shot, imprisoned and went on hunger strike in 1923 for assisting Republicans.[78] A mover and shaker in the County Kerry branch of the union, she wrote to the *British Journal of Nursing* and remarked that although the other nurses' organisations did good work, they did not represent the mass rank-and-file and declared that the INU's function was to 'let down the net for the multitude of fishes'.[79] In a shot across the bow of the Irish Nurses' Association, she concluded: 'I trust that our other Associations may not attempt to stand in the way, as elder Associations so often do.'[80]

The INU was quite unique among nurse-representative organisations, both nationally and internationally. Conceived amid a heady labourist, nationalist and feminist backdrop, it found a degree of acceptance among a workforce whose historic aversion to trade unionism had been temporarily suspended. The union's auspicious beginning emboldened its ambition and outlook, but a range of challenges beset it. Syndicalism waned, recession set in, some doubted women's ability to reap change in nurses'/midwives' working conditions and others were either sickened or spooked at the prospect of joining up. Tensions also emerged between the union and other nurse-representative bodies of the day – particularly the rival Irish Nurses' Association.

Both factions shared some of the same goals; however, the Nurses' Association was opposed to trade unionism as a strategy to achieve its ends. This opposition was largely borne from the association between trade unions and striking; the evolving labour context, with its focus on sympathetic strike action, merely added to the INU's woes. The prospects of a strike also supplied the union's detractors with sufficient ammunition to damage and disparage it, and the union's liaisons with the IWWU made a bad situation even worse. Along with imaginative and tenuous links between the INU and 'syndicalist wild man' James Larkin (who had long since left Ireland for America), they represented clear and successful attempts to dissuade nurses/midwives from joining, many of which played on their prevalent service-obligation and posed major problems for the union in the years ahead.[81]

CHAPTER 3

The Early Years of the Irish Nurses' Union, *c.*1919–24

The INU had a challenging beginning, and things were not about to get easier. Within Ireland, different working conditions prevailed in different geographic regions, and this made it difficult for the union to achieve standardised terms. Furthermore, the new Irish government was unwilling to accede to workers' demands, as its priority in the 1920s was reducing expenditure with an 'almost penitential zeal'.[1] This meant that the nurses' union had to content itself with gaining piecemeal improvements, which set the tone for the painstakingly slow progress that characterised the union's achievements in the years ahead. The continued presence of uncertified practitioners in midwifery, in spite of the establishment of the Midwives' Roll, also exercised the union. Crucially, too, employers were growing aware of nurses'/midwives' duty of service and of the INU's aversion to strike action. The results of this awareness could not help but delay progress even further.

I. Representing Midwives

The INU was a misnomer and belied the fact that midwives outnumbered nurses in the fledgling union. The relatively large number of midwives may be partly explained by the fact that other organisations, such as the Irish Nurses' Association, excluded them from membership.[2] A handful of the union's midwife members were employed on private duties. Their small number owed to the fact that they were mobile and difficult to liaise with. Private duty midwives' tenuous employment status and their lack of guaranteed income may also have rendered them unable to afford the union's yearly subscription. The union's representation on behalf of this sector mainly concerned standardising their fees. The INU set a minimum fee of 25 shillings per case and implored midwives not to accept cases for less than this fee.[3] The union also sought to direct business to its members and published the names of local INU members in the press, asking other trade unionists to choose from among these midwives 'when their wives require [one]'.[4]

Dispensary midwives comprised the majority of INU members. The dispensary service came under the control of the Poor Law in 1851 and, comprising over 700 dispensary districts, provided 'outdoor', or community medical relief to the poor. Essentially, dispensaries were clinics, and there was a dispensary located in each district. One or more midwives were employed at each dispensary under the auspices of the Board of Guardians of the Poor Law Union, in which the dispensary was located. The INU attributed its success in organising dispensary midwives to the fact that they had a postal address at their workplace and were easy to liaise with. They were also independent practitioners and not under the watchful and disapproving eye of matrons. The union's claim on behalf of dispensary midwives was modest, and it sought an increase in midwives' salaries to £75 per year and a month's annual leave.[5] The INU sent this claim to the Board of Guardians of almost eighty Poor Law Unions. The union's priority was to effect a nationally standardised salary, but this was not going to be easy.

In 1920, the Board of Guardians in Nenagh, County Tipperary, received a telegram from Marie Mortished. Mortished cut to the chase: 'Strongly urge guardians favourably consider midwives [*sic*] application for salary scale adequate to present cost of living and arduous and important work … Situation will become intolerable unless speedily relieved.'[6] Six midwives were employed in the Nenagh area and it is clear from the board's deliberations that it considered a number of factors when deciding their salaries. Some midwives who were relatively new to their position earned more than others with established tenure.[7] The board also appears to have taken into account fringe benefits when deciding on salaries, such as whether or not the midwife lived in the dispensary premises. The number of cases a midwife attended also influenced the board. One midwife based in Nenagh was described as having a greater workload than the midwives in all the outlying districts combined; yet the midwives in the outlying districts had to negotiate 'mountainy districts' when attending to cases, and this was factored into consideration.[8] Mortished's telegram was somewhat successful, and one of the board members remarked: '[the midwives] like all others … had their association and their fixed fees, and their rules [and] the Board should fix a salary.'[9] A standardised salary was introduced for some of the midwives in Nenagh, and all received salary increases.

Setting a standardised salary was further complicated by dispensary midwives' involvement in private case work. Some midwives who worked in the Poor Law (or public) system topped up their small income with revenue from private case work. This was an economic necessity for midwives based

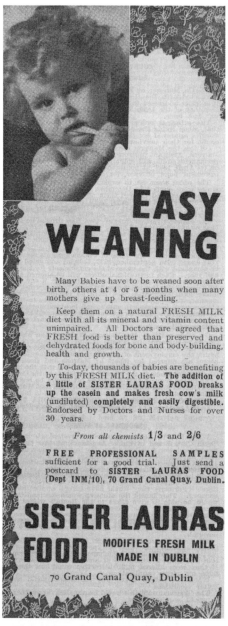

The iconic and eponymous baby food founded by Laura Smith, Ward Sister at Glasgow Children's Dispensary at the turn of the century. Digital content created, published and reproduced courtesy of Digital Library, UCD.

in districts with an insufficient number of Poor Law cases to sustain their earnings. The records of some boards, such as the Loughrea Board of Guardians, County Galway, suggest that this did not work in their favour, as the salary midwives earned for their work in the Poor Law system came to be viewed as just one of their sources of income and was titrated accordingly.[10] The INU took issue with this when, in June 1922, it wrote to the Macroom Board of Guardians, County Cork in relation to what it perceived as an insufficient salary increase: 'The [salary increase] gave great dissatisfaction to the midwives concerned, as it was apparently not calculated on the value of the work given, but on certain midwives [sic] private means, which should not, of course have been taken into consideration at all.'[11] The assumption that midwives blended work in the Poor Law system with private case work was not always correct. A midwife in County Kildare personally wrote to that county's Board of Health after INU representation on her behalf had failed to secure a salary increase in 1928. The midwife noted that her district was large and densely populated and that the high volume of patients she attended to meant that she did not have the time to engage in private case work.[12] Seemingly unimpressed, a board member remarked: 'It appears she has plenty of time to write letters.'[13] She was awarded a bonus of £5.

It seems that some employers were also suspicious that midwives were accepting money from Poor Law patients, and this too impacted on their remuneration. Under the Poor Law system, a patient deemed unable to pay for midwifery services was issued with a ticket by the Board of Guardians. A black ticket entitled the holder to free assistance at the dispensary and a red ticket, referred to as a 'scarlet runner', entitled the holder to free home visits by the midwife. The patient 'paid' the midwife with the ticket and midwives, in turn, were paid for producing these tickets to the board. A notable case arose in Castlebar, County Mayo in 1921, in which the Board of Guardians sought to remove four midwives from their posts.[14] It was alleged that the midwives in the district seldom produced tickets which, in turn, suggested that they were either not attending women in labour, in which case their services were no longer warranted, or, that they were receiving payments from the poor for midwifery services, a practice that was not permitted.

The midwives complained and were represented by the INU, which wrote to W.T. Cosgrave, the then Minister for Local Government at Dáil Éireann, on the matter. The minister wrote to the Board of Guardians, suggesting that, over time, a tradition had evolved where the poor were either asked for or donated a 'small fee or present' to a midwife for delivering a baby.[15] As a result, some pregnant women had stopped asking for tickets, as they felt that they had effectively paid the midwife. The practice spawned an ad hoc system of payment, referred to as a 'no ticket and small fee' system, which militated against a proper system of remuneration.[16] The minister sought, successfully, to have the proposed dismissal of the midwives overturned and decreed that, in the future, the public pay midwives with a ticket. The INU, realising the practice was injurious to midwives' salaries, also sought to stem the practice and reminded midwives to urge pregnant women to obtain a ticket at least one month in advance of childbirth and not to be 'too easy-going' with women who did not do so.[17]

Midwives' enduring service-obligation also played a role in their remuneration. The County Cavan Board of Health inquired into the production of tickets by midwives in 1928, to which one midwife responded: 'I attended several cases during the twelve months where parties called on me in a hurry, saying they would procure tickets later on, but never do so when the case is over. I am always ready and willing to attend the poor, whether presented at the time with a ticket or not.'[18] Another midwife remarked that she sometimes attended urgent cases, regardless of whether or not the patient had a ticket, for fear that 'the waiting to procure such tickets might have proved fatal.'[19]

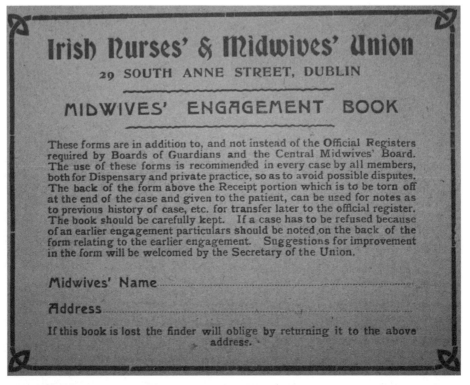

A Midwives' Engagement Book was instituted by the Irish Nurses' Union in order to help midwives keep an accurate record of the cases they attended. Courtesy the author.

In some cases, the INU's claims for better terms and conditions were successful. At the Navan Union in County Meath in 1920, all of the INU's requests were conceded. Conversely, in Armagh, the union's claim for a salary of £75 was only partially conceded, and salaries rose from £40 to £50 per year.[20] The main reason underlying the state's reluctance and inability to grant improvements in conditions at the time was economic. The Poor Law system was funded by local taxation, including a tax paid by local landowners known as the Poor Rate. Following the War of Independence, the Free State government concentrated much of its efforts on improving the competitiveness of Irish agricultural exports – a strategy that involved keeping landowners' taxes low. The ramifications of this strategy were commented on by the INU, when a nurse, who was also expected to perform midwifery duties, was sought in Sneem, County Kerry, in 1928: '[It is] very nice for the ratepayers, but we wonder how the nurse would enjoy it.'[21] In keeping with concerns over an increase in local taxation, some local authorities were also reluctant to grant pay increases as they feared a knock-on effect. A meeting of the Loughrea Board of Guardians in County Galway in July 1920 considered an application by the INU for an increase in salary. A board member responded: 'Of course, if you grant an increase in this case, they will all want it later on.'[22]

The changing Irish political landscape also determined the union's success. The Local Government Board for Ireland, formerly known as the Poor Law Commissioners, was the authority that governed public health services. The board was also a vestige of Westminster rule. After Sinn Féin's resounding victory in the 1918 general election, the establishment of Dáil Éireann in 1919, and the success of Sinn Féin in winning control of almost all Poor Law Boards of Guardians in local elections in 1920, the fledgling Irish parliament sought to undermine the authority of the Local Government Board. W.T. Cosgrave attempted to convert the allegiances of local authorities from the board to Dáil Éireann and by 1921, had much success. In retaliation, the British government decreed that Poor Law Boards of Guardians must recognise the Local Government Board in order to receive further funding. In addition, in 1920, as the War of Independence continued, the British government diverted exchequer grant funding away from local services and toward meeting the costs of claims for injuries sustained in the ongoing war. Bereft of these grants, Dáil Éireann needed to find savings if it was to assume responsibility for local services, including health services.[23]

This prompted the setting up of a Commission on Local Government in 1920, which recommended widespread rationalisation of local health services to include the closure of some workhouses and hospitals. The diversion of funding and the proposed rationalisation of the services was a source of great concern to the INU. Indeed, the first motion at the union's inaugural conference in 1920 called that any cuts to the health services be 'strenuously' resisted.[24] The union also sent a deputation to Dublin Corporation to protest. Marie Mortished railed against this: 'It will be little use establishing a Republic to rule a rachitic, adenoidal, tubercular and mentally deficient people.'[25] The cuts were also poised to affect INU members' conditions, with one member of the Commission on Local Government noting that he would 'make it a strict condition, by arrangement with Trades Unions or otherwise, that no increased expenditure be incurred by way of wages or salaries.'[26]

Nor was its members' devotion to duty helping the INU's case. A representative of the union put forward a case for an increase in midwives' salaries to the board of the Leitrim County Home in 1924. The representative detected some ambivalence on behalf of the board and inquired whether her efforts were 'only to see the wastepaper basket'; upon doing so, a board member derided her, and to the laughter of those present, remarked: 'Let the Union call them all out'.[27] The board did not accede to the pay claim. An implied no-strike policy now characterised the union, and this clearly left it in a weak bargaining position, of which Mortished observed: 'I am not at all sure that the authorities do not take advantage of the nurses' devotion to duty'.[28]

II. Opposition to the Handywoman

The First World War provided a new impetus to address some of the shortcomings in the health services in Ireland, including infant and maternal services. A heightened interest in these services was attributed to a number of factors including the high mortality rate inflicted by the war, the declining birth rate and a relatively slow rate of decline in Ireland's infant mortality rate. Maternal mortality, largely caused by puerperal septicaemia, which was associated with poor hygiene measures at childbirth, was also a concern. The state increased the funding for infant and maternal health measures and the *Midwives (Ireland) Act* of 1918, which provided for the establishment of the Central Midwives' Board and the Midwives' Roll, was passed. Nonetheless, progress was slow and in 1920, Marie Mortished, for the INU, wrote to the *British Journal of Nursing* and recounted an incident in which a farmyard manure cart was despatched by a Poor Law Guardian in County Meath to relay a midwife to a woman who required her services.[29] The midwife declined the offer of a jaunt in a veritable cesspit and made other arrangements to attend the woman, but the guardian's devil-may-care attitude was a reasonably good reflection of the state's overall detachment from public health issues at the time.

One area in which progress was especially slow was in the eradication of uncertified midwifery practitioners. The provisions of the *Midwives Act* forbade uncertified practitioners, often referred to as 'handywomen', from practicing as midwives. Handywomen carried out midwifery, and sometimes laid out the dead in their own communities. The INU had concerns over the quality of handywomen's practice and alleged that they were 'responsible for much of the terrible infant mortality in Ireland'.[30] At a meeting of the board of the Leitrim County Home in 1924, Miss Gloster, for the INU, reprimanded a local doctor for working with handywomen and implored him to desist from working with them in the future. The doctor's response suggested that he used the services of handywomen for fear of having to 'wash babies, etc.' himself.[31] Under the act, certification as a midwife was open only to those who held a certificate in midwifery from the Royal College of Physicians of Ireland or a lying-in hospital, those who already held a position as a midwife and those of 'good character' already engaged in 'bona fide' midwifery practice.[32]

The act also stipulated that no uncertified woman shall attend birthing women 'for gain'.[33] Thus, in County Leitrim, the doctor's defence was that the handywoman did not take any payment. Miss Gloster seemed dubious, however, and remarked that such women 'have their hand out for the fee all the same'.[34] Another stipulation in the act was also problematic as it decreed that uncertified women had to attend births 'habitually' in order to contravene the law.[35] This posed problems for the INU, as it meant that uncertified women were still permitted to attend to birthing women in emergencies. Therefore, successful prosecutions of uncertified women rested not only on proving that they were paid for their services but also on proving that such women attended births regularly and that such births were not emergencies; a sizeable burden of proof. One of the INU's primary aims was the introduction of a unique uniform and badge in order to differentiate certified practitioners from uncertified practitioners, and it lobbied the Central Midwives' Board of Ireland in this regard.[36] The union even went so far as designing a badge for the purpose; it was round, minted in silver, with a Celtic cross in the centre and four small shamrocks on its outer border. It bore the inscription 'CMB Saorstát Éireann'.[37] The board, however, maintained that it was unable to institute a uniform or badge until the *Midwives Act* was amended.[38]

The INU reported handywomen to the relevant local health authority and to the Central Midwives' Board in the hope that they might be prosecuted and, on occasions, wrote to local handywomen with a 'warning'.[39] Some 'quacks' stopped practicing on receipt of such letters.[40] The INU also published the names of uncertified midwives in its *Gazette*. One woman from County Laois received multiple warnings from the union and was reported to her local authority.[41] Some local authorities took action following the union's intervention, including Donegal County Council, who wrote to handywomen identified by the INU and warned them that they would be 'drastically dealt with' should they continue attending births.[42] The INU also convened public meetings and issued press notices informing the public of the importance of engaging only certified midwives to attend at childbirth. The union was unwavering in its hostility toward uncertified midwives. One provision of the *Midwives (Ireland) Act* of 1918 permitted 'bona fide' practitioners of 'good character' to have their names entered on the Midwives' Roll. These women were generally experienced midwives in receipt of good references from a doctor.[43] This did not placate the INU and, following a ballot, membership of the union was restricted to midwives certified by examination only. This resulted in one midwife being shown the door.

In its efforts to eradicate handywomen, the INU showed vigour and vitriol and referred to handywomen as 'dirty old women' lacking 'the remotest idea of aesepsis [*sic*]'.[44] Was this the case? Evidence certainly suggests that some handywomen were gruff and crotchety: One handywoman recounted her dealings with birthing women: 'Course you can get [the baby] out ... Don't be stupid. I'll put your head in a bucket of water if you don't shut up ... You've 'ad yer sweets, now you must 'ave yer sours.'[45] Birthing women also recounted some dubious practices by handywomen:

> When Maureen was born, I had to have a doctor ... [but] an old lady of 70 came. Oh God, she nearly drove me crackers! And d'you know what she did with our Maureen? She believed in bringing a baby up hardy, you know, in the country way. Maureen was born on the sixth of December. We had a big barrel of rain water outside and she brought in a bath from it. She had to break the ice on the water![46]

But the INU's allegation that handywomen were unhygienic is not fully supported: '[Our handywoman] always had a pure white apron on. And she actually turned it up at the corners and tucked it into her belt to keep the inside clean till she got to you ... your house had to be spotlessly clean before she'd enter. Scrubbed out with carbolic ... I can remember seeing her scrubbing her hands.'[47] Indeed, the union's pursuit of handywomen on occasions resembled that of a witch-hunt. At a meeting of the Cavan Health Board, the Secretary of the INU wrote: 'I am directed to write to you with reference to the death last month of a young woman ... We understand that this poor woman lost her life through being "attended" by an unqualified person [and] we consider that at least this woman should be prosecuted.'[48] The board did not entertain the request and remarked: 'If blame attaches to anybody it is to the woman's husband, who didn't go for a doctor until the eleventh hour.'[49]

The eventual passage of the *Midwives Act* of 1931 was welcomed by the INU as it embodied the union's long-sought aim of providing a distinct badge to midwives.[50] Other stipulations in the act also found favour. The legislation dispensed with the 'habitually and for gain' stipulation that had allowed handywomen to evade prosecution, and the activities of handywomen decreased from that point on. In spite of this, it was 1937 before a sustained downward trend in maternal mortality from puerperal sepsis was achieved: a trend

The long-awaited badge that would differentiate certified midwives from handywomen. It bore a shield with the Cross of Cong set on a green enamel background. A symbol representing the tree of life, in blue enamel, formed the crest of the badge. *Irish Nursing and Hospital World*/Image courtesy of the National Library of Ireland.

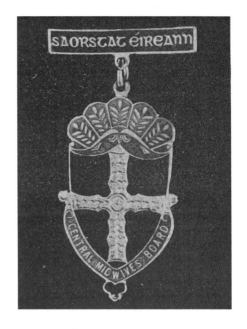

that appears largely as a result of the introduction of antimicrobial drugs.[51] The INU's campaign to eradicate handywomen formed part of a suite of measures that it, and organisations such as the 18,000-strong Women's National Health Association, took in order to improve the quality of maternity welfare. One account of district midwifery at the time referred to a woman who gave birth in a shack on an earthen floor, all the while harassed by chickens who flew in through a hole in the wall to shelter from the rain. The only other room in the woman's home was occupied by eight other children and a calf.[52] In another account, a doctor recalled attending women in 'dark, filthy, smelly slum[s] … Delivery was carried out in the family bedroom, from which we were continually shooing the children and pets. Once I caught the cat eating the placenta.'[53]

The INU's campaign against handywomen also doubled as a protectionist labour strategy that increased the employment prospects of certified midwives. This was evident to some, and in 1926 a member of Cavan County Council suggested that the union was not acting in the interest of patients and was 'only' seeking to 'safeguard the Nurses' Union'.[54] The union's eventual success regarding the abolition of handywomen was bittersweet. County medical officers were employed from 1927 onwards as part of increasing preventive health measures instituted by the state. They were responsible for maternity and child welfare and also sought the abolition of handywomen.[55] Although the nurses and midwives of the INU had been campaigning for over a decade in this regard, the doctors, the majority of whom were male,[56] campaigned for just a few years before the law was changed. This inequitable distribution of power and influence between men and women, doctors and nurses/midwives, would become a familiar theme in the years ahead.

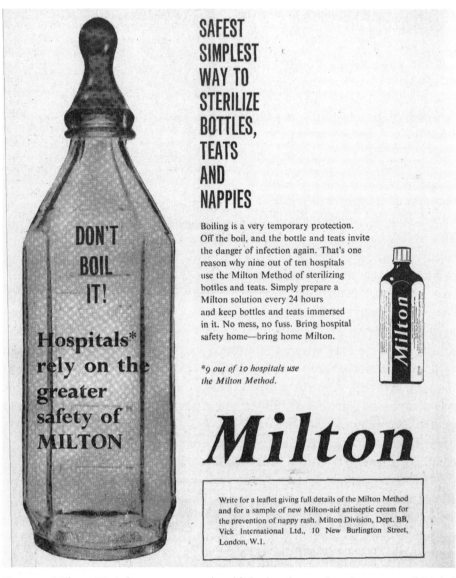

Courtesy Milton. Digital content created, published and reproduced courtesy of Digital Library, UCD.

III. Representing Nurses

The INU represented private practice nurses as well as nurses working in Poor Law hospitals, voluntary hospitals, sanatoria and the Jubilee district nursing service (precursors to today's public health nurses). The union sought improvements in the salaries and decreases in the working hours of its nurse members, in a similar fashion to that of its midwife members, by submitting a single claim to multiple employing authorities at once. The claim submitted was for a salary of £75, rising to £100.[57] The INU also put forward a motion for the implementation of a 48-hour work week at the Labour Party and Trade Union Congress meeting in Cork in 1920.[58] The reduction in nurses' working hours was resisted from both within and outside nursing. Miss Burkitt, Matron at Mercer's Hospital, Dublin, was asked her opinion regarding an 8-hour working day for nurses:

> I do not think that under present conditions it is practicable … it would mean a very big increase in the staff, and very few – if any – hospitals could afford that. Also, I do not think it would be good for the patient. I believe that changing the nurse during the night might have a bad effect in some cases, and after all, the patient must always come first.[59]

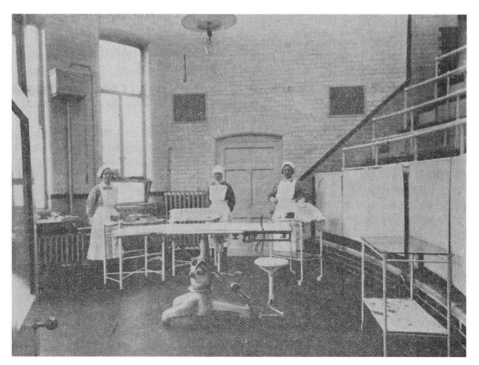

Nurses pictured in the operating theatre of Dublin's Richmond, Whitworth and Hardwicke Hospital in the early 1930s. *Irish Nursing and Hospital World*/Image courtesy of the National Library of Ireland.

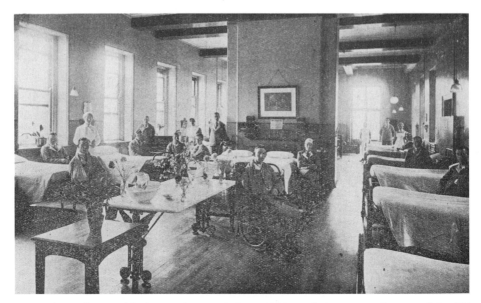

Surgical Ward at Dublin's Meath Hospital in 1931. *Irish Nursing and Hospital World/* Image courtesy of the National Library of Ireland.

Burkitt was not alone in her opinion. Senior Medical Officer, Sir Lambert Ormsby, of the National Children's Hospital, Dublin, argued that a shorter working week was applicable to the 'artisan or builder's labourer' but was incompatible with nursing.[60] According to Ormsby, a nurse's day was spread out and could not be captured in a set shift. He noted that nurses spent half their day 'reading a book, writing a letter or doing needlework' but needed to be 'within hail to answer a bell or call'.[61] A vexed Marie Mortished issued a swift rejoinder: 'Very few matrons would be satisfied to find a nurse reading a novel in her ward … Indeed, few nurses would dare even to sit down … Moreover, any time during which a nurse is bound to be on duty, to attend a call or answer a bell, cannot be considered as rest time.'[62] The idea of a shorter working week was also seen as unfeasible in the case of district nurses and midwives: 'By the very nature of her work she must be always ready to go out on duty. An accident or case of sudden illness calls her at any hour. Could she refuse to go by saying that she had already done her eight hours that day?'[63] The INU was not necessarily assured of support from the wider labour movement in its quest for a shorter working day.

Marie Mortished took issue with William O'Brien of the ITGWU, who had allegedly remarked that an 8-hour day for nurses working in Dublin hospitals was 'impossible'.[64] Mortished, never backward in coming forward,

A poem contributed to the *Irish Nurses' Journal* in 1938. Digital content created, published and reproduced courtesy of Digital Library, UCD.

Ode to an Nurse

The world grows better year by year,
Because some Nurse in her little sphere
Puts on her apron and cap and strings,
And keeps on doing the same old things.

Taking the temperatures, giving the Pills
To remedy mankind's numerous ills
Feeding the baby, answering the bells
Being polite with a heart that rebels.

Longing for home and all the while
Wearing the same old professional smile
Blessing the newborn baby's first breath
Closing the eyes that are still in death.

Taking the blame for the doctor's mistake
Oh dear! what a lot of patience it takes,
Going off duty at eight o'clock,
Discouraged and tearful and ready to drop

Called back for a "special" at eight fifteen
With woe in our hearts but it must not be
    seen.
Morning and evening, noon and night
Just doing it over and hoping it's right

reminded O'Brien that nurses were as entitled to a reduced working week as were the manual workers that his union represented. She continued that long working hours were a 'disease' and that O'Brien's talents 'would be better devoted to advocating remedies for the disease rather than to insisting that the victims of the disease should continue to suffer'.[65] The INU would return to the topic again and again. While a lack of support and solidarity from other trade unionists was clearly problematic for the INU's aspirations, it did not have to look as far as the wider trade union movement for evidence of waning solidarity. A schism was also developing among the INU's own members.

IV. Tensions Among and Between Nurses and Midwives

The first evidence of division between nurses and midwives in the INU appeared in 1920 when members stipulated that the union's badge for nurses be different to its badge for midwives.[66] In addition, in 1920, the Irish Nurses' Union changed its name to the Irish Nurses' and Midwives' Union, reflecting the fact that over half of its members were midwives. However, in 1925, at the behest of the Limerick branch, the union's name reverted to the original title,

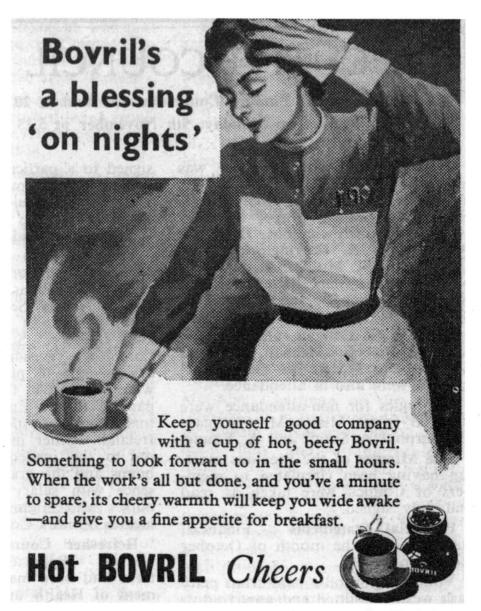

Bovril's a blessing 'on nights'

Keep yourself good company with a cup of hot, beefy Bovril. Something to look forward to in the small hours. When the work's all but done, and you've a minute to spare, its cheery warmth will keep you wide awake —and give you a fine appetite for breakfast.

Hot BOVRIL Cheers

Revenue from advertising played a vital part in keeping the union's periodical afloat. Courtesy Unilever. Digital content created, published and reproduced courtesy of Digital Library, UCD.

as this was believed to be 'less clumsy'.[67] This is scarcely credible considering the lengthy names of other unions, such as the Irish Transport and General Workers' Union, and suggests that, in reality, some members found the inclusion of midwives in the union's title as unpalatable. Issues with regard to the union's badge and title were manifestations of deeper discord.

By the late 1920s, membership of the INU was dwindling. INU representatives surveyed the reasons underlying this trend and discovered that general nurses were not inclined to join because of the presence of midwives in the union.[68] The precise reason for nurses' objection to midwives was not made explicit; however, the union did note a tendency to 'regard some branches of nursing as inferior'.[69] In the early 1900s, only a fraction of midwives were also nurses, and midwifery training lasted six months. In contrast, nurse training lasted three years. This, for some, diminished the midwife's professional status. The INU once made a representation to the Board of Health in County Cavan seeking pay increases for midwives, whom it noted were one of the 'worst paid professions in the country'.[70] One board member remarked: 'Would you call it a profession? It takes them only a short time to qualify'.[71] There were also industrial tensions between nurses and midwives as each sector competed for cases. The union issued a statement in 1926 to the effect that it was sure that no members of the INU would 'poach' anybody else's patient but cautioned: '[Do not] expect the Union to act as a kind of policeman ... [as] no Union can make an unprincipled person act fairly and decently: it can only ... shame the guilty nurse into more loyal behaviour in future'.[72]

The fact that the topic was raised again in 1929 suggests that the problem persisted, and a resolution was passed at that year's Annual Council Meeting, imploring midwives not to take on general nursing cases, and general nurses not to take on midwifery cases.[73] The issue prompted an editorial in the *Gazette* in 1930 which asked: 'What good is our Nurses' Union if it doesn't join us together?'[74] Some members were outright in disobeying the union's rules. In 1934, a midwife asked the INU for help in recouping fees owed to her for some general nursing cases she had taken on. When the midwife was informed that general nursing cases were outside her remit, she snapped that she would engage in any general nursing work she could find and would recover the fees herself.[75]

The lack of unity evident between nurses and midwives was also evident within each group. The union discouraged nurses from applying for positions it considered underpaid – one position as a public health nurse in the 'Kingdom' of Kerry paid a 'beggarly' £100, for which nurses would reportedly be 'tumbling over each other' to fill.[76] It also bemoaned midwives who were willing to fill underpaid positions as maintaining the problematic status quo: 'Unfortunately midwives are so disloyal to one another ... The Cavan midwives have only

" To Destroy or to Build, that is the Question "

It is easy to destroy.

It is so hard to build.

You would like to destroy this Organisation ?

1. Don't be a member;

2. Be a half-hearted member; only pay your Sub-scription when you have received several reminders;

3. Threaten to resign the moment a difficulty is experienced in solving some particular prob-lem on your behalf.

4. Keep on pointing out what the Organisation has not achieved and forget the good things it done;

5. Insist to yourself and to everyone else that you would have got ALL that you have without any Organisation;

6. Enjoy your fool's paradise—while it lasts—let someone else pay the bill.

The union and organisation made frequent calls for nurses and midwives to take a more active role in membership. Digital content created, published and reproduced courtesy of Digital Library, UCD.

£35 a year, and yet if every district was vacant to-morrow, there would be ten applicants in every case.[77] Petty provincialism also featured. On one occasion, the union was forced to censure its Limerick branch for victimising a member from Dublin who had taken up a position at a local hospital.[78] The Limerick branch believed that local positions should be awarded to local nurses, some of whom were unemployed. The branch took exception to being reprimanded by the INU's executive and began withholding subscriptions.[79]

The parochial manner in which health services were administered and funded proved a significant impediment to the INU's attempts to establish standardised working conditions. The severe economic backdrop also meant that public monies needed in order to accede to the union's demands were scarce and rendered the union's successes as gradual. Considering the straitened economic times, all alternative means of improving its members' conditions were exploited, and this is clear in the union's campaign to

SAVE POSTAGE

★ Why not attend your Branch Meeting ?

★ Why not pay your Membership Contribution at that meeting ?

★ Does this save Postage ?

YES. The Branch Secretary sends contributions in bulk to Head Office, having given you your receipt BY HAND.

★ Head Office sends a single receipt to the Branch Secretary.

★ Please help us to save both time and postage.

eradicate handywomen, which doubled as a public health strategy. Unwilling to exercise its industrial muscle by means of strike action, the union advised members not to apply for positions that it considered underpaid. Unflinching adherence to this strategy was crucial, yet when solidarity was most needed, it was found wanting, and the trend in INU members violating core trade union principles and applying for underpaid positions partly explains the modest successes the union achieved in its early years. Nurses and midwives were seemingly a labour force with a loose commitment to trade union principles and were willing to sacrifice such principles in favour of pragmatism when necessity dictated.

The nature of nursing and midwifery work also influenced progress. The exigencies of patient care led matrons to rule out the possibility of shorter working hours for nurses, and midwives proved willing to attend birthing mothers free of charge where clinical necessity dictated. This informed the union's de facto no-strike policy, and it was only a matter of time before employers recognised that, for nurses and midwives, the obligation to serve was sacrosanct. Once they did, they capitalised upon it – evident in County Leitrim where an employer refused to accede to the union's claim and, amid laughter, goaded an INU representative into calling a strike, knowing how remote that possibility was. Considering the multitude of challenges it faced, the INU would not last long in its current guise.

CHAPTER 4

New Name, Familiar Aim: From Trade Union to Professional Association, 1925–37

Hopes that the late 1920s might bring some respite from Ireland's challenging economic times would soon be dashed. Economic depression and unemployment took root in the early 1920s and necessitated draconian austerity measures; government expenditure was almost halved from £42 million in 1923 to £24 million in 1926;[1] the advent of a six-year economic war with Britain in 1932 resulted in an increase in taxes and in the price of goods and, as if things were not bad enough, from 1932 onwards, the effects of the global economic depression were widespread. Signifying a lack of faith among workers in their trade unions' ability to effect improvements in their working conditions, membership of the ITUC plummeted from 189,000 in 1922 to just 95,000 in 1933.[2] The country's dire economic situation meant that the state soon 'largely ignored' the trade union movement.[3] This was the heady backdrop to the INU's most significant decision to date: to leave the trade union fold entirely.

I. Rethinking Trade Unionism: Becoming a Professional Association

The INU's transition from trade union to professional association commenced in 1925 when it sought to affiliate to the ICN. The ICN was founded in 1899 and aimed to establish a global network of nurses – its core concerns were internationalism, professionalism and the standardisation of nursing. Affiliation to the international council was on a country-by-country basis, and the establishment of the Saorstát in 1922 meant that Ireland was no longer affiliated to the ICN in tandem with Britain. This prompted the Irish Matrons' Association to investigate the establishment of a National Council of Nurses for the Irish Free State in 1924.[4] Individual nurses' associations wishing to affiliate to the ICN would firstly affiliate to the National Council, which would, in turn, affiliate to the ICN on their behalf. The INU's enthusiasm to affiliate to the ICN may have been prompted by the international actions of other women's groups: in the same way that the National Council of Nurses was considering being affiliated to the ICN, a National Council of Women in Ireland had been formed in order to affiliate to the International Council of Women in 1924.[5] The INU's parent, the IWWU, was among the members of that council.

The INU was deemed unable to affiliate to the National Council of Nurses for the Irish Free State because the union comprised 'lay' persons among its 'officers'.[6] The most prominent 'lay' person in the INU's fold was Louie Bennett who, in response, cordially relinquished the INU Presidency in 1925 and was made Honorary Vice-President. The union attempted to replace Bennett with Annie Smithson. Smithson was a nurse and midwife and had an exemplary employment record. Her reference from the Edinburgh Royal Infirmary describes her as 'thoroughly reliable, clever, and capable, extremely pleasant … and most efficient in her ward management'.[7] Her nursing and managerial prowess was not the only feather in her cap. Smithson had a very successful sideline as an author and, by 1925, was one of Ireland's most celebrated novelists. Kathleen Nora Price, for the INU, wrote to Smithson: 'the meeting elected you as President … They all thought it would be most valuable to have you, and it need not entail your attending meetings regularly: just if you can put in an appearance now and again.'[8] Smithson was not taken in by Price's advances and declined the position due to pressure of work: she was still working as a health visitor and 1925 alone witnessed the publication of three of her novels. Instead, Mrs Mary McCarry, a nurse at the Dublin Union Hospital, assumed the role of President of the INU, initially in an acting capacity but, thereafter, in a standard capacity. The union now had its first nurse President and its application to affiliate to the National Council was successful. Thereafter, the National Council, on behalf of the Irish Free State, affiliated to the ICN.

Transition continued in May 1928 when, at the Annual Council Meeting, the INU decided to disaffiliate from the IWWU. Disaffiliation was felt to be necessary as 'it was thought that the Nurses' organisation [*sic*] standing on its own might be an incentive to keenness on the nurses' part' and because of fears that 'the general body of nurses will not join an organisation which is not entirely owned and controlled by nurses'.[9] Mrs McCarry also noted, with good reason, that the INU had become a 'drag' on the IWWU.[10] The INU was in a state of near-constant financial embarrassment and benefitted enormously from financial guidance and handouts from the IWWU. Things changed in 1923. That year, the INU promised to make a donation of one penny per member to the Association of Blind Workers. When it found itself unable to

NURSES' UNION ANNUAL MEETING

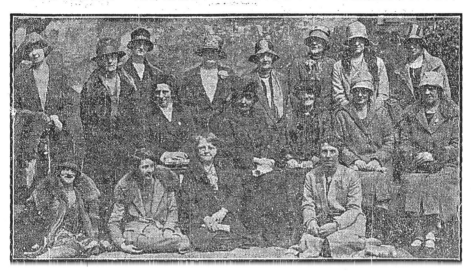

In this photograph, taken yesterday at 34 St. Stephen's Green, Dublin, the names read, left to right, front row:—Miss A. Guinane, Miss Price (Sec.), Mrs. Cann (Dublin), Mrs. Price (Finglas). Middle row, left to right:—Mrs. Hannelly (Loughlinstown Hospital), Miss Guinane (Dublin), Miss Porter (do.), Mrs. McGarry, President (Dublin), Mrs. Foley (Waterford), Mrs. McCarthy (Dublin), Mrs. Richardson (do.) Back row, left to right:—Miss O'Connor (Loughlinstown), Miss Rafferty (Roscommon), Miss Jordan (Dublin Union), Mrs. Donovan (Child Welfare), Miss Ryan (Galway), Miss Kenny (Dublin).—"I.I." Photo.

Members at the union's 1928 Annual Meeting where the decision was taken to leave the Irish Women Workers' Union. With thanks to Irish Newspaper Archives and the *Irish Independent*.

afford to do so, it asked the IWWU to pay the money on its behalf – only to be turned down.[11]

Two months later, the INU was informed that the IWWU would no longer pay it any surplus expenditure over and beyond income.[12] The threat resonated and the INU was forced to conceive of all and any strategies to keep the cash-strapped organisation afloat. A stopwatch competition was one of the schemes hit upon: a valuable watch was procured, wound and placed in a locked box. Members then bought tickets, with each ticket pertaining to a particular time on the watch. After a number of days, the locked box was opened and the watch, which had invariably stopped, was examined. The member whose ticketed time was closest to the time at which the watch had stopped won a prize – generally the watch itself.[13] Desperation really did breed ingenuity!

The INU attributed much of the blame for its financial difficulties to members' reluctance to pay their subscriptions. By June 1921, a total of 263 members out of a membership of 576 were in arrears, and over 150 members had their membership discontinued for non-payment of fees.[14] Many women, considering their paltry salaries, were unwilling to pay modest trade union subscription fees,[15] and it is easy to see why. A midwife from County Clare contacted INU headquarters at the time and complained that a farmer refused to pay her any more than £1, 10 shillings from a total bill of £11, which he had accrued for daily post-operative dressings.[16] Cases such as this kept the union's solicitor busy throughout the 1920s and illustrate that INU members and, in turn, their union, experienced the same financial difficulties as the patients they tended. It is little wonder that the INU's early meetings were partly funded by members who held whist drives, a type of card game where players competed against one another, and kindly sent the proceeds to headquarters.

The union's decision to disaffiliate from the IWWU was not unanimous[17] and was arrived at during the union's Annual Council Meeting, which was attended by just twenty delegates. The IWWU perceived this to be 'undemocratic'[18] and wrote to the INU, noting that it had 'misunderstood' its status, which was that of a 'woman's organisation permanently attached to the I.W.W.U.'[19] The significance of the IWWU's position will become clear in time, but the break-up, which was more amicable than it sounds, proceeded. The divorce did result in the Nurses' Union having to find a new office and, in 1930, it moved to a space on Dublin's main thoroughfare, 28 Upper O'Connell Street – beside the renowned Findlater's grocery store. It soon moved once again to 24 Nassau Street, where it shared its premises with a car parts dealer and an architect. An extension in its office hours from 9:30 a.m. to 1 p.m. and 2 p.m. to 5 p.m. demonstrated its increasing activity levels.

Following its breakaway from the Women Workers' Union, the INU sought to affiliate independently with the Labour Party and Trade Union Congress.[20] This gives lie to speculation that the INU broke ties with the IWWU in order to placate general nurses who had, a year earlier, indicated that the INU's association with the party and congress dissuaded them from joining.[21] Nonetheless, disquiet within the union regarding its association with the Labour Party and Trade Union Congress soon manifested. A motion at the Annual Council Meeting in 1930 read: 'In view of the fact that this is a Union of Professional Women, would it be desirable in the interests of the Union that it remain no longer affiliated to the Unions [?]'[22] Another motion called that the word 'Union' be removed from the INU's title altogether.[23] Neither motion was carried, but it was becoming clear that the INU's unionateness was coming under increasing scrutiny. The Labour Party and Trade Union Congress separated in 1930 and became the Labour Party and Irish Trade Union Congress, respectively. The Labour Party invited the INU to affiliate to it following the separation.[24] This necessitated the INU reaffirming its status as a trade union, which had been interrupted following its separation from the IWWU in 1928.

The INU did so and had its status as a trade union reaffirmed in 1933 by the Registrar of Friendly Societies.[25] Although the union balloted its members on whether or not to affiliate to the Labour Party, the ballot was judged as void on account of a technicality and no evidence exists as to its outcome. Affiliation to the Labour Party never took place, and the union adopted the mantle of being 'non-political' from then on.[26] The INU would no longer countenance affiliating to a political party, but nevertheless, its political activities continued. The union rose on the crest of new unionism and attempted, unsuccessfully, to have a member of its executive elected as a Poor Law Guardian in Dublin shortly after its establishment.[27] In the 1930s, it requested that a nurse be appointed to the Department of Local Government in order to advance a nursing perspective on policy issues[28] and extensive lobbying of politicians also continued unabated.

The INU was still affiliated to the ITUC – but not for long. In 1935, the ITUC sent a communication to the Nurses' Union with regards to the designation of 1 May, May Day, as a national holiday. The Nurses' Union's Executive marked the letter: 'read'. Congress appears to have been miffed by the response and its Secretary requested that the INU be 'kind enough' to explain what it meant by marking the letter as 'read'.[29] The ITUC's Secretary, who apparently exited from the wrong side of the bed that morning, continued that the ITUC took 'serious notice' that the INU should treat the resolution in 'so offensive a manner'.[30] The INU assured the ITUC that any offence was unintended but reminded it, cynically, that it 'did not think that the matter applied to the nursing profession, the majority of whom could not avail of the existing bank holidays [hence] an additional one would be of little use to them'.[31] The incident was the last straw, and a few weeks later, at its Annual Meeting, the INU decided to disaffiliate from the ITUC.[32] The transformation of the INU into a professional association was complete in 1936 when it was decided that the 'union' moniker would be dropped altogether in favour of a new title: the Irish Nurses' Organisation (INO).

The INU was established as a trade union amid the potent labourist atmosphere of 1919. Trade union membership was falling by 1936, and the INU's decision to leave the trade union fold marked a move with the times. Considering its members' rumblings about trade unionism being incompatible with nurses'/midwives' professional status, the Nurses' Union's decision to join an avowedly professional organisation like the ICN and its decision to leave the

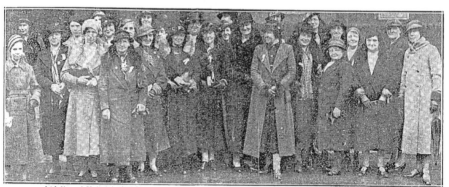

Irish Nurses' Union Annual Meeting at 24 Nassau St., Dublin, yesterday.   From the left: Mrs.
Millar, Mrs. Nicholson, Miss Clinton, Mrs. Hickey, Miss Griffin, Miss A. Smithson (Secretary),
Miss Kiely, Mrs. Jones, Mrs. Joyce, Miss Condon, Miss Healy (President), Mrs. O'Brien, Miss
Hannelly, Miss O'Callaghan, Miss Corless, Miss O'Connor, Mrs. Cann, Mrs. Bonass, Mrs. T. Nix-
and Miss Murphy.   —*Irish Independent* Photo. (McM.).

Members at the union's 1936 Annual Meeting where the decision was taken to leave
the trade union movement entirely. With thanks to Irish Newspaper Archives and the
Irish Independent.

IWWU and Trade Union Congress can be viewed as an attempt to appease and
attract into membership those nurses and midwives for whom trade unionism
had never been palatable. From that point onwards, the INO increasingly
blended both industrial and professional matters in an effort to appeal to a
wide membership base and to blunt the perceived gulf that separated nurses'
and midwives' industrial and professional aspirations.

The transformation from trade union to professional association
coincided with some key personnel changes: Louie Bennett's departure as
President of the INU in 1925 was the first. Bennett later became the first
woman President of the ITUC. Although she adopted largely conciliatory
methods, she led a successful fourteen-week-long strike of women laundry
workers in the 1940s. Her ability to remain conciliatory yet utilise strike
action when absolutely necessary may have served the INU and its successor,
the INO, better than the dogged aversion to strike action that soon became
the Nurses' Organisation's hallmark. Some forty years after it left the congress,
the INO found itself severely disenfranchised because its position outside of
congress rendered it unable to influence national wage agreements. Had the
INO remained a trade union and remained within congress, this would not
have been the case. Yet analysis of whether the INU's decision to leave the
trade union movement was wise is largely pie in the sky. Membership of the
INU was low and falling lower, and had the union not altered its status, its
continued existence was unlikely.

There were also other key personnel changes at this time. Marie Mortished resigned her post as Secretary of the INU in May 1921. It appears that she was pregnant and 'family ties prevent[ed] her from giving the time and attention she would like to the Union'.[33] This was the second occasion on which Mortished tried to resign but, on the previous occasion, had been persuaded to stay by the union, who were fearful of losing her expertise and extensive connections. Mortished was replaced by Kathleen Nora Price, the INU's erstwhile clerk. Price suffered an even worse fate than Mortished in the acknowledgement stakes, and it is largely through fleeting references in the histories of her renowned brother, the judge and antiquarian Liam Price,[34] and his wife, the prominent tuberculosis doctor Dorothy Stopford Price,[35] that anything at all is known of her. Indeed, prior to the extensive genealogical inquiry undertaken as part of this book, Kathleen Nora Price was known only as 'KN Price', as her first name remained unknown. Price was a member of the Socialist Party of Ireland and served as Secretary of the Irish Section of the Friends of Soviet Russia.[36] In a letter to Bennett following the INU's decision to disaffiliate from the IWWU, she added a postscript: 'I need hardly say that I myself am very sorry that this decision was come to.'[37]

She resigned her position thereafter. The INU arranged a function at Clery's Restaurant, Dublin in her honour, at which she was presented with a suitcase. The gift was a fitting one as Price was soon bound for Leningrad where, at the invitation of the Russian trade union movement, she formed part of a delegation from the Dublin Trade Union and Labour Council.[38] Price all but disappeared from public life after her departure from the INU. She died in 1949; the crumbling disrepair of her grave at Dublin's Mount Jerome Cemetery belies a memorable life. Her departure from the INU in 1928, in her mid-thirties, suggests that, as a committed trade unionist, she foresaw and disliked the direction in which the union was headed. Albinia Brodrick was also aggrieved at developments and wrote a letter in which she protested that the term 'Union' had been dropped in favour of 'Organisation'. Her request that the letter be published in the organisation's periodical was not entertained,[39] and Brodrick resigned from the organisation's County Kerry branch.[40] The union's 'old guard' was changing, but certain core principles remained the same. This was especially the case in relation to strike action.

II. 'No nurse would leave her patient, even if she were never paid for her work': The Service-Obligation in Action

The 'new' INO referred to itself as 'purely professional' and cultivated a new image.[41] This was most evident in the organisation's increased focus on nurse

THE IRISH NURSES' UNION.

A POST GRADUATE COURSE FOR MIDWIVES.

WILL BE HELD AT

The ROTUNDA HOSPITAL, DUBLIN

(by kind arrangement of the Master and Matron of the Hospital).

Tickets, price, 5/-. Obtainable from either the Matron, Rotunda Hospital, Dublin, or Miss Price, Secretary, Irish Nurses' Union, 29 South Anne Street, Dublin.

Single Lecture Tickets, price, 1/-.

Applications to be made by October 1st. Syllabus supplied on request.

Advertisement for the union's first refresher course for midwives held at Dublin's Rotunda Hospital in 1928. Digital content created, published and reproduced courtesy of Digital Library, UCD.

education. The INU organised lectures at the Dublin Nurses' Club on topics such as diabetes, puerperal sepsis and radium from as early as 1924. In 1928, after leaving its parent IWWU, the *Gazette* began to incorporate educational articles. Before long, the union also began organising refresher courses for midwives. The first such course was held at Dublin's Rotunda Hospital in 1928. The course commenced on Saturday 6 October with tea. Subsequent activities included a practical demonstration on how to bathe babies and trips to the infants' dispensary and antenatal clinic. A lecture on gynaecological surgery and venereal diseases was also held, and the course concluded on Saturday 13 October with a written examination.[42] Lecture notes were reprinted in the union's periodical which, in 1936, changed its name to the altogether more scholarly *Irish Nurses' Journal*. Lectures addressed issues of concern such as record keeping and the importance of reporting cases of sepsis; these were two issues over which the Central Midwives' Board sometimes investigated midwives.

Refresher courses were state-supported, with the Department of Local Government and Public Health meeting attendees' expenses and paying for a substitute in their absence. A course for nurses, organised by the INU, in 'housewifery and storekeeping', 'as an aid to the management of large institutions' was held at the Rathmines Technical Institute, Dublin in the same year.[43] Education courses were partly responsible for increasing the

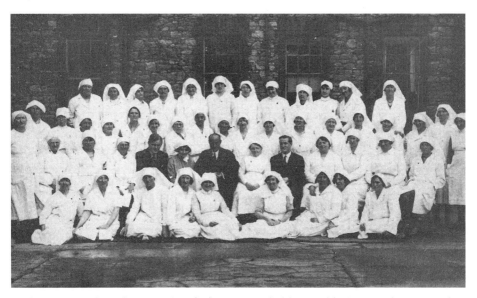

Midwives attending the union's refresher course held at Dublin's Coombe Hospital in 1930. Courtesy INMO.

organisation's membership. Of the twenty-five midwives who joined the INO in October 1936, seventeen had been sourced at a refresher course at Dublin's Coombe Hospital.[44] INU membership had fallen to perilously low levels in the late 1920s. In 1929, the union had just 437 members.[45] However, as the INU evolved into the INO, membership increased. In 1930, membership amounted to 220 general nurses and 324 midwives,[46] but by 1936 there were 937 members;[47] the INO clearly commended itself to members in a manner that the INU had not.

The organisation's decision to rescind its trade union identity reinforced its disinclination to take strike action. Kathleen Nix, earnest INO organiser and former tuberculosis nurse in County Clare, attended a meeting of the North Tipperary Board of Health in 1937 and made a representation requesting improvements in members' conditions. In replying to Nix, a board member remarked 'if you were organised in a trade union you would be in a position to compel what you now ask as a favour'.[48] The remark was a veiled reference to strike action but appeared to go over Nix's head. Instead, she responded that, if necessary, nurses would work 168 hours per week, as nurses 'could not go on strike [as] no nurse would leave her patient, even if she were never paid for her work'.[49] On first consideration, the wisdom of Nix's statement is questionable; if nurses could not bring the pressure of strike action to bear on their employers, then there was little incentive for employers to accede to their demands. However, as Nix gave expression to what was previously a de facto no-strike policy, INO membership reached almost 1,000, its largest ever, suggesting that nurses and midwives, in keeping with their service-obligation, were commended to the organisation because of its aversion to strike action.

The organisation's aversion to strike action was given its first practical expression that same year when, at the Ardee Mental Hospital, County Louth, nursing staff, who were members of the ITGWU, threatened to strike. The dispute concerned salaries, allowances and demands for a 48-hour week. The hospital's Medical Superintendent took grave issue and reported:

> Service must be continuous. [The hospital] cannot be closed down like an industrial concern during a dispute ... No organisation of nurses could so far forget the principles of the nursing professions to suggest that the patients should be let suffer for want of skilled attention, and that such suffering should be used as a lever to bring pressure on their employers.[50]

In response to the threat, the hospital's managers decided to hire temporary staff and to fire those who took strike action.[51] Having turned down the

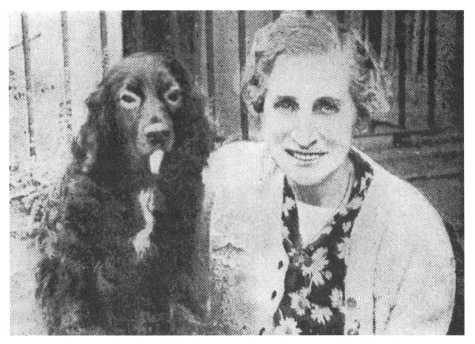

Annie Smithson pictured with her favourite dog Judy. Copyright Talbot Press.

Presidency of the INU in 1925, Annie Smithson was appointed Secretary of the union following Kathleen Nora Price's departure in 1929. Smithson's celebrity preceded her; she was popular with rank-and-file members and put her penmanship to use. Writing in the *Irish Independent*, she questioned whether the strikers were trained nurses as, if they were, 'there could be no question whatsoever of a strike'.[52] For Smithson, a striking nurse was clearly an oxymoron, and she asked: 'Why should the mentally afflicted patients be allowed to suffer through the employment of untrained "nurses" who do not scruple to sacrifice them to their own material ends? With nurses the patients always come first.'[53] Smithson lauded the hospital's managers for their attempts to replace the strikers with temporary nurses who, it appears, were INO members. The local Branch Secretary of the ITGWU wrote to the Registrar of the General Nursing Council at the time:

> In view of the fact that many of those presently participating in the lock-out strike at Ardee Mental Hospital are on the register of the General Nursing Council, does that body consider it proper that these nurses should be unfairly ousted from their positions by other nurses who are presumably

on the Register of the General Nursing Council, and are, we understand, all members of the Irish Nurses [*sic*] Organisation[?][54]

A spokesperson for the ITGWU also wrote to the press, noting '[that] neither the attendants and nurses of the Mental Hospitals throughout the Saorstat [*sic*], for the great majority of whom we speak, nor the general nurses, for the great majority of whom the Irish Nurses' Organisation does not speak, will thank Miss Smithson for her virtual encouragement of an attempt at strike-breaking.'[55] Smithson's refusal to countenance striking endeared the INO to the institution's managers and, following the strike, membership of the INO was made a compulsory precondition of employment there.[56] A small number of mental nurses, thirty-seven in total, subsequently appeared on the organisation's roll books, for a short period of time, in the early 1940s.[57]

III. The Quest for Pensions Begins

There was no end to the issues that nurses and midwives implored the INU/INO to address. A midwife wrote to the organisation bemoaning the fact that one of the rooms in her 'condemned' two-room 'château' had water coming through the floor, necessitating the other room's use as a combined kitchen, bedroom, bathroom, dining room, waiting room and antenatal and postnatal clinic.[58] The midwife's sentiments kick-started a long-running campaign by the INO to secure better accommodation for the sector. The organisation also found itself campaigning for the addition of sufficient tea, butter and vegetables to nurses' meagre food rations. But the organisation's efforts to secure improvements in its members' conditions were none more evident than in its campaign to establish adequate pension arrangements, which began in 1929. The decision to establish a pension scheme was timely, as the Nation's Tribute Fund to Nurses, a charitable fund, was encountering financial difficulties owing to the fact that its capital had ceased earning sufficient interest.

Nurses who worked in state-run institutions and dispensary midwives had pensions, as provided for under the 1925 *Local Government Act*.[59] These pensions were small, and the union had fears over their adequacy. Worse off was the sizable number of nurses and midwives who worked in voluntary hospitals or in private practice, who had no pensions at all. This had far-reaching ramifications, as unemployment and the absence of a comprehensive pension scheme were cyclically related, with the lack of a pension scheme meaning that older nurses could not retire when they should, which diminished turnover and deprived younger nurses of jobs. The pension scheme envisaged by the

INU was one which would supplement nurses/midwives who were in receipt of small pensions and would provide a pension of at least £1 per week to those with no pension.

The union established a fund known as the Irish Pension Fund for Nurses in 1930. The fund's aim was to 'get together a sufficient sum of money to enable [it] to give pensions to all nurses in every branch of the profession.'[60] The union proposed that each nurse pay 5 shillings initially and 5 shillings per year thereafter and envisaged that, in time, the state would augment the fund with grant aid.[61] The INU received all subscriptions to the fund at its headquarters. It also began to explore the possibility that a pension scheme could be funded by sweepstake lotteries. Sweepstakes had been used to fund various Irish hospitals throughout the 1920s. Up until the early 1930s, such sweepstakes had been run under questionable legal circumstances. Indeed, the Nurses' Union once received a visit by detectives who informed it that a sweepstake it was running to benefit its pension fund was illegal[62] due, it appears, to the fact that the sweepstakes' prize money exceeded that which was permitted and because the tickets were sent outside of the Irish Free State.[63] As a result, all monies had to be returned to subscribers and the Minister for Justice ordered that the union's mail be placed under surveillance for a period.[64]

Ireland's recession in the 1920s gave way to global depression in the 1930s. The country's economic circumstances caused grave difficulties for voluntary hospitals and in 1930, due mainly to the financial embarrassment of Dublin's National Maternity Hospital, where part of the ceiling in the hospital's gynaecology ward was teetering on the brink of collapse, sweepstakes received legal legitimacy and were earmarked as a manner in which funds could be raised for impoverished hospitals. Annie Smithson welcomed the development:

> Hospitals have risen Phoenix-like from the ashes of debt, and now stand strong and secure with satisfactory finance and a feeling that their future will not be hampered through lack of funds ... [However] brick and stone and slate and steel will be kept in good repair, but the human side to the hospital cannot look to the future with the same sense of security.[65]

The idea that a nurses' pension fund would be financed by charitable means was not new. The Jubilee Nurses' Institute, which provided community nursing services, funded its nurses' pensions with a £100,000 gratuity, which it received from an anonymous philanthropist. Kilkenny Castle sometimes opened its gardens to the paying public in order to fund district nurses' pensions. Not everybody believed that sweepstakes were a fitting means to fund a nurses' pension scheme. A member of the public, Ita O'Shea, wrote to the *Irish Independent* in 1931 and took issue with Smithson's hopes to have pensions funded from a sweepstake lottery. O'Shea believed that nurses should be pensioned in the same way as other state employees, as opposed to 'picking up the crumbs from someone else's feast'.[66]

The Nurses' Union was not put off by these sentiments, but Smithson's efforts to divert sweepstake monies to a nurses' pension fund soon hit a brick wall. A response from the sweepstakes' trustees was curt and dismissive: 'I hope some philanthropist will soon come your way'.[67] Further correspondence between the INU and the Hospitals Trust, which administered the sweepstake, identified the impasse. Joseph McGrath, Director of the Trust, wrote to the INU, informing it that it was outside the remit of the legislation upon which the sweepstake operated to fund a nurses' pension scheme.[68] McGrath had once worked for the ITGWU but, by the time he assumed management of the Hospitals Trust, 'his days as an advocate of workers' rights were behind him'.[69] Indeed, the INU's former parent, the IWWU, expressed concerns regarding working conditions among the sweepstakes' workforce and, consequently, some unions considered shunning the sweepstake entirely.[70] In the sweep's early days, nurses loaded sweepstake tickets into the drums. Blind children then chose the winning tickets from the drums in an effort to ensure impartiality.

Nurses were responsible for drawing the winning tickets in later years. The experience was exhilarating, as recalled by a nurse from Dublin's National Maternity Hospital in 1931: 'I was literally shaking! ... I never closed my eyes all Tuesday night ... [the person in charge] explained the routine of the Draw to us; telling us not to talk amongst ourselves, and to be very careful in every way while we were on the stage.'[71] Although this nurse's appraisal was, overall, a positive one – indeed she was treated to lunch at the Gresham Hotel and given a ticket to a show at the Gaiety Theatre (she narrowly missed out on a box of chocolates) – it was not long before questions regarding how they were treated also arose. In 1932, Dublin surgeon William Taylor complained: 'Some of [the nurses] had been sent [to the draw] after being on night duty all night. That was nothing short of a scandal, and those who sent them there in those circumstances had not a particle of human kindness in them.'[72] Worried at damaging the prospect of its pension fund becoming a beneficiary of the sweepstakes, Annie Smithson kept quiet.

The INU persisted and notified all general nurses on the Register of the General Nursing Council and all midwives on the Roll of the Central Midwives' Board of the Irish Pension Fund for Nurses and invited them to subscribe. The response was poor, and by 1933 only 475 had joined, some of whom were already in arrears.[73] Many of those who applied were also aged. One called personally to the union's headquarters: the woman in question was eighty-two years of age and remarked: 'You must forgive me – I am rather deaf. Is this the place where we are to come about the nurses' pensions? ... Do you think we will get it before I die?'[74] Ultimately, the low number of subscribers and the ineligibility of the fund to become a beneficiary of sweepstake monies resulted in the failure of the Irish Pension Fund for Nurses, and subscribers had their contributions returned in 1937.

The age profile of those applying for pensions suggested that a Benevolent Fund also needed to be established, as older applicants were not likely to gain significantly from late entrance to a pension scheme. The INU established such a fund in 1939 which considered applications for financial relief from destitute members each month. The fund was financed by a range of measures including donations and raffles for prizes such as tea chests and cakes. 'Fancy fairs' (jumble sales) were also held, at which the union sold turkeys for Christmas and at which nurses could have their fortunes told – yet even the most gifted psychic could not have foreseen that the INU's pension campaign would become one of the most tortuous in its history. Hardly a month passed in which the Benevolent Fund did not render assistance to a needy member, some of whom were dependent on selling their furniture in an effort to make ends meet[75] and others who sought financial assistance to meet the cost of tooth extractions and dentures.[76]

As it became clear that the Irish Pension Fund for Nurses was on its last legs, the INU sought strength in numbers and began to work in unison with the Irish Guild of Catholic Nurses and the Irish Nurses' Association; the three bodies established a joint committee known as the Irish Nurses' Pension Committee. The INU took the lead and its President, Mrs McCarry, acted as Committee President. The Committee was encouraged when, in 1933, Sir Edward Coey Bigger, a Senator and Chairperson of the General Nursing Council and Central Midwives' Board, recommended to the Parliamentary Secretary to the Minister for Local Government,[77] Dr Ward, that a national pension scheme for nurses be funded from the proceeds of the sweepstake. Ward reportedly 'did not receive the suggestion with wholehearted enthusiasm'.[78] Nonetheless, Senator Dowdall, with the support of Coey Bigger, was successful in having an amendment to the 1933 Public Hospitals Bill passed in the Senate. The amendment sought to provide that the sweepstake would fund a nurses' pension scheme.

The amendment looked set to proceed to the Dáil and, on behalf of the Irish Nurses' Pension Committee, the INU's President, Mrs McCarry, wrote

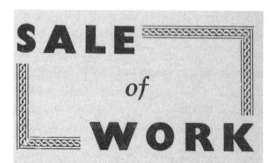

SALE of WORK

Will there be a Sale of Work this year?

1 bottle of Perfume.	1 Cardigan.
Costume Jewellery.	1 Matinee Coat.
Ear Rings.	1 Child's Frock.
Hair Clips.	1 Cushion.
A jar of Vanishing Cream.	Fruit—Fresh or Tinned.
A jar of Cold Cream.	One Sandwich.
A Powder Puff.	One Apple Tart.
Nail Varnish.	One Fruit Cake.
Cotton Wool.	Brown Bread.
Elastoplast, Flexoplast,	Scones.
Bandages, Pins.	One Box of Biscuits.
A bar of Soap.	Cheese.
1 box of Talcum Powder.	1 packet of Peas.
Flowers (Real or Artificial).	1 lb. of Rice.
Pencils.	1 lb. of Sultanas.
Pens.	1 lb. of Raisins.
1 Pair of Nylons.	1 lb. Candied Peel.
1 Pair of Gloves.	1 lb. of Cherries.
1 Pair of Socks.	Mixed Spice.
1 Necktie.	Almonds.
1 Scarf.	1 lb. of Tea.
1 Handkerchief.	1 lb. of Sugar.
Toys—Soft or Hard.	1 lb. of Butter.
1 Woollen Sweater.	1 lb. of Margarine.

Books and Magazines, First-hand—Second-hand.

These are the things we dream about. They are the ingredients of the Sale. We haven't got any of them yet. That is why we say **Will there be a Sale of Work this year ?** One item from the list we have given from each of the 5,000 nurses on our membership rolls—how will we find enough stalls to accommodate all the gifts. **YOU** provide the goods—Leave it to us to provide the accommodation.

The accommodation Address is :—

**THE SOCIAL SECRETARY,
IRISH NURSES' ORGANISATION,
20, LOWER LEESON STREET,
DUBLIN.**

The date of the Sale is **TUESDAY, NOVEMBER 2, 1954.**
The venue : **SUPPER ROOM, MANSION HOUSE.**

All donations gladly received. Digital content created, published and reproduced courtesy of Digital Library, UCD.

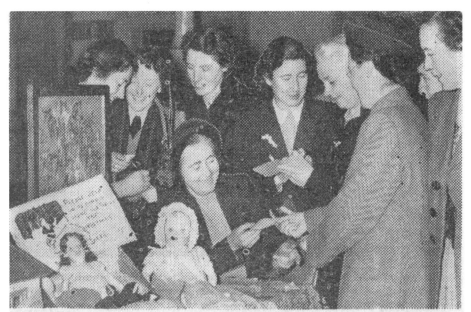

Miss Kathleen Sweeney, Tutor Sister, Peamount Sanatorium, did a brisk business
at the Raffle Ticket Stall at the Irish Nurses' Organisation Sale of Work in the
by courtesy]   **Mansion House, Dublin.**   [" Irish Press."

An INO Fancy Fair at Dublin's Mansion House in 1949 that aimed to raise money for
the organisation's Benevolent Fund. Digital content created, published and reproduced
courtesy of Digital Library, UCD/Courtesy *Irish Press*.

to every TD in the country and asked them to support it. McCarry envisaged
that a sweepstake grant could comprise a basis for a pension scheme, which
would be augmented by nurses', midwives' and employers' contributions.[79]
The amendment was, however, withdrawn before reaching Dáil Éireann,
when Dr Ward undertook to 'ascertain what could be done to formulate a
pensions scheme for nurses, and when a satisfactory scheme was forthcoming,
[to] introduce if necessary special legislation to have it passed'.[80] Ward also
undertook to liaise with the various nurses' associations in this regard. A
successful end to the pension campaign appeared to be in sight.

The following year, Mrs McCarry reported that the Pension Committee
had yet to be contacted by the government, as anticipated.[81] This caused
disquiet, with one nurse noting:

> There is a great deal of truth in the old saying: 'a bird in the hand is worth two
> in the bush,' ... I feel that it would have been better if [the] amendment had

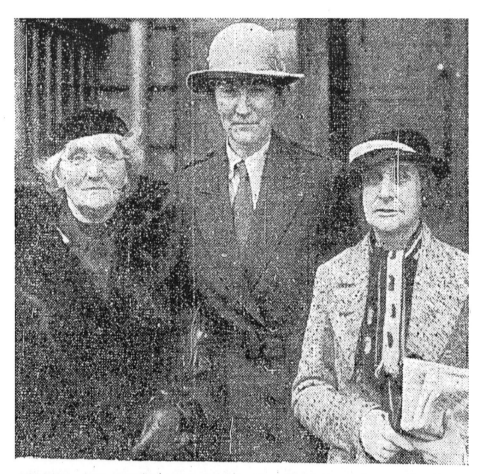

Members of the Irish Nurses' Organisation deputation who saw Mr. S. T. O'Kelly, Minister for Local Government, at the Custom House, Dublin, yesterday. (L. to R.)—Councillor Mrs. K. Nix; Miss N. Healy (President), and Miss A. M. Smithson (Secretary).
[I.P. Photo (S.H.)

INO Deputation to meet Sean T. O'Kelly, Minister for Local Government, at the Custom House, Dublin, in 1937. From left: Kathleen Nix, Nellie Healy and Annie Smithson. With thanks to Irish Newspaper Archives and the *Irish Press*.

been carried, because that would have made sure of something, whereas now we have nothing except the hope that Dr Ward will live up to his promise.[82]

Further similar attempts were made in the Senate in 1935 to introduce a Nurses' and Midwives' Pensions Bill. Although the bill was passed by the Senate in late 1935, in response to questions in Dáil Éireann, the Minister for Local

Government and Public Health, Sean T. O'Kelly, stated that the government did not intend to adopt it.[83]

Why the hold-up? The Matron of Dublin's St Ultan's Hospital suggested that a pension fund would benefit if nurses gave up smoking and diverted their cigarette money to the scheme.[84] Perhaps this was true, but the overarching issues were a little more complex. Firstly, although membership was growing steadily, in 1936 the INO represented only about 13 per cent of the country's nurses and midwives,[85] and McCarry's successor as INO President, nurse, midwife and Lady Superintendent of the Child Welfare Centre on Dublin's Lord Edward Street, Nellie Healy, noted that the Hospitals Trust 'had taken the attitude that the nurses did not want pensions or more of them would be members of [the INO]'.[86] The organisation's lack of success, on account of a lack of members, is notable because the INO (while still the INU) passed up the opportunity of potentially increasing its membership. In 1933, the rival Irish Nurses' Association expressed an interest in amalgamating with the INU.[87]

This was one of a number of times the association sought to amalgamate with the union. But the association's proposals came with a caveat: after amalgamation, the new body should refer to itself as an association, organisation or federation and not a union.[88] The Irish Nurses' Association argued that it predated the Nurses' Union and that international nurses' organisations were generally referred to as associations. The proviso was yet more evidence of the unpalatability of the title 'union' to many nurses. The INU declined the request and members of the Irish Nurses' Association were encouraged to join the Nurses' Union as individuals, if they so wished. A pension scheme may have been realised sooner if such petty rivalries had been laid to one side.

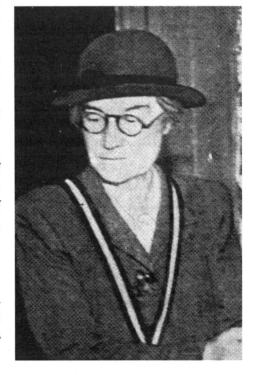

Nellie Healy, INO President 1934–54. Digital content created, published and reproduced courtesy of Digital Library, UCD.

Secondly, some nurses and midwives, depending on whether or not they were employed by the state or by a charitable institution, were already accruing a pension, meaning that there was little incentive for mass mobilisation of the workforce in pursuit of a pension scheme. Thirdly, nurses received mixed messages with regard to financial reward, which subtly reinforced a view that nursing and financial gain were an ill-fit, and this may have contributed to their ambivalence in relation to joining the Pension Fund. The INU suspended production of its *Gazette* in 1931 and its Secretary, Annie Smithson, was appointed as editor of a popular, new, non-union publication, the *Irish Nursing and Hospital World*. Smithson's editorials were laden with mixed messages which faintly reinforced the view that nursing and monetary reward were incompatible.

In 1932, she wrote: 'Nursing is more a vocation than a career, and those who embrace it think less of the remuneration than of its responsibilities ... They give of their best ... with little thought of measuring their services by the amount of remuneration they receive.'[89] Even after Smithson's (acrimonious) departure from the *World*, and in spite of the fact that the *World* overtly supported efforts to secure improved working conditions for nurses, the publication too relayed mixed messages. A feature piece directed at nurses appeared in 1937, entitled: 'Fun Without Money'.[90] As if preparing its readers for the frugal life that awaited them, the piece satirically advised them to get a hobby which did not cost any money such as gathering stones, 'counting crooked noses' or collecting soap advertisements.[91]

Other factors also militated against the establishment of a pension scheme. Sweepstake funding revolutionised many hospitals but caused a drop in philanthropic funding to some voluntary hospitals and in grant funding to some state-run institutions. This meant that the funds became a vitally important source of revenue for hospitals – some £110,000 of sweepstake funding had permitted a major upgrade to Dublin's Sir Patrick Dun's Hospital alone.[92] The idea that monies from the funds might go to a pension scheme for nurses was unpalatable, especially considering that amid the global economic depression in 1933, the INU estimated that the proposed capital necessary to institute a pension scheme for nurses exceeded one million pounds.[93]

The vast majority of nurses were women and efforts to improve their conditions were also impacted by the gender order and, in particular, by the overriding view of men as the breadwinners. In 1920s' Ireland, only 6 per cent of married women held occupations.[94] Social expectations of women as homemakers and mothers were soon formalised and, in 1933, a marriage bar was introduced for women primary school teachers, which necessitated their

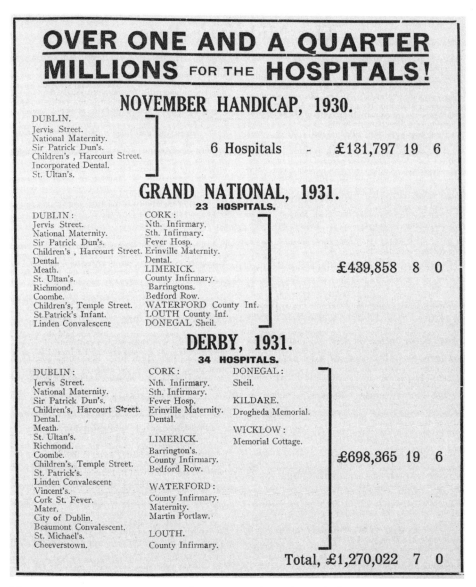

OVER ONE AND A QUARTER
MILLIONS FOR THE HOSPITALS!

NOVEMBER HANDICAP, 1930.

DUBLIN.
Jervis Street.
National Maternity.
Sir Patrick Dun's.
Children's , Harcourt Street.
Incorporated Dental.
St. Ultan's.

6 Hospitals   -   £131,797 19   6

GRAND NATIONAL, 1931.
23 HOSPITALS.

DUBLIN :   CORK :
Jervis Street.   Nth. Infirmary.
National Maternity.   Sth. Infirmary.
Sir Patrick Dun's.   Fever Hosp.
Children's , Harcourt Street. Erinville Maternity.
Dental.   Dental.
Meath.   LIMERICK.   £439,858   8   0
St. Ultan's.   County Infirmary.
Richmond.   Barringtons.
Coombe.   Bedford Row.
Children's, Temple Street. WATERFORD County Inf.
St.Patrick's Infant. LOUTH County Inf.
Linden Convalescent   DONEGAL Sheil.

DERBY, 1931.
34 HOSPITALS.

DUBLIN :   CORK :   DONEGAL :
Jervis Street.   Nth. Infirmary.   Sheil.
National Maternity.   Sth. Infirmary.
Sir Patrick Dun's.   Fever Hosp.   KILDARE.
Children's, Harcourt Street. Erinville Maternity. Drogheda Memorial.
Dental.   ,   Dental.
Meath.   WICKLOW :
St. Ultan's.   LIMERICK.   Memorial Cottage.
Richmond.   Barrington's.
Coombe.   County Infirmary.
Children's, Temple Street. Bedford Row.   £698,365 19   6
St. Patrick's.
Linden Convalescent   WATERFORD :
Vincent's.   County Infirmary.
Cork St. Fever.   Maternity.
Mater.   Martin Portlaw.
City of Dublin.
Beaumont Convalescent. LOUTH.
St. Michael's.   County Infirmary.
Cheeverstown.

Total, £1,270,022   7   0

Money, money, money: propaganda posters such as this one from 1931 illustrate just how much money the sweepstakes were garnering for needy hospitals. *Irish Nursing and Hospital World*/Image courtesy of the National Library of Ireland.

retirement upon marrying.[95] The trend of restricting women's ability to remain in gainful employment following marriage soon spread to other employment sectors both informally, through sector specific rules, and formally, through legislation. In 1941 the *Local Government Act* stipulated that the Minister for Local Government and Public Health may, if he so wishes, make it a prerequisite for certain jobs that women be unmarried.[96] Some nurses agreed with the spirit of the marriage bar. A letter to the *Irish Nursing and Hospital World* in 1931 went:

> No woman has any right to keep on her work after marriage. If she is a conscientious wife and mother, then her marriage will be a whole time job. One of the greatest errors made by the so-called 'modern woman' is this one of working after marriage. Her home, her husband and her children are bound to suffer in consequence.[97]

Societal expectations of women workers as brides in waiting explains some of the more unusual correspondence received by women's trade unions. A 38-year-old man of 'fair appearance, sound and healthy' once wrote to the IWWU – the INO's former parent: 'I wonder if you could get me an introduction from among your union members to any country girl … who would fancy a farmer husband. The only qualification I would ask for is that the lady should be able to milk a cow as we are all dairy farmers here in Co. Limerick.'[98] The INO was on the receiving end of similar correspondence and, in 1939, received a letter from an earnest American suitor who was seeking a wife. The organisation chose to entertain the man's request and wrote in its *Irish Nurses' Magazine*: 'We do not run a Matrimonial Bureau, but all the same we have been asked by a gentleman in the U.S.A. to find him a young nurse … He assures us of his honourable intentions, and says he is aged 39, fairly good-looking, and of average height … his people came from Mayo, and he wants an Irish wife.'[99] Whether or not these intrepid swains found the *cailíns* they so desired (and whether or not the cows of County Limerick got milked) is not known. But stories in this vein are legion: another man described how his recovery from illness was hampered when he found out that his nurse, to whom he had taken a shine, was already spoken for.[100]

So why all this talk of love and marriage? In 1926, prior to the marriage bar, 10 per cent of female nurses were married.[101] By 1936, the number of married female nurses fell to just 5 per cent.[102] Combined with the requirement for many nurses to live at their place of work, nursing was largely a profession for single women and upon marriage, most nurses left the job entirely. The first *Report of the Irish Free State Hospitals' Commission*, published in 1936, noted that 'a considerable number of girls do not take up nursing as a permanent profession. Many of them do not intend to devote thir [sic] whole lives to nursing and so would be difficult to organise' for the purposes of a pension scheme.[103] Essentially, nurses did not view nursing as a long-term pursuit and many, in response, did not unduly concern themselves with efforts to establish a pension scheme.[104] The multitude of issues that impinged on attempts to institute adequate pension arrangements for nurses and midwives ensured that the INO's pension campaign would continue. But one finding in the report gave the organisation reason for hope. The report suggested collating the demographic and employment details of the country's nurses as a first step in the establishment of a pension scheme.[105] This was the first exercise of its kind, and the INO hoped that it would yield results.

The demise of the INU and emergence of the INO signified as much continuity as it did change as, by the 1930s, its de facto no-strike policy moved toward a more actualised form. This was remarkable for an employee representative association, as it effectively gave employers free rein over members' working conditions, however dire. Yet, to suggest that the remedy to nurses' and midwives' suboptimal working conditions lay in the INO increasing its militancy is far too simple. An increase in the organisation's militancy was likely to clash with the service nature of nursing/midwifery work and to dissuade nurses/midwives from joining; in effect, a militant INO was likely to perish, leaving members in an even weaker position. Nor was nurses'/midwives' aversion to strike action the only factor that militated against improvements in their working conditions; their status as women workers and the gendered inequalities that characterised women's work were also beginning to emerge. A reappraisal of that particular inequality remained some forty years away.

CHAPTER 5

War and Wage Rounds, 1938–47

My day begins with opening the correspondence. All monies are entered up and acknowledged. These will comprise the Organisation [*sic*] fees from the members; subscriptions to the Nurses' Journal [and] Benevolent Fund ... The office correspondence consists of every kind of query and request. We are asked to apply to the various Local Authorities for increases in salary for nurses and midwives; shorter hours [*sic*] uniform allowance, and so on ... Other nurses require legal assistance and these letters are referred to our long suffering [*sic*] honorary legal adviser. When we are arranging about the Post Graduate Courses for Midwives ... we receive questions relating to same. Some nurses want us to find them places to stay while in Dublin ... There are letters from would-be nurses asking for full information as to how they may enter the nursing profession. And often enough, comes an application for help from our Benevolent Fund – some poor soul is ill or in need, and if she is a member we do what we can for her ... I return to my letters. Here is one asking for a list of nursing homes where a nurse may get work ... Another knock at the door. A nurse from the country, up in Dublin for her holidays. She has come to thank us for certain concessions the Organisation has obtained for her from her Board. There was once a notice in the office: 'If you have a moment to spare, don't worry the man (or woman!) who hasn't.' But it is only when I am extra busy that I feel like that. And even if I am busy, I am always glad to see the nurses – they are always welcome. My heart warms to them, let them be old or young, the elderly nurse with her years of service behind her, or the young nurse with her career just beginning. The telephone rings. It is a trunk call from the Branch Secretary of one of our Provincial Branches, and she tells me that it is necessary that our Organiser should attend at the next meeting of the Board of Health in that county. Very likely the meeting is in a couple of days' time, and another call must be put through to the Organiser to ask her to call at once to the office. My day varies. It has not the monotony of many offices because I never know what problem will be sprung upon me at a moment's notice. A telephone call may summon me to the Offices of the Hospital Trust in connection with the Pension Scheme ... Now and then, we even have a Deputation to the Minister and sit and look at him and think, that if I were but in his place for even twenty-four hours, what work I could do for my fellow nurses. But somehow, he never sees my point of view – not being a nurse himself ... Twice in the month we have our own Executive Committees and then the office is not closed until fairly late; and again on another day, I attend the meeting of the Council of Nurses at Dr Steevens' Hospital when, in that wonderful old building we discuss the nursing problems of today. Do some of the old nurses, dead and gone these years and years, sometimes hover round us as we talk [?] Sometimes an unwelcome visitor comes to my office. It happened not long ago, just when I was busily working at our Nurses' Journal, in order to have the copy ready for the printers. This caller was an irate lady to whom we had written asking her to pay the fee to which one of

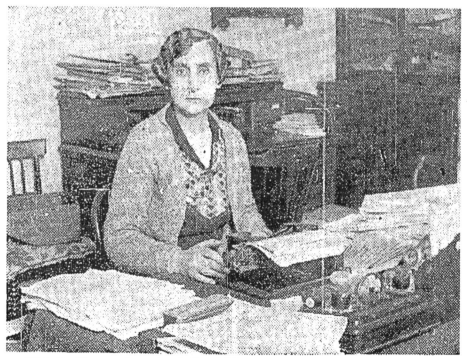

Miss Smithson at work at the Offices of the Irish Nurses' Union, of which she is Secretary.

Hard at it! Annie Smithson at work at the office of the Irish Nurses' Union in 1935. With thanks to Irish Newspaper Archives and the *Irish Press*.

our members was entitled. She had called to let us know just what she thought of all nurses, their Organisation, and everything connected with them, and this she did in no uncertain terms. But it is not only nurses or those connected with them, who call here. Oh, not at all! … we have the ex-Service man who addresses me as sister and gives the military salute while alcoholic fumes are wafted around; the travellers for various firms, who all assure us that their firm is the only one who can supply us with what we want … But there was one traveller once whom I will not forget. He was an exceedingly handsome Austrian with little English but a great deal of charm, as I know to my sorrow. He was selling pencils and there must have been some witchery about him, as I paid him twenty shillings for what I could have got anywhere for about half a crown … But there is the day of days, and it comes just once a year. It is the day of our Annual Meeting, when I sit in an office that does not seem to be mine and listen to the accents of every county in Ireland reaching me through a haze of tobacco. (Need I say that I am a non-smoker?) This re-union is pleasant but strenuous [*sic*] But even the most strenuous time must come to an end, and when at last it is over and I close the office and go to bed, I certainly can call it a day.[1]

This was an account by INO Secretary Annie Smithson of her typical working day. Smithson was no shrinking violet. A one-time member of Cumann na mBan, she once recalled how little she thought of the Queen of England when, one day, a road closure to facilitate the Monarch and her entourage delayed a bus trip Smithson was taking in London. She also recalled that, as a trainee nurse, the Matron of the Chelsea Hospital for Women, London sent her to her room for refusing to 'remove that weed' in response to a sprig of shamrock she donned on her nurses' uniform on St Patrick's Day.[2] Little did the Matron know that Smithson would later base herself in Moran's Hotel, Dublin during the Civil War where she tended to injured republican insurgents. It also appears that she stored arms during the war, as when her home was raided by Free State Forces in 1923, one confiscated letter read: 'Will you please lend me your .45 tonight for an arms class. I guarantee you will get it back in perfect condition.'[3] In her autobiography she remarked: 'Looking back now, I can remember how I hated the very name of Free State.'[4]

But for all her fighting spirit, life at the INO was beginning to take its toll and amid acrimony, a falling out with her colleagues and a warning from her doctor that she was approaching a nervous breakdown, she resigned in 1943: 'Owing to certain conditions then prevailing in the office, life was made intolerable for me, and I had no option but to leave … the wound which I had received had been deep – so deep that, although it is healing, the scar will remain for ever.'[5] Smithson's stress levels are understandable. The 'purely professional' INO that emerged in the mid-1930s faced many challenges. The *Report of the Free State Hospitals' Commission* suggested collating the demographic and employment details of nurses in Ireland as a first step in establishing a pension scheme. This work proceeded against a bleak and unpromising economic backdrop. The Great Depression and Ireland's economic war with Britain gave way to the Second World War. Ireland's neutrality did not spare it the harsh economic consequences, which included a shortage of imported goods, rampant inflation, rationing of commodities and severe austerity measures. A wage freeze was introduced and attempts to effect improvements in nurses' and midwives' working conditions were stifled.

The period was mainly one of preparation for the post-war period. Enthused by developments in Britain and by soaring public support for improvements in nurses' working conditions, the INO increased its efforts to secure a standardised national salary scale for members. The organisation was also granted excepted body status under the provisions of the *Trade Union Act* of 1941. This concession secured the INO's status as a negotiating body and, outside the trade union movement, assured its emergence as the pre-eminent nurse and midwife representative body in the country. It also ruled out the possibility of strike action by the organisation for some forty years to come.

I. The Path to Standardised Salaries

The outbreak of the Second World War had a number of consequences for the INO. Ireland suffered an acute shortage of imported commodities including tea, flour and fuel and the shortages resulted in the price of these commodities spiralling upwards. The cost of living rose by 70 per cent between 1942 and 1946,[6] and nurses and midwives found themselves increasingly hard-pressed to make ends meet. A number of equally hard-pressed retailers reneged on the organisation's long-standing discount scheme, which had offered cut-price goods and services to members since 1921; this made matters even worse. The government established a Department of Supplies and began a system of rationing and, in an effort to curb inflation, instituted strict salary controls and wage freezes. The Mayo Board of Health wrote to the INO in 1941, refusing to grant a pay increase: '[The Board] do not think that the present is an opportune time for the granting of such an allowance and the present increase in the price of foodstuffs would not justify same. If you repeat your application in say 6 months [*sic*] time the Board would be prepared to consider it.[7]

A pay freeze in a time of inflation had the anticipated effect: one midwife reportedly took the next train home after arriving in a provincial district to take up a post only to find that the cost of her board and lodging exceeded her salary.[8] The INO had to content itself with achieving non-salary-related concessions. Petrol rationing meant that district nurses were restricted in the use of their cars, and this hindered their ability to tend to patients. The organisation successfully lobbied the Department of Supplies on petrol allowances in 1944, and district nurses were granted a special allowance in order that they be able to continue with their duties.[9] Bicycles also became the primary means of transport, and representatives of the INO met with the Department for Bicycle Tyres and Tubes and successfully requested that its members receive preferential treatment in the rationing of these scarce commodities.[10] The organisation also raffled a bike among its members and directed the proceeds toward its Benevolent Fund.[11] The war, for all of its austerity, was also a time of preparation for brighter days. Up to then, the INO's efforts to improve members' conditions had been moderately successful. Salary increases had been achieved in some areas but the national standardisation of salaries had not. A surge in wage claims was anticipated when the wages freeze was lifted as workers' demanded restitution. If nurses and midwives were to keep pace with other occupational sectors, the INO had a lot to do.

I.I. Support Grows

INO members received public support for improvements in their working conditions during the war. One correspondent to the *Sunday Independent* noted: 'If this country were plunged into war the indispensability of our nurses would become painfully evident.'[12] In January 1942, Jean Sheridan, a columnist at the same newspaper, wrote an article entitled 'A Nurse's Lot is Not a Happy One'.[13] Sheridan's article was informed by interviews she conducted with a number of nurses. One trainee nurse recounted the £50 entrance fee she paid to train at a Dublin hospital, for which she often worked thirteen hours per day. A night nurse recounted how she got just two days off each month and another remarked:

> You can't dress yourself smartly and go many places on £6 a month ... Do [doctors] know how difficult it is to dress as prettily as we want to when we discard the stiffness and the starchiness on such a pitifully small pittance ...

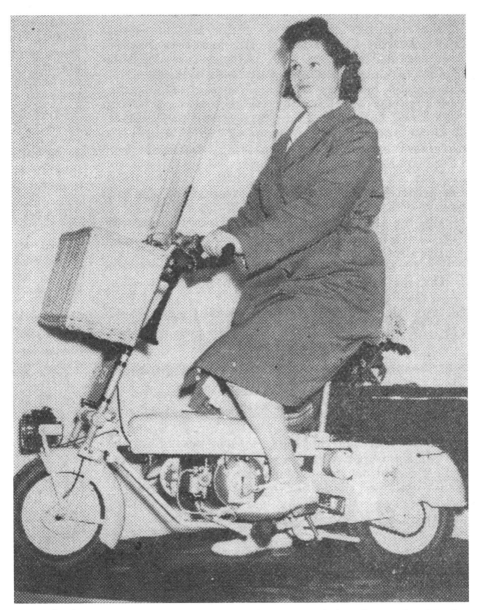

'Of midwives and motorbikes': this motorcycle was unveiled at the London Nursing Exhibition in 1948 and may have provided a remedy to rural midwives' transport problems. The contraption was a motorcycle originally invented for paratroopers but modified for midwives, could travel at up to 35 miles per hour and was even equipped with gas-air apparatus to provide pain relief. Digital content created, published and reproduced courtesy of Digital Library, UCD/Courtesy *Irish Press.*

How can we ever feel contented, not to mention secure, when we cannot
enjoy ourselves as trained shop assistants [do]?[14]

Sheridan's article resulted in a flood of correspondence to the newspaper. This
provided impetus to the INO and exerted what the organisation referred to
as 'moral force' to its campaigning.[15] One of the most notable aspects of the
correspondence in the *Sunday Independent* was the degree to which doctors
expressed their support for nurses. Indeed, Sheridan's article was prompted
by disquiet, expressed by a Dublin doctor regarding nurses' conditions.
Nurse correspondents also indicated their reliance on doctors to lobby for
improvements in their conditions. One nurse implored doctors to visit their
hospitals' nurses' home: 'Take a thermometer with you. See how many degrees
below zero it will register. See how many of your nurses have done six months'
night duty – because they look strong enough for it … You are the only people
who can really help.'[16]

    One doctor who expressed particular support for improvements in nurses'
conditions at the time was Max Millard. Millard was a fifth-year medical student
at Trinity College, Dublin, and was sympathetic to the need for improvements
in nurses' conditions. He conducted interviews with the INO's Secretary and
with a number of hospital nurses regarding their terms of employment. He
presented his findings and recommendations to an audience of 500 nurses
at a 1944 meeting of Trinity's Biological Association, in a paper sarcastically
titled, 'See Florence and Die: Wanted – a Gale-in-the-Night Nursing Reform'.[17]
Millard suggested that nurses should join their representative organisation
and not back down from efforts to achieve better working conditions. He later
recounted in his memoir how he was chastised for having made the speech.

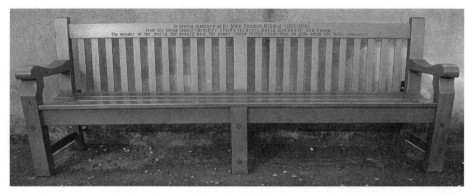

A bench dedicated to the memory of Max Millard in Trinity College, Dublin. Courtesy
Lisa Moyles/INMO.

His Obstetrics and Gynaecology professor, and the Master of Dublin's Rotunda Hospital, Nigel Faulkner, told him: 'It's lucky you have already passed your Ob-Gyn finals, because otherwise you never would have.'[18]

Nurses' working conditions also entered the public domain at the time when the Irish Jesuit journal, *Studies*, incorporated a symposium entitled 'The Nursing Profession and its Needs', in which contributor after contributor put forward their view that improvements in nurses' conditions were needed.[19] The spate of publicity succeeded in nurses receiving a measure of political support. Speaking in Dáil Éireann, William Norton of the Labour Party remarked:

> It is nothing short of a scandal that we allow young, energetic, promising, well-educated girls to go into the nursing profession … and pay them probably the lowest scale of wages … I had a letter during the week from a nurse in a western hospital who told me that she is obliged to work 84 hours per week … and her scale of pay was the customary scale for nurses in district hospitals – £60 rising by increments to £70, sometimes £80.[20]

Deputy Norton's comments were possibly as much political rhetoric as real support, but they provided reason to be optimistic. One of the assumed reasons the pension scheme had yet to come to fruition was because of the relatively low membership of the INO, but this was about to change.

I.II. Membership Grows

The INO was wise in spreading its appeal to an increasingly wide membership base. In 1938, the organisation convened its first refresher course for general nurses at Dublin's Richmond, Whitworth and Hardwicke Hospitals. The course comprised visits to the wards of the hospitals and dispensaries and lectures on theatre technique, medical and surgical nursing, ophthalmology, otorhinolaryngology, radiography and electrocardiography.[21] The following year, INO membership exceeded 1,200 and, for the first time, comprised equal numbers of general nurses and midwives.[22] The former were now joining the organisation in large numbers. Matrons were not in favour of the INU when it was founded, but the provision of refresher courses, which were held in a different Dublin hospital each year, necessitated the organisation to develop close relations with these senior hospital managers. The change in the organisation's relations with matrons was soon remarkable and, by the 1950s, eight out of ten of those who represented hospital nurses on the organisation's Executive Council were matrons or assistant matrons, and the INO requested

FEBRUARY, 1938   THE IRISH NURSES' JOURNAL   79

Richmond, Whitworth & Hardwick Hospitals
North Brunswick Street, Dublin, C.11.

PROPOSED SYLLABUS FOR POST-GRADUATE NURSES
FROM FEBRUARY 14th TO 19th (INCLUSIVE), 1938

Monday

10—11 a.m. Surgical Wards.

11 a.m.—1 p.m. Operations.

LUNCH

2.30—3.30 p.m. Lecture (Theatre technique)

4 p.m. Surgical Lecture.

TEA

Miss Healy, President, will speak to the Post Graduates.

Tuesday

10—11 a.m. Medical Wards.

11.30 a.m.—1 p.m. Skin Dispensary.

LUNCH

2.30—3.30 p.m. Lecture

4 p.m. Lecture (Medical)

TEA

Wednesday

10—11 a.m. Wards.

11 a.m.—1 p.m. Operations.

LUNCH

2.30—3.30 p.m. Lecture (Tutor Sister)

4 p.m. Lecture (Surgical)

TEA

Thursday

10—11 a.m. Wards.

11 a.m.—1 p.m. Eye Dispensary

LUNCH

2.30—3.30 p.m. Lecture.

4 p.m. Lecture (Eyes)

TEA

Friday

10—11 a.m. Wards.

11 a.m.—1 p.m. Operations.

LUNCH

2.30—3.30 p.m. X-Ray and Electro Cardiograph.

4 p.m. Lecture (Nose and Throat)

TEA

Saturday

10—11 a.m. Wards.

11—1 p.m. Nose and Throat Dispensary.

Local Appointments Commission

NURSING POSITIONS VACANT

Application forms for and particulars of the following vacant posts may be obtained from the Secretary of the Commission, 45 Upper O'Connell Street, Dublin.

1. Trained Nurse, St. Brigid's Sanatorium, Portlaoighise, Laoighis. Salary: £65-£5-£90 a year with board and residence.
2. Trained Nurse. Co. Hospital, Croom, Co. Limerick. Salary: £65-£5-£80 a year with emoluments.
3. Matron, District Mental Hospital. Letterkenny. Co. Donegal. Salary: £120-£5-£180 a year with allowances. Age Limits: 25-40 years with extension in certain cases.

Latest date for receiving completed Application Forms: 1st February, 1938.

Syllabus for the INO's first-ever refresher course for nurses held at Dublin's Richmond, Whitworth and Hardwicke Hospitals in 1938. Digital content created, published and reproduced courtesy of Digital Library, UCD.

the Irish Matrons' Association to co-opt its members onto the organisation's Executive Council.[23]

The liaison was a transformative one; in 1937, only 169 INO members out of a total membership of 1,025 were based in Dublin.[24] This suggests that INO membership in the Dublin voluntary hospitals was low. Yet in the 1940s, nurses from prestigious Dublin voluntary hospitals such as the Adelaide, the Charitable Infirmary at Jervis Street, the Meath, Mercer's and Sir Patrick Dun's joined the INO and, on occasions, up to 200 new members joined the organisation each month.[25] Matrons even started to facilitate the INO to organise in their hospitals; in 1941, the Matron of Mercer's Hospital permitted INO personnel to address probationers and proposed that the Sister Tutor of the hospital help organise its probationers.[26] The INO's professional remit acted as a Trojan horse, facilitating the organisation in accessing hospitals and increasing its membership in a manner that its industrial remit had not. Ulterior motives may also have lain behind the matrons' sudden acceptance of the INO; a nurses'/midwives' strike was not in the matrons' best interests, and membership of the strike-averse INO imposed a degree of social control over the rank-and-file nursing/midwifery workforce.

It was becoming clear that education endeared nurses and midwives to the INO, and the organisation established a committee to pursue higher education in 1942. The committee comprised matrons and sister tutors from many of the largest hospitals in the country. The organisation wrote to UCD and to Trinity College, Dublin to enquire about the feasibility of post-registration university courses, namely a diploma in nursing and a sister tutor's course, which would equip nurses to work in administrative, teaching and specialist positions. Education was necessary to keep members abreast of the many advances in healthcare. The late 1930s witnessed a number of developments in medicine: the discovery of a link between excessive sun exposure and cancer,[27] and the discovery that cancer was not contagious being just two that made the pages of the organisation's journal.[28] The organisation's journal also carried stories that spoke to advances in treatment such as the case of Kelvin Rogers. Rogers was a 3-year-old boy who swallowed a nail and was forced to travel 8,000 miles, by boat, from his home in Melbourne, Australia to Philadelphia, USA in order to have it removed by an early pioneer of bronchoscopy: 'Kelvin, who enjoys being at sea, is a pink-cheeked youngster who looks none the worse for the presence of the nail.'[29]

The INO was also beginning to associate improved education with increased remuneration: 'The better educated the nurse is, the higher her qualifications, so much the better should be her status and rate of remuneration.'[30] Frustratingly

IRISH NURSES ORGANISATION

♣

A Grand Concert

will be held at

The Aberdeen Hall Gresham Hotel Dublin

on

Sunday, January 17
1954

Among the artistes taking part will be :
EILIS MULVEY, Soprano; KAY MAHER, Soubrette; MOLLIE HICKEY, Monologues; MARTIN DEMPSEY, Bass; PATRICIA VICTORY, Piano Solos; ANGELA and JACK O'CONNOR, Vocal Duets; P. J. HENRY, Entertainer; CHRIS. F. BRUTON, Compere; LUCY LEENANE, Accompanist.

♣

COMMENCING at 8 p.m.

ADMISSION 5/-, 3/6, 2/6

IT'S A DATE . . . .

NURSES' SECOND ANNUAL
DANCE
HARRISON HALL, ROSCOMMON
6th January, 1947.

THURLES & DISTRICT
NURSES' DANCE
(In Aid of Nurses' Benevolent Fund)
CONFRATERNITY HALL, THURLES
January 14th, 1947.
MUSIC: MICK DELAHUNTY'S NO. 1 BAND.
Catering by Mrs. Forster.

IRISH NURSES' ORGANISATION (BENEVOLENT FUND)
STUDENT NURSES' DANCE
OLYMPIC BALLROOM, DUBLIN
Wednesday, 22nd January, 1947.
NEIL KEARNS AND HIS BAND.
Dancing : 8 p.m.—Midnight.   Spot Prizes.
Tickets, 3/- (payable at door).

IRISH NURSES' ORGANISATION (BENEVOLENT FUND)
A DANCE
(in aid of above) will be held in
CITY HALL, CASHEL
Tuesday, 11th February, 1947.
MUSIC : MICK FOGARTY AND HIS BAND.
Tickets, 10/- and 12/6 (including sit-down Supper).
Dancing, 10—4 a.m.

STUDENT NURSES' DANCE
OLYMPIC BALLROOM, DUBLIN
Wednesday, 12th February, 1947.
NEIL KEARNS AND HIS BAND.
Dancing, 8 p.m.—Midnight.   Spot Prizes.
Tickets, 3/- (payable at door).

WHIST DRIVE
MANSION HOUSE, DUBLIN
Wednesday, 26th February, 1947.
At 8 p.m. sharp.   M.C. : Mr. R. A. Owens.
TOP SCORE, £10
Numerous Valuable Prizes.   Scoring Cards, 2/6

Digital content created, published and reproduced courtesy of Digital Library, UCD.

No shortage of 'socials': an extensive list of the INO's forthcoming dances and social activities in 1947. Digital content created, published and reproduced courtesy of Digital Library, UCD.

for the organisation, neither of the colleges that it approached had the resources to accede to its request.[31] Irish colleges experienced financial hardship during the 1930s and 1940s, but other factors may have been at play. Colleges were predominantly male spaces; at Trinity College, Dublin, women comprised less than one quarter of the student body at the time and female students were subject to a range of exclusionary sexist practices.[32] Could this have been a factor in the colleges' failure to institute courses for nurses?

The INO's Benevolent Fund remained as important as ever and, poignantly, Annie Smithson became a benefactor in the period before her death. She died at her home in Rathmines, Dublin, from heart failure, aged seventy-four, in 1948.[33] The social activities that financed the fund were diverse. The organisation inquired into the possibility that counties Cavan and Roscommon could hold a football match at Croke Park in 1947 and donate the proceeds to the fund. Ballroom dances in aid of the fund were especially successful and became a defining feature of the organisation, solidarising members at local level and providing relief from the arduous world of work and austerity. Two bands and an 'Irish Hour' attracted 1,617 dancers to a 'powerful' INO dance in Cork's City Hall in 1950,[34] and it was only the collapse of the roof of the Olympic Ballroom, Dublin, under the weight of snow, that scuppered the organisation's plans to host a dance there in 1947.[35] The existence of the Benevolent Fund even prompted the INO to take legal advice as to whether it could claim tax exemption as a charity.

Education and socialising aside, one other event was also to the benefit of the INO at the time. In the late 1930s, Linda Kearns, Secretary of the INO's main rival, the Irish Nurses' Association, began a campaign to establish a holiday and convalescent home for sick and convalescing nurses. The home, christened 'Kilrock', and located in Howth, County Dublin was the first of its kind and was considered necessary, owing to nurses' small salaries and meagre pension arrangements.[36] It was expected that the position of matron at the home would be awarded to a nurse; after all, there were few promotional prospects in nursing. This did not occur, and the post was ultimately awarded to a lay person, a turn of events that caused a furore among nurses, who inundated the INO with letters of complaint. The organisation reprinted many of these letters in its journal, wrote in protest to Kearns, and spearheaded a campaign against the appointment, which it believed amounted to a 'belittling of the Profession'.[37]

The INO may have expected to find a sympathetic ear in Kearns: it had gone out on a limb for her some years beforehand. In 1921, during the War of Independence, Marie Mortished, for the INU, requested that a conviction against Kearns for transporting men and munitions be quashed. Kearns was

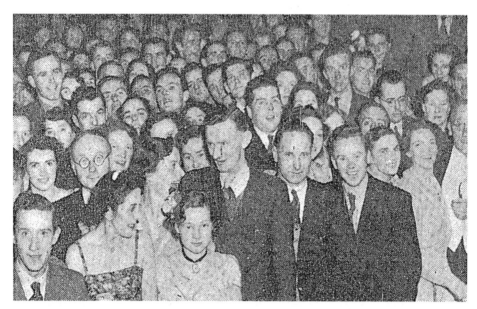

Large attendance at a 'nurses dance' organised by the Cavan Branch of the INO and held in the Town Hall, Cavan, in 1950. With thanks to Irish Newspaper Archives and the *Irish Press*.

NURSES' CONVALESCENT AND HOLIDAY HOME
(INCORPORATED)

"KILROCK," HOWTH, CO. DUBLIN
Telephone : HOWTH 61

OPEN TO NURSES ALL
THE YEAR. BATHING,
TENNIS, CROQUET, GOLF.
EXCELLENT CUISINE.

Terms :

2 GUINEAS

weekly

a prominent figure in Republican circles and relied on her status as a nurse to deflect suspicion from her Republican activities at the time.[38] When apprehended, her car contained three men, four revolvers, ten rifles and 500 rounds of ammunition. Mortished wrote to the British Prime Minister, Lloyd George, indicating that Kearns (who was seemingly a member of the union at the time[39]) had accidentally left her purse in the Shamrock Hotel, Sligo and was returning to retrieve it when she happened upon the men:

> The whole case against her [rests] on the fact that the arms, etc., were found in a car belonging to, and driven by her. It is common knowledge that Nurses, in the pursuit of their calling, do not hesitate … in just such matters as the giving of a 'lift on the road' … I need hardly point out that the difficulties of Nurses in country districts, already great, will be made unendurable if the exercise of ordinary civility on the road is to render them liable to the risk of such treatment as Nurse Kearns has received.[40]

In spite of former favours, Kearns refused to reconsider the appointment.[41] Her response to the INO was written under the letterhead of the Irish Nurses' Association, and its strategic reproduction in full in the INO's periodical in 1944 was all it took. The Irish Nurses' Association existed only in name from then on. With its nearest rival on the ropes, INO membership surged. In 1937, membership stood at 1,025.[42] By 1940, possibly assisted by the cult of celebrity that surrounded Annie Smithson, membership was at 1,376 members, comprising 699 general nurses, 640 midwives and 37 mental nurses.[43] In 1943, membership was 2,223; in 1944, 2,834; in 1945, 3,422; in 1946, 4,047 and by 1947 was 4,552.[44] The increase in membership put the organisation's office staff and administrative and accounting practices under enormous strain, and it was necessary to ask members to pay their subscription annually rather than monthly as a result. When considered in light of the census returns of 1946, which show that there

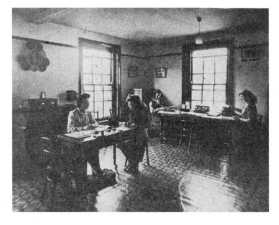

The INO's office at 15 Dawson Street, Dublin, in the late 1940s. This image is reproduced courtesy of the National Library of Ireland.

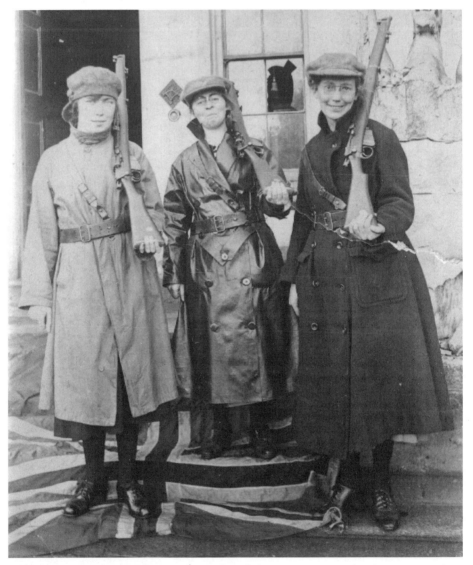

Linda Kearns pictured here on the right of the image at Duckett's Grove, Carlow, in 1921. Also present are, from left, Mae Burke and Eithne Coyle. Courtesy Delia McDevitt.

were 1,079 midwives and 8,874 nurses in Ireland, the INO now had a density of some 41 per cent.[45] Nurses and midwives had now amassed support, and the INO had amassed a vastly increased membership. The organisation now needed to formulate a comprehensive claim for improvements in members' conditions. The impetus in doing so came from Britain.

I.III. *The Rushcliffe Report*

The British government anticipated up to three million casualties as a result of air raids during the Second World War and was keen to ensure sufficient numbers of nurses were available to tend to the injured. It recommended increases in, and the standardisation of their salaries in order to ensure an even geographic distribution of the nursing workforce.[46] The government's intervention was an interim one, and a committee, chaired by Lord Rushcliffe, was established in 1941 to make further recommendations. It issued its seminal *First Report of Nurses' Salaries Committee*, often referred to as the *Rushcliffe Report*, in 1943.[47] The report recommended annual salary increments, the provision of sick pay, twenty-eight days paid annual leave and a 96-hour working fortnight 'subject always to the requirements of the service'[48] – clearly service-obligations problematised nurses' working conditions internationally, not just in Ireland. The INO took great interest in the *Rushcliffe Report* and reminded Irish nurses that it was 'LOYALTY' to the Royal College of Nursing[49] that inspired it [original emphasis].[50]

The reminder was a revealing one. Membership of the INO was increasing, but the vast rank-and-file of members were of the apathetic variety, evident in frequent calls for more active membership; in the high turnover of roles; and in the very small number of members who ordered the organisation's new badge in 1945.[51] INO activists ploughed a lonely furrow and probably found themselves rolling their eyes skywards in resigned disbelief with an editorial in the organisation's *Irish Nurses' Magazine* in 1945: 'When the history of the struggles of the nursing profession comes to be written, we are sure that those who sowed the seed, whereof the present developments are the flower, will be given their due meed of praise.'[52] It was likely that they considered an often reproduced verse that appeared in the journal in 1957 as more fitting:

Twelve Straight Tips [on] How to Kill an Association:

1. Don't attend the meetings.
2. If you do attend, come late.
3. If the weather doesn't suit you, don't dream of attending.
4. If you do attend, find fault with the officers and other members…
5. Never accept office, it's so much easier to criticise than to do things.
6. Get sore if you are not appointed to a committee, but if you are appointed, then don't attend the meetings.
7. When asked by the Chairman for your opinion, just tell him you have nothing to say; then after the meeting tell everyone how things ought to be done.

8. Do nothing more than is necessary (absolutely) but when other members roll up their sleeves and do it all, howl about the Association being run by a clique.
9. Hold back your subscription as long as you can …
10. Start a whispering campaign about the Association's finances.
11. Don't bother about getting new members. Let someone else do it.
12. Never contribute to the Association's Journal. This bucks up the Editor no end …[53]

Annie Smithson regularly put her talents as a writer to use in defence of her members' conditions. Early in her tenure as INO leader, she wrote a satirical letter to the Editor of the *Irish Independent* regarding a post for a dispensary midwife in County Mayo, which attracted a salary of just £20 per year: 'Surely this is too liberal a salary for a nurse who only has to be on duty, ready for calls, every hour of the twenty-four … For such an easy and unimportant position would not £10 per year, or, at the most, £15, be ample?'[54] Smithson's successor, Eleanor Grogan, a nurse and midwife from Bansha, County Tipperary, was no less gifted a wordsmith. The INO's journal printed the average salaries paid to nurses in Ireland and compared these salaries with those recommended for nurses in England. The contrast was a stark one, and Grogan remarked: 'This foolery has got to stop! … The salaries of nurses in Ireland are an absolute disgrace … [and are akin to] the remuneration of serfs.'[55]

The INO requested a meeting with Seán MacEntee, Minister for Local Government and Public Health, in order to debate the points raised in the *Studies* symposium, the report of which it had sent him. A meeting was granted in October 1943. The minister requested that the deputation submit a 'tabulated' report of its grievances to his office.[56] For the next four months, the INO surveyed a cross section of members in order to ascertain working conditions nationwide. The organisation compiled its findings, made a number of recommendations and sent its report to the minister in April 1944. Members were clearly very aggrieved as the 'tabulated' report ran to over forty pages in length. The organisation's hard work was about to pay dividends.

I.IV. The Standardisation of Salaries

The minister responded with a range of circulars recommending improvements in working conditions. Circular M.15-44 recommended standardisation of the salary scale for dispensary midwives at £60–£80 per year in February 1944.[57] Circular M.105/44 followed in November and recommended standardisation of general nurses' salaries at £75–£90 per year.[58] The move toward standardised salary scales represented a victory for the INO, but the scales fell short of those the organisation had hoped for. The INO had requested a salary scale of £80–£100 per year for dispensary midwives[59] and £100–£140 per year for general nurses.[60] Some members were already being paid the government's recommended scale and did not benefit at all. Public health nurses were especially upset as their salary increase was fully inclusive and did not allow for increases in the rate of emoluments (incidental expenses, uniforms, etc.), meaning that some ended up less well off than their hospital nurse counterparts. The fact that nurses' stated salaries often excluded consideration as to the value of their emoluments leads some authors to question whether their poverty was real or imagined.[61] Closer inspection suggests the former, as the minister's recommended salary for a newly qualified staff nurse, including the allowance for emoluments,[62] totalled £163 per year at a time when the average industrial wage was some £20 higher.[63] Poultry instructresses, whose job it was to instruct rural inhabitants on how to rear chickens and ducks, in fact, enjoyed a higher salary than public health nurses.[64]

I.V. Wage Rounds and Working Hours

With the emergency and its associated wage freeze over, 1946 marked the beginning of the 'wage round' era. The wage round era witnessed employee representative associations and trade unions applying for salary increases, in keeping with the increases awarded to other groups. This was of dubious benefit to nurses and midwives, as they commenced the wage round era earning less than the average industrial wage, and a system that increased their salary to the same extent as it increased the salary of other occupational groups did little to address the contentious issue of salary relativity. In keeping with the male breadwinner model, women workers also tended to receive about 60 per cent of the salary increases awarded to men under the wage round system.[65] This trend perpetuated INO members' positions as lowly paid and, in the years ahead, the organisation had its work cut out in seeking redress. The inherent sexism that played such a large role in deciding its members' salaries went, for the time being, unacknowledged by the INO and, in 1946, under the wage round system, nurses and midwives received another pay increase. Circular P.143/46 from the Minister for Local Government and Public Health met with many of the organisation's requests and recommended a salary for dispensary midwives and nurses of £80–£100 and £100–£120 per year, respectively.[66] The INO lauded the circular but stopped short of wholeheartedly endorsing it as it provided for a 96-hour fortnight in 'so far as [it was] practicable' for employers.[67]

Irish Nurses' Meeting In Dublin

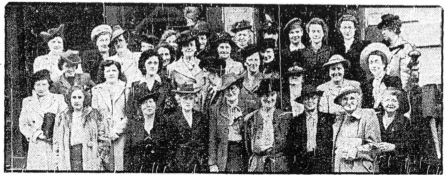

Irish Nurses' Organisation Annual General Meeting, at the Hibernian Hotel, Dublin.—The group includes: Miss N. Healy, President; Miss E. G. Grogan, General Secretary; Miss C. Meehan, Assistant Secretary; Miss E. Russell, Organiser. Branch Secretaries: Miss A. Hourihan (Cork) Miss McLaughlin (Donegal) Miss Feely (Roscommon), Miss Culhane (Waterford), Miss Flood (Monaghan), Miss Clinton (Cavan), Miss McGowan (Sligo), Miss Duffy (Mayo), Miss Creed (Tipperary N.R.), Miss Daly (Wexford), Miss Ward (Wicklow), Mrs. Miller (Carlow), Mrs. Hickey (Kilkenny); with members of the Executive Council: Miss Considine, Mrs. Nix, Miss Crowley, Miss O'Rourke, Miss Hannelly, Miss Sweeney, Miss Fagan, Miss Murphy, Mrs. Hawkins, Miss Clarke, Mrs. Finn, Miss Farrell, Miss Reddy, Mrs. Cann.—*Irish Independent* Photo. (R.).

Members of the INO who attended the organisation's Annual Meeting in 1947. With thanks to Irish Newspaper Archives and the *Irish Independent*.

The INO had been largely successful in lobbying for an end to continuous night duty, but long working hours remained a blight. Newspapers in the 1940s were littered with commentary on the shortage of nurses; no applications at all were received for a vacancy for a staff nurse at the Meath Infirmary in 1946.[68] In addition, not all local authorities instituted new salary scales in a timely manner, and the INO had fears that their failure to do so militated against their ability to recruit nurses which, in turn, militated against the ability to reduce working hours. The Galway County Manager wrote to the organisation in 1947: 'I agree that [nurses'] hours should be reduced when possible, but effect cannot be given to a 48-hour week while the supply of nurses is inadequate.'[69] The nature of nursing work also impacted on working hours. Ireland experienced an unusually cold and protracted winter in 1947. Icy conditions resulted in an increase in mortality, partly as a result of slips, trips and falls. Hospitals struggled to cope with the deluge of patients with fractures, including to the back and skull, and exhausted nurses who had already finished long shifts were instructed to return to their wards to help ameliorate the situation.[70] It is little wonder that prospective nurses were advised to have 'a very thick skin'; 'sound organs, a good constitution'; 'no flat feet, hammer toe, bunions or corns'; guard against constipation; have no varicose veins and, if necessary, have a cold bath and 'vigorous rub down' before starting duty each morning.[71]

II. The Quest for Pensions Continues

Industrial motions far outnumbered all other motions at the INO's annual meetings. Among the wide and varied scope of its industrial activities at the time, the organisation lobbied that army nurses be redeployed to local authority hospitals and have their army service reckoned for pension purposes when the Second World War ended; the organisation rendered assistance to a member who had been suspended from her job in County Sligo following an allegation that she had accidentally burned a patient with a hot water bottle. It also lobbied for salary increases to occupational health nurses employed in sugar beet factories. Nor was the pension issue going away. The first *Report of the Irish Free State Hospitals' Commission* signalled that no pension scheme could be instituted without first collating the demographic and employment details of the country's nurses. This was necessary as there were concerns regarding how private nurses could contribute to a pension scheme considering that many of them experienced episodic unemployment. There were also accounting and actuarial challenges with regard to members, such as dispensary midwives, who blended income from public and private practice.

In total, 12,000 questionnaires were issued to nurses and midwives by the INO, eliciting their employment and demographic details but, in keeping with members' apathy and ambivalence, only about one quarter of the questionnaires were returned to the organisation and many of these were poorly completed. The poor response rate ultimately resulted in the scheme's demise. By 1939, impatience was growing with regard to pensions, and the INO wrote to every member of Dáil Éireann on the subject. The letter reminded politicians of nurses and midwives who were 'destitute after many years of service for others' and asked:

> How many lives have these women saved during their years of service? How many hours have they spent fighting for those lives by day and by night … the Midwife has the care of two lives … the nation allows many [nurses and midwives] when their work is done to end their days in semi-starvation, or even to die in County Homes and similar Institutions … Since we have been trying to start the Scheme, many an old Nurse has passed away after living in hope for several years – a hope which was not destined to be realised.[72]

The INO attributed the ongoing failure to establish a pension scheme to a lack of co-operation from nurses. Some disagreed. A nurse from County Cork wrote anonymously to the *Sunday Independent* in 1942 and took issue with the organisation for ascribing blame to nurses for not having returned their questionnaires: 'A good excuse bound with red tape for the Government to shelve something they didn't want to face.'[73] Both were correct. INO members did fail to co-operate but did so because the prospect of a pension was irrelevant considering that many would resign upon marriage. Equally, there was no impetus at political level to redress sexual inequalities, and even those who may have been expected to defend INO members' employment conditions failed to do so. As the Nurses' and Midwives' Pensions Bill was being debated in the Senate in 1935, Thomas Farren, a trade unionist, Labour Party member, one-time President of the ITUC and, ordinarily, a staunch supporter of workers' rights, refused to support it: 'I see a grave objection to giving pensions to a number of people who will be included in the scope of this Bill. Take for example a married woman whose husband is in a position to keep her and who, for a hobby or for some other reason, takes up the profession of midwifery.'[74]

In 1943, a delegation from the Irish Nurses' Pension Committee met with Seán MacEntee, Minister for Local Government and Public Health. MacEntee reminded the delegation of the paltry return of demographic questionnaires some years earlier and urged the committee to again collect the necessary data but issued a caution: the government was willing to consider the matter, but the state's finances might hinder progress. The Pension Committee engaged a representative to tour the country in earnest in 1944 to collect the appropriate demographic details. The involvement of the Matrons' Association in the committee was crucial as matrons facilitated the committee's representative to address nurses/midwives in their hospitals. The response rate in returning questionnaires was better on this occasion but challenges remained. Many questionnaires were poorly completed. Whether they could not remember, or would prefer to forget, some nurses/midwives pleaded ignorance as to their date of birth; others returned the first demographic questionnaire which had been issued seven years earlier. The Pension Committee forwarded 5,228 completed questionnaires to the Department of Industry and Commerce in 1945.[75] The tabulated data showed that one third of practitioners were already in pensionable positions and that one third were engaged in private case work.[76] In spite of the INO's best efforts, it appears that no immediate action was taken and in 1947, Dr James Ryan, Minister for Health, noted that the pension scheme had been 'deferred', pending considerations regarding the introduction of a system of social insurance by the Department of Social Welfare.[77]

The minister's intention to defer consideration of suitable pension arrangements after a campaign that was almost twenty years in progress,

IRISH NURSES' PENSION SCHEME

LAST CLARION CALL TO ACTION !

Are you going to allow the Pension Scheme to fail through your own indifference or that of your colleagues. Don't think you have your duty done when you have your own form completed. To have completed one form is certainly a praiseworthy act. To persuade some of your indifferent colleagues to complete THEIR forms is more praiseworthy still. So don't rest on your oars. ADVERTISE THE PENSION SCHEME. You are our most powerful publicity agent. You can, if you choose, be more effective than any Radio or Press propaganda could ever be. See that every nurse of your acquaintance completes a Pension Form, on or before 31st January, 1945, which is the latest date for receiving completed Registration Forms for the Irish Nurses' Pension Scheme.

May we remind you for the very last time, that forms may be had on application to the Hon. Secretary, Joint Pension Committee, Irish Nurses' Organisation Offices, Dawson House, 15 Dawson Street, Dublin.

A concerted effort to enlist members' help in advancing the pension scheme in 1945. Digital content created, published and reproduced courtesy of Digital Library, UCD.

suggests that the state's apathy toward the establishment of a pension scheme matched that which the INO attributed to its members. This apathy remained gendered in nature. The organisation urged nurses, especially young nurses, to co-operate in returning the requisite data, and an editorial in the *Irish Nurses'*

Magazine remarked that nurses wrongly comforted themselves with a belief that a 'young knight with gleaming sword and waving plume' is on his way to propose marriage.[78] The Editor drolly reminded readers that, although growing old was inevitable, marriage was not. But marriage appears to have been a certain enough eventuality in the minds of many nurses. Census returns for 1946 indicate that of the 8,703 female nurses in Ireland, just 425, or 5 per cent, were married.[79] Indeed, the trend of married nurses leaving their positions was a central concern for nurse managers. A provincial organiser for the INO wrote of a visit to the County Hospital in Kildare in the 1950s. Employing language more consistent with that of infection control, she noted: 'Sister Dellastrada, Matron, and her nurses are very happy. Their only worry at times is the outbreak of matrimony amongst the nursing staff.'[80] As the 1940s came to an end, the INO was seemingly no closer to instituting adequate pension arrangements than it had been twenty years earlier, but the organisation maintained its steadfast moral opposition to strike action. Burgeoning events were about to reify this opposition.

III. Rhetoric, Reality and Reification: Achieving 'Excepted Body' Status

The evolution of the INU into the INO brought with it a change in the content of its official publication. The *Irish Nurses' Journal* was replaced by the *Irish Nurses' Magazine* in February 1939. The narrative in these publications differed from that of the organisation's first periodical, the *Gazette*. Light-hearted pieces began to appear in an effort to appeal to a wider readership. A piece on folklore commented on a trend by birthing mothers to remove their wedding rings in order to render labour easier and noted that any woman who sat on the bed of a mother and infant may herself expect to fall pregnant by the end of that year;[81] another piece warned readers that if a dead family member was placed in a coffin while still 'limber', another family member would also soon die.[82] Such items were most likely attributable to Annie Smithson whose autobiography, referring as it does to ghostly apparitions, the banshee and a close encounter with 'hungry grass', suggests she was extremely superstitious.

A humorous feature appeared in the *Irish Nurses' Magazine* regarding the town of Westport, County Mayo, in 1939. It remarked on an incident in which a goldfish had been found in a local river and commented on the townspeople's newest fashion accessory – ankle watches.[83] Another piece addressed onion juice as a means to remove rust from knives and commented on Vaseline as an aid to brighten up door knockers.[84] Accounts of nurses' weddings also began to command front-page coverage.[85] Insightful articles related to nursing and midwifery customs and traditions also appeared. A piece written by a former Jubilee nurse, who, on horseback, attended birthing mothers, went:

> During labour a woman friend or neighbour would roast an egg hard and give it to the patient in order to hurry the labour ... To get the placenta away quickly it was the custom to put a candle in the patient's mouth ... She was also made to wear some article of clothing belonging to her husband ... Any box in the house which happened to be locked had to be unlocked during the labour ... On the day of the Christening, before the child left the house, a piece of coal or burned turf was put into the corner of the christening robe.[86]

The organisation's journal retained an occasional penchant for grandstanding. The view that nurses were partly compensated for their work by the mere fact that they were engaged in humanitarian labour was a popular one and is referred to as intrinsic reward. In 1953, Minister for Health, James Ryan, noted: '[Nursing] has its compensations, of which the greatest, perhaps, is the satisfaction of relieving suffering.'[87] Whether Ryan was reassuring or deluding himself is not clear, but his sentiments perhaps partly explain the state's meagre response to the INO's pay claims. The INO was not impressed by such sentiments, and Eleanor Grogan struck a militant note in response:

> [The public] look upon nursing as a self-dedicatory calling ... [nurses] are supposed to consider themselves more than compensated by the good they are doing. From this handy springboard the people who are getting the nurses' services for next to nothing, and under conditions that in former days would be a reflection on a colony of slaves, go on to sentimentalise about the nurse; drag in Florence Nightingale and her lamp ... and then go on to disguise their lazy and selfish and cowardly attitude with other pseudo-historical and pretty-pretty embroideries hoping ... that the Nurse ... will accept their metaphorical bedizzened bonbons as the equivalent of the substantial recognition to which all honest and arduous work is entitled.[88]

Grogan was never one to say in a sentence what could be said in a paragraph, but another commentator put her diatribe a little more succinctly: 'Too many have been the bouquets; too few the rewards.'[89] An editorial in the INO's

Irish Nurses' Magazine in 1944 continued with the militant slant: 'If anyone, anywhere took us for an afternoon tea club, or a school of etiquette or for a harmless debating society ... then all we say is that the sooner that illusion is got rid of the better.'[90] But the tone of the INO's rhetoric was not matched by its actions and, however forthright its protestations were in print, the organisation remained opposed to strike action. Up to then, this opposition was of the moral kind, but in the early 1940s, a seminal piece of legislation placed this opposition on a legal footing. The 1941 *Trade Union Act* sought to limit the right to collectively bargain to 'authorised' trade unions in possession of a negotiating licence.[91] This presented a problem for the INO: it was no longer a trade union and, if deprived of the ability to collectively bargain, its utility and continued existence was questionable. However, the 1941 act provided that certain organisations could be regarded as 'excepted bodies'; a status which allowed them to bargain collectively in the absence of a negotiating licence.[92]

The INO requested and was granted excepted body status under the 1941 *Trade Union Act*, but this status came with a caveat: that the INO did 'not carry on negotiations in the ordinary way in which negotiations are carried on by a Trade Union with employers'.[93] The organisation's solicitor explained: 'Really what the [government] mean is that, as they are confident that nurses would never take strike action, you will get the full benefit of exemption from the Act and you are not likely to be ever deprived of it.'[94] Essentially, state-stipulations now deprived the INO of the ability to strike and the government retained the right to 'revoke the exemption if the Irish Nurses' Organisation takes action of such a kind as may be described as normal Trade Union action'.[95] These stipulations did not perturb the INO; they simply codified the organisation's moral opposition to strike action. Drawing on military metaphors consistent with the unfolding war in continental Europe, the INO referred to striking as a 'drastic measure of social warfare'.[96] The organisation soon set forth its stance on strike action in its constitution. Bye-law number five of the INO's constitution, which was formulated in the best interests of 'patients, [nurses'] professional status and ... the community', read 'The Organisation shall not, either directly or indirectly, suggest or approve of strike action. Any member or members of the Organisation who choose this method of solving their professional problems shall be expelled.'[97]

The INO now had a narrow and often ineffective range of protest strategies available to it, and lobbying, by means of letter writing to employers and state representatives, became the organisation's primary way of kicking up a stink. This was a strategy that was all too easily dismissed, and a representative of the Department of Local Government and Public Health wrote to the INO in 1945, scolding it for its 'ill-considered verbiage', reminding it that nursing reform took time, owing to the 'multiplicity of other equally urgent duties' and requested the organisation to keep its future correspondence 'moderate in its volume and expression'.[98] Many of the organisation's representations were dismissed outright, marked as 'read' or put on the long finger indefinitely. Certainly, militancy did not achieve the desired result in all circumstances, evident in primary school teachers' futile seven-month-long strike in 1946, during which some invaded the playing pitch at Croke Park during the All-Ireland Football Final,[99] but the compound result of years of non-militancy by the INO put the organisation on the back foot.

The Second World War was a time of ferment for the INO in which growing public and political support, the support of the medical profession and unbridled media coverage of members' poor working conditions propagated the necessary conditions for a vast increase in membership. This necessitated the move of the organisation's premises from Nassau Street to a larger building, Dawson House, on Dawson Street in 1943. The state bowed to the momentum behind the INO's claim for improvements in conditions but, similar to its success in relation to the eradication of handywomen, the INO's success in the establishment of standardised salary scales was a qualified one. The interruption to the system of free local bargaining by the austerity of war, the propensity on the state to standardise salary scales in anticipation of the era of wage rounds and increasing concerns over the shortage of nurses played as much a role in the process as had twenty years of lobbying by the INU/INO. Yet a success it was, and this added to the mood of optimism at a silver jubilee dance, convened by the INO, to mark its twenty-fifth anniversary at the Metropole Ballroom in 1945. A commemorative *Souvenir Book* was published in 1947 – a little behind schedule due to war-related paper shortages.[100]

The organisation's efforts to effect a reduction in members' working hours and to institute a pension scheme continued throughout the 1940s. Considering the longevity of these campaigns, it is arguable that a more militant stance by the INO was warranted. Yet, paradoxically, the INO's opposition to strike action was reified and became part of the organisation's constitution at the time. The granting of excepted body status represented a means of control by the state over nurses/midwives, as it statutorily ruled out any militant recourse by the organisation in the future. The local trend of granting suboptimal improvements in INO members' working conditions, knowing that they lacked any militant option to challenge it, now became a national one.

THE END OF A NURSE'S DAY

Seven o'clock ! And the Nurse's work
  Was done for another day !
She heaved a sort of tired sigh
  And put the charts away.
Then sat for a moment and bowed her head
  Over the little white desk—
" I wonder," she said to herself, " after all,
  Am I really doing my best ? "
" Perhaps I could have begun the day
  With a brighter, cheerier smile,
And answered the bells with—' Right away '
  Instead of ' After a while.' "
" And I might have listened with sweeter grace,
  To the story of Six's woes ;
She may be suffering more, perhaps,
  More than anyone knows."
" And I might have refrained from the half-way
    frown,
  Although I was busy then,
When the frail little girl, with sad blue eyes
  Kept ringing again and again."
" And I might have spoken a kindlier word,
  To the heart of that restless boy,
And stopped a moment to help him find
  The missing part of his toy."
" Or perhaps the patient in Eighteen A,
  Just needed a gentler touch ;
There are a lot of things I might have done
  And it wouldn't have taken much."
She sighed again and brushed a tear,
  Then whispered—praying low,
" My God, how can You accept this day,
  When it has been lacking so ? "
And God looked down—He heard the sigh,
  He saw that shining tear ;
Then sent His Angel Messenger,
  To whisper in her ear . . .
" You could have done better to-day,
  But, oh ! the Omnipotent One,
Seeing your faults, does not forget,
  The beautiful things you have done."
" He knows, little nurse, that you love your
    work,
  In this house of pain and sorrow,
So gladly forgives the lack of to-day,
  For you will do better to-morrow."
The Nurse looked up with a grateful smile,
  " To-morrow I'll make it right,"
Then added a note in the order book,
  " Be good to them to-night."

From a Reader.

A poem from the *Irish Nurses' Magazine* in 1943. Digital content created, published and reproduced courtesy of Digital Library, UCD.

CHAPTER 6

Religion and the Religious:
Roots and Repercussions, *c.*1948–59

In Britain, the seminal 1942 report, *Social Insurance and Allied Services*, better known as the *Beveridge Report*, established the basis for increased state intervention in the welfare of citizens.[1] The report proposed a system of social security and a comprehensive, preventive and curative health service for all; six years later, the National Health Service (NHS) was established. These measures were innovative and exerted pressure on the Irish government to do likewise. As the government set about the task, it could not have foreseen that it had embarked on one of the most contentious plans in Irish history. Not only did the Irish Medical Association oppose the plan, but the Catholic Church did as well. The INO supported both factions throughout the debate on the matter.

This chapter examines the INO's activities at the time, including its response through a range of newly formed member sections, to the proposed changes to the health services. The chapter's timeline begins in 1948 with the appointment of a government minister for health who, within a few short years, sensationally resigned. It ends just prior to the launch of a new campaign by the INO to effect conciliation and arbitration machinery in 1960. Yet, in order to better understand the organisation's activities and approach at the time, the chapter returns to the organisation's early days and examines relations between the INU and the religious. The chapter also briefly moves ahead to the 1980s and examines the organisation's position regarding two divisive social issues in Irish society and the extent to which that position was infused by Catholic teaching.

I. The INO and the Rise of Vocationalism

The Parliamentary Secretary to the Minister for Local Government and Public Health, Dr Conn Ward, instituted a plan to radically overhaul health service provision in 1945. Ward's plan, detailed in the 1945 Public Health Bill, concerned the treatment of infectious diseases and proposed what became known as the Mother and Child Health Scheme, in which local authorities would provide a free maternity service for mothers and compulsory free medical inspections for children up to the age of sixteen.[2] The bill also anticipated devolving responsibility for educating mothers and children in relation to healthcare to the local authorities and met with opposition from the Catholic Church, who viewed families as institutions in which parents were obliged to take responsibility for the welfare of their children. Some amendments to the bill were proposed by Ward in order to assuage concerns but, shortly afterwards, he was replaced by Ireland's first Minister for Health, Dr James Ryan.

The amendments were incorporated into the 1947 Health Bill, which decreed that children would not have to undergo compulsory medical inspections provided that their general practitioner was satisfied with their overall health status. Nonetheless, the 1947 bill retained plans for the provision of the Mother and Child Health Scheme. The provisions of this scheme remained unpalatable to the Catholic hierarchy, who had concerns regarding the 'danger posed to the morals of women and children' should they be educated by the state with regard to contraception, abortion and sexuality.[3] The provisions also became increasingly unpalatable to some doctors, who feared the erosion of their livelihoods under a system of free healthcare provision.

The INO also began to express its reservations about the scheme. The organisation arranged its first refresher course for public health nurses in 1947. The course included a visit to Vergemount Fever Hospital, lectures on tuberculosis and bedside teaching related to orthopaedics at St Ann's Hospital, Clontarf. It also included instruction regarding dichlorodiphenyltrichloroethane, better

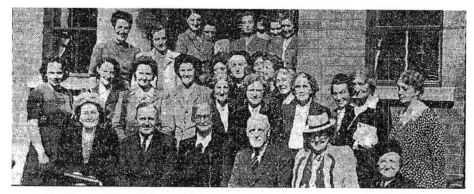

INO members attending the first Refresher Course for Public Health Nurses in Dublin in 1947. With thanks to Irish Newspaper Archives and the *Irish Independent*.

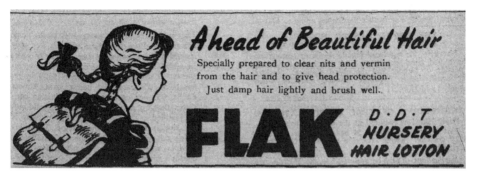

A head of Beautiful Hair

Specially prepared to clear nits and vermin from the hair and to give head protection. Just damp hair lightly and brush well.

FLAK D·D·T NURSERY HAIR LOTION

Digital content created, published and reproduced courtesy of Digital Library, UCD.

known as the insecticide DDT, and lectures on bugs, scabies and 'disinfestation' at the Iveagh Baths, Dublin; after all, Irish emigrants were deloused before emigrating to Britain in the 1940s for fear of what they might take with them.[4] The Chief Medical Officer at the Department of Health, Dr James Deeny, addressed those attending the course and indicated that nurses were crucial in the government's 'crusade' to improve the health of the Irish population.[5] In line with the Church's misgivings, a subsequent commentary in the INO's *Irish Nurses' Magazine* pulled no punches: 'This crusade will have to be carried out by [the public health nurse] without any violation of the unalterable and inalienable rights of that social institution, the family.'[6] This was the INO's first public utterance on the scheme and it was clear which side the organisation was taking.

In spite of opposition, in 1947, the *Health Act*, including provisions for the Mother and Child Scheme, was passed.[7] This was followed by a general election in 1948, which witnessed the election of a coalition in which Noël Browne, a medical doctor, was appointed Minister for Health. Browne's tenure was a short one. Amid conflict with the Irish Medical Association and a lack of support by his government colleagues, some of whom harboured concerns about the scheme's cost and some of whom were reluctant to defy the Catholic Church's teaching (not to mention the challenge of reaching a consensus in a five-party coalition), Browne resigned in 1951 when the Church judged that the Mother and Child provisions of the act were in breach of Catholic social teaching.[8] Browne was a loss. Both his parents had died of tuberculosis and he himself developed the condition as a young man. In his time as minister he championed TB, and the INO paid tribute to the significant advances in the eradication of tuberculosis made under his tenure. Nonetheless, the organisation lauded the Irish Medical Association following his resignation, which it noted had 'every right to fight for the independence and integrity of the Medical Profession'.[9]

Overall, Browne was an advocate for nurses/midwives, but his words sometimes contradicted his actions. While addressing the Annual Meeting of the INO in 1948, he remarked: 'When you are blaming people for your conditions of service, don't forget to blame yourselves.'[10] There is an element of victim blaming here. Nurses and midwives had a loose commitment to trade union principles, and their solidarity was fractured along multiple lines, but their apathy in relation to certain issues, such as pensions, was gendered and infused by the marriage bar. This was a political construct over which Browne had more influence than the nurses and midwives he chose to scold. In addition, not all nurses passively accepted their conditions of service. A number from the Limerick County Infirmary threatened to resign and 'go to England' in a pay dispute in 1950.[11]

Nor was Browne always receptive to nurses' claims to improve their conditions. In 1950, the INO received reports that a new nurses' home at Mallow Chest Hospital, County Cork, was to be used to accommodate thirty-two tuberculous patients and that the nurses were to be moved from the home to the trainee nurses' quarters.[12] The hospital's nurses were disgruntled at the proposal: they found the trainees' quarters too small and lacking in kitchen facilities.[13] The INO wrote to Minister Browne on the matter but did not find a sympathetic ear. Instead, the minister played the (by now familiar) card of portraying improvements to nurses' working conditions as being detrimental to patient welfare:

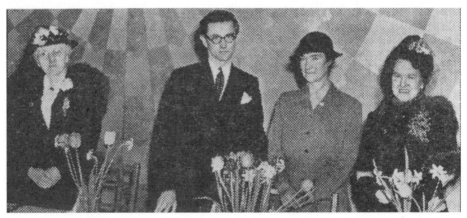

Minister for Health Noël Browne with, from left, Kathleen Nix, Nellie Healy and Eleanor Grogan at the INO's Annual Meeting in 1948. Note the body language. Digital content created, published and reproduced courtesy of Digital Library, UCD.

the action of the nurses in not being willing to suffer the small inconvenience involved in the change from one home to another is likely, if persisted in, to jeopardise the chance of recovery of at least 30 sick persons ... and is also likely to endanger the health of their families who are exposed to the continued risk of infection.[14]

Leaving events in Mallow aside, Browne had long since shown a concern for nurses and, in one example, while working at Dr Steevens's Hospital, Dublin, he had approached the Matron (in vain) in an effort to improve their conditions.[15] Browne also remarked that he was unhappy with the number of Irish nurses who had emigrated and believed that improvements in their working conditions might halt this.[16] He was most interested in improving nurses' living quarters, which sometimes consisted of refurbished stables. This was by no means the worst example: proposals were afoot to accommodate nurses at the County Surgical Hospital, Cavan in a room atop a morgue and coal shed,[17] and at the Boyle District Hospital, County Roscommon, nurses were obliged to pay for their room in the nurses' home whilst on holidays – despite the room being simultaneously sublet, in box and cox fashion, to another nurse.[18] Meanwhile, a sister at the County Home in Mullingar, County Westmeath, reported being 'heartily sick of the discomfort' of having no sanitary facilities; this resulted in nurses having to bathe in an outhouse in a nearby field.[19] Browne issued a circular to all local authorities in 1948 in which he implored them to institute improvements in nurses' sleeping, living and dining conditions. He also requested that the introduction of a 96-hour fortnight be expedited and that any discipline not considered 'reasonable' be relaxed.[20] It was also under Browne's tenure that one of the INO's long-sought goals was achieved: the appointment of a nursing supervisor to the Department of Health. The position was filled by Margaret Reidy, a nurse, midwife and member of the INO.[21]

The INO clearly proved itself willing to sacrifice pragmatism in favour of principles and lost an ally in Browne. The General Secretary of the organisation, Eleanor Grogan, identified the crux of the issue: '[The] struggle of the Medical Profession to preserve its integrity and independence was of supreme significance for all the free professions. We trust that its triumph will represent the beginning of recognition by the State that it will lose nothing by providing opportunities for the development of vocationalism in Ireland.'[22] Vocationalism increased in popularity in Ireland following the publication of the Papal Encyclical *Quadragesimo Anno* by Pope Pius XI in 1931.[23] At the core of vocationalism lay the concept of 'subsidiary function',

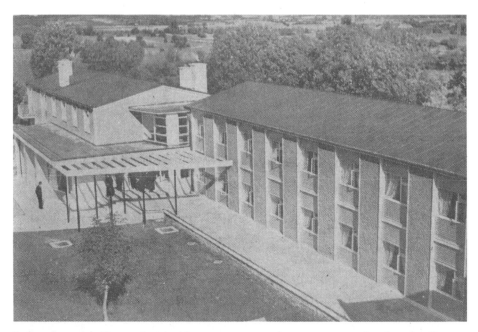

In keeping with Browne's priorities, a new nurses home was completed at the County Hospital, Mullingar, Co. Westmeath, in 1953. It slept fifty nurses in bedsit-style accommodation. Digital content created, published and reproduced courtesy of Digital Library, UCD/Courtesy *Irish Independent*.

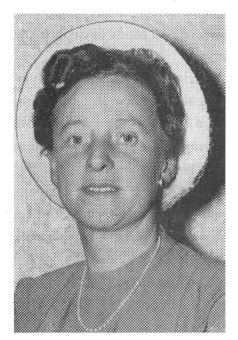

Margaret Reidy on her appointment to the Department of Health. Digital content created, published and reproduced courtesy of Digital Library, UCD.

wherein the state devolves responsibility for a range of services, such as healthcare, to a number of non-governmental organisations. Vocationalist principles were already evident in Ireland in the activities of the voluntary hospitals, all of which ostensibly functioned independently of the state. The Encyclical added fuel to the fire and witnessed the rise of what is referred to as the 'Catholic social movement', which aimed to put its principles into increasing effect.[24]

As the Catholic social movement reached its peak in the late 1940s, its philosophy collided with the idea of increasing state involvement in health service provision. Adherents to papal teaching had much to be wary of. The influence of the *Beveridge Report* saw Ireland establishing the structures and passing legislation consistent with what became known as 'the welfare state', most notable in the introduction of the Children's Allowance in 1944, the establishment of the Department of Social Welfare in 1947 and the passage of the *Social Welfare Acts* of 1948 and 1952.[25] The INO was unimpressed and implored individuals and voluntary hospitals to co-operate and form a 'bulwark against the growing interference of the benevolent state'.[26] In keeping with *Quadragesimo Anno*, the INO also began marketing itself as an organisation without which 'we cannot give effect to Christian social teaching'.[27]

The particular Christian teaching which the INO espoused was Catholicism, and an editorial in the *Irish Nurses' Magazine* in 1950 commented on a recently published white paper on social security: 'No reference is made to the fundamental principle of Catholic philosophy governing the subsidiary function of the State which is charged, not with the duty of suspending individual and group activities, but with "directing, watching, stimulating and restraining" those activities.'[28] The organisation expressed similar sentiments following Browne's resignation:

> The family ... is the primary unit of society ... The projection of Catholic Social Philosophy into politics or economics constitutes no threat to essential human liberties [but rather] would provide genuine safeguards against excessive state control ... It cannot be questioned that the Hierarchy of Ireland ... are well qualified to decide whether or not any State Scheme militates against the rights of the family as set out in Catholic Social teaching.[29]

A general election was held shortly after Browne's resignation. Fianna Fáil returned to government and Dr James Ryan reassumed the health portfolio. Ryan returned to office intent on instituting reform despite the continued opposition of the Catholic Church, the Irish Medical Association and the

THE WHITE PAPER
on HEALTH SERVICES

STATE MEDICINE IS BAD MEDICINE

The Government White Paper, if adopted, will mean a great step forward in the control of medical services by the State. It would be foolish to suppose that, while your doctor may worry about this trend, it is none of your affair. A State stranglehold on the practice of medicine places the whole structure of family life in the same immediate peril. In exchange for heavier taxation, loss of privacy and chaotic services, you will be deprived of the very keystone of your individual liberty.

SOME VIEWS ON THE WELFARE STATE

His Eminence Cardinal D'Alton : "Increased State services tend to lessen responsibility of parents and to undermine their spirit of independence."

Most Rev. Dr. Browne : "State control results in monopolies which give worse service at higher cost. It also leads to a greate increase of Government patronage with great risk of corruption."

Most Rev. Dr. Lucey : " . . . The State whose citizens cannot afford to own their own house, pay their own doctor and hospital bills, feed and clothe their own children is failing in its primary duty to them: the very extent of its "free" services is proof of its failure as a Government for the common good."

Most Rev. Dr. Gregg : "The Welfare State weakens self-reliance and initiative. Its beneficiaries become lost behind the workings of what is, for all its apparent benevolence, an almost inhuman machine."

Rev. Fr. Phelim O'Briain : "I challenge the Minister to produce a single moral authority in defence of his scheme."
Extract from Report of the American Medical Association on the working of the National Health Act in Britain :
"Abuses of the Service are evident everywhere, and they must lead to more and more regulations, tighter enforcement, greater penalties for violation, further limitation on freedom and further deterioration of the quality of Medicine. In the end the great consumer group will suffer most. What is most to be deplored is the present and future effect on the quality of medical care received by the English people."

Sir Earle Page, formerly Minister for Health in Australia :
"There have been various attempts in different countries to nationalise medical treatment or to give 'free' treatment at the taxpayers' expense. These over-simplified solutions have proved wasteful in their administration, disastrous in their effect on the quality of treatment and destructive of the morale of the people."

WHAT DOES THE WHITE PAPER OFFER ?

1. Treatment only in public wards of hospitals (para. 26).
2. Birth of your children in public maternity wards (para 24 (c)). Your own doctor may not attend you unless he accepts State control (para. 27).
3. Private treatment ? Yes)! If you pay for it yourself (para. 24C and 26).
4. Your health and sickness recorded by the local authority in its files (para. 21).
5. Your doctor ordered around by lay officials (para. 21).
6. Queues for such beds as are avilable (para. 38).
7. The "Red Ticket" goes—and the "Coloured Card" comes in its place (para. 34).
8. End of assistance to insured persons for private or semi-private maintenance in hospital (para. 39).
9. And, inevitably—wire-pulling and political influence in access to "benefits" (para. 24 (f)).

Facilities for existing services are deplorably inadequate. Yet the Government talks glibly of extending the medical services.

There are no proper facilities for existing services; where are the facilities for extended services ?

WHAT WILL IT COST ?

Read what the Minister said :

Dail Debate—30th October, 1952 : "It is not possible at this stage to estimate the annual cost of the new Health Services when fully in operation. . . . I have no reliable estimate."

At Sligo, Mr. Kennedy (representing the Minister) said : "I cannot guarantee that it will not cost more than 2/- on the rates."

And remember, the increased rates will cover only half the cost !

A lesson from Britain : The original estimate for the cost of the British Health Scheme was 178 millions. Five years later the cost reached 460 millions. Withdrawal of certain benefits was needed to reduce the cost of the present "ceiling" of 400 millions.

THE SAME SORT OF THING WILL HAPPEN HERE

(Issued by the Irish Medical Association).

The Irish Medical Association trounced the White Paper and its reservations were reprinted in the *Irish Nurses' Magazine*. Digital content created, published and reproduced courtesy of Digital Library, UCD.

INO. The organisation reprinted a lengthy critique from the *Irish Ecclesiastical Record* in 1950 that commented on the advent of the NHS in England. The piece concluded: 'We must observe the principle of subsidiary function …

the evolution of medical services should begin not with Leinster House,[30] but with the medical profession [and] the voluntary hospitals.'[31] Ryan made some further concessions to the 1947 act, but these were considered insufficient to placate its detractors and the Irish Medical Association countered in 1951 by drafting its own voluntary health insurance scheme. The INO reproduced details of the scheme in the *Irish Nurses' Magazine* and applauded it.

Minister Ryan published a white paper on health in 1952. The paper's proposals guaranteed free or subsidised healthcare depending on recipients' means. Once again, an editorial in the *Irish Nurses' Magazine* expressed opposition to the White Paper and concluded: 'It is hoped that wiser counsels will ultimately prevail to prevent Ireland's domination by the Welfare State.'[32] In spite of protest, following some further minor concessions, the White Paper was embodied in a bill that ultimately formed the basis of the *Health Act* of 1953.[33] All that the INO could do was express its relief that the Mother and Child Health Scheme provided for in the 1947 act did not feature and that no person would be obliged to avail of the services proposed.

I.I. Ulterior Motives

Could the INO's stance in opposition to statism have been infused with concerns for its members' welfare? Many nurses in Ireland were from middle-class backgrounds and commentary in the *Irish Nurses' Magazine* suggests that the organisation was concerned that the tax burden of the emergent welfare state would fall unevenly on the middle class.[34] In addition, the 1940s and early 1950s witnessed marked changes to the distribution of sweepstake funding between voluntary and state-run institutions, the former of which used to enjoy the bulk of the monies.[35] This concerned the INO for two reasons. Firstly, the remuneration for a nurse working in a state-run hospital in Ireland in the 1950s was £340–£400, minus a maximum of £140 for emoluments. The remuneration for nurses employed in some voluntary hospitals was £100–£160 plus £41 living expenses.[36] The organisation had long since requested redress of this anomaly and feared that any interruption to voluntary hospital funding might stifle its progress. One voluntary hospital, Dublin's Meath Hospital, wrote to the INO in 1953, indicating that although it was 'favourably disposed' to adequate nurses' salary scales, the timing for the introduction of such scales was 'inopportune.'[37]

Secondly, although a number of voluntary hospitals had introduced pension schemes by the 1950s, only a minority (three in total) had established federated or reciprocal pension schemes which enabled nurses to accumulate

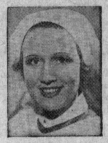
their pension entitlements if they transferred employment. The diversion of sweepstake funding from the voluntary sector did not augur well for the INO's efforts to see this arrangement extended, and it became clear that the organisation was going to have to take measures to implement such a scheme without the state's assistance.

In 1952, the organisation invited Norwich Union Life Insurance Society to address its members on the subject of its endowment scheme for nurses. The scheme allowed nurses to contribute a small sum from their salary on a monthly basis, leading to a lump sum upon retirement. The endowment scheme was an interim measure. The INO continued to lobby the voluntary hospitals to adopt a federated pension scheme with great success. A total of ten voluntary hospitals were operating the federated scheme by the end of 1953, and a total of seventeen Irish hospitals subscribed to it by 1957.[38] But what of the INO's broader relations with the Catholic Church and its teachings?

II. From Defiance to Deference: The INO and the Catholic Church

The INO supported, endorsed and disseminated the position of the Catholic Church at every critical juncture in the debate on the proposed changes to the health services. The organisation's stance can be located in its broader deference to the Church and its teachings. However, things had not always been that way. In its early days, the INO vocally challenged the Catholic hierarchy when it had concerns over members' working conditions. This was most apparent in relation to nursing nuns. Nuns were highly sought after as caregivers. A member of the County Mayo Board of Health surveyed patients' opinions regarding whether they wanted the County Home staffed by lay nurses or nuns: 'For God's sake give us the nuns' went the response.[39] The reputation of nuns as excellent carers meant that they were frequently appointed to staff and manage hospitals. This tendency had the potential to displace lay nurses from their jobs, caused much disquiet and may even have been instrumental in the establishment of the INU.

Nurse Bridget Doyle was the first person to approach Louie Bennett with regard to establishing a trade union for nurses in 1919.[40] Doyle trained at Dublin's Mater Hospital and qualified as a nurse in 1910. She later took a job at the city's Pigeon House Road Tuberculosis Hospital. Four nursing nuns from the Sisters of Charity, including a sister superior, were appointed to the tuberculosis hospital two years prior to Doyle's approach to Bennett,[41] and it is possible that Doyle feared displacement by the nuns and sought protection by means of trade unionism. Nursing nuns colonised institutions, and subsequent appointments were made to other nuns merely on the recommendation of the Mother Superior. Marie Mortished questioned if this practice was fair and noted that nursing in some institutions was being 'taken out of the hands of lay trained nurses'.[42] In 1919, when fears arose that Dublin's Crooksling Sanatorium was being 'taken over' by nuns, the INU sent a deputation to Dublin Corporation to protest.[43]

The INU also defiantly called into question the educational credentials of nursing nuns in its early days. Kathleen Nora Price contrasted lay nurses with nursing nuns, some of whom, she argued, were not properly trained, 'never make a bed, and have no idea (never having been taught) how to treat a helpless patient'.[44] The union's questioning of the standard of nursing nuns' training was shrewd. One nun corresponded with the General Nursing Council in 1922, having been refused registration as a nurse because part of her training had been conducted in a hospital that was not an officially recognised training school. The nun requested, without success, that discretion be shown in her case: 'It would surely be very anomalus [*sic*], especially as my life will be devoted to nursing the sick poor in Workhouse Infirmaries … that I should be discarded while my position is rendered capable of being filled … by Nurses possessing far inferior qualifications'.[45]

The most acrimonious clash between the fledgling INU and the Catholic Church occurred in 1922. That year, the union publicly challenged the Catholic Bishop of Killaloe, Dr Edward Fogarty, when questions arose over nursing nuns' ability to undertake night duty at a hospital in County Clare. The bishop wrote to the County Clare Board of Health, forbidding the nuns from undertaking night duty for fear that it would hinder their 'spiritual exercises'.[46] It is not clear what constituted 'spiritual exercises', but a similar case at Waterford Fever Hospital in 1935 suggests that night duty was unpalatable to nuns because they fasted by night in anticipation of receiving Holy Communion; indeed, it was a 'great danger' and caused havoc among the nuns.[47] Nor could some nuns undertake night duty because it interfered with their choir duties.[48] In sum, and much to the INU's annoyance, night duty was largely the responsibility of lay nurses – some of whom had been on continuous night duty for up to thirty years.[49]

Bishop Fogarty continued by reminding the Board of Health that nuns worked out of a sense of 'Christian charity' and not for 'gain or pleasure' and remarked that if the nuns were 'turned out' of the institution and replaced by lay nurses, then may 'God help' the patients who would be left to 'rot neglected and uncared for by Divine love'.[50] Bishop Fogarty does not appear to have envisaged his letter being published in the *Clare Champion* but, when it was, it attracted the ire of the INU. Kathleen Nora Price, for the union, requested that Bishop Fogarty withdraw his 'totally unjustifiable and uncalled for insinuations' and, in a letter to the same newspaper, asserted:

> If members of Religious Orders wish to enter the nursing world, they should do it fully, as some Orders do, and be prepared to perform all the duties connected with that profession. If, as Dr Fogarty states … Nuns undertake the care of the poor, and infirm for Christian charity, it is hardly consistent with such Christian charity to condemn a fellow creature to such an unnatural life as continuous night duty, which they will not undertake themselves.[51]

The fledgling INU was clearly not averse to vocally challenging the Church when it came to defending the employment conditions of lay nurses, but as the Catholic social movement took hold, it soon found itself singing a different tune. At the Annual Council Meeting of the INU in 1933, it was alleged that nuns were 'ousting' lay nurses from their jobs and that any critics of the practice were labelled 'Bolshevists and Communists'.[52] A decision was taken at the meeting to write to the Catholic Archbishop, Edward Byrne, on the matter. Annie Smithson, for the INU, informed the cleric that the press had been asked not to publish reports on aspects of the meeting, which concerned nursing nuns. Some newspapers apparently disregarded the request, and their reporting of the matter caused 'offence' to nuns from one particular order.[53] In later correspondence, Smithson assured Archbishop Byrne that the union did not 'wish to interfere with the Religious Sisters, nor do we want to appear in anyway [*sic*] anti-Catholic for the vast majority of our Members are Catholics', but asked that lay nurses be considered to fill at least half of any nursing positions which would arise in the future.[54] The tone of Smithson's correspondence contrasted with that which characterised the Bishop Fogarty case a decade before and hinted at a less belligerent attitude toward the Church by the INU. Belligerence was replaced by deference in the late 1940s and, in his autobiography, Noël Browne recounted that when he proposed that nuns and lay nurses be promoted on equal merit, the INO 'made no attempt to defend the proposals'.[55]

The change in the organisation's stance, from defiance to deference, may have been owed to changes in its leadership. The union's first President, Louie Bennett, was a Protestant. Its first Secretary, Marie Mortished, who served until 1921, came from Protestant lineage, as did Kathleen Nora Price, her successor. Price was succeeded by Annie Smithson. Smithson's life was often as dramatic as those of the characters in her novels. Born in Sandymount, Dublin (where she shared her home with a pet monkey called 'Jacko'), Smithson was left a sizable sum in wills following the death of both her father and grandfather – some of which she spent frivolously and the rest of which she spent clearing her family's debts. Broke, her aunt advised her to become a nurse: 'As you have little education and do not appear to be blessed with much in the way of brains, I think that nursing is the best career for you', she said.[56]

And the drama did not end there. After qualifying, Smithson, an incurable flirt, fell in love with a doctor whilst serving as a Jubilee nurse in County Down in 1901. A passionate affair followed, but in light of the fact that the doctor was married, Smithson considered the relationship wrong and ended it by moving to Scotland in 1904. She sought succour for her broken heart in religion and, in 1907, converted from Protestantism to Catholicism under the tutelage of nuns from the Sisters of Charity order who were attached to Dublin's Harold's Cross Hospice in 1907. She was extremely devout, and an analysis of her bestselling novels concluded that, for Annie 'in the fictional world … as also in real life, the One, True Church is Roman Catholic'.[57] Smithson found like-minded company at the INU as, in 1934, Nellie Healy, past President of the Irish Guild of Catholic Nurses, was elected President. Catholics now comprised the organisation's leaders.

After Smithson assumed leadership of the union, items concerning the possibility of Ireland hosting a Catholic Nurses' Congress appeared in the organisation's periodical, as did accounts of the 1937 Congress of Catholic Nurses in London. The organisation invited members to donate to the construction of an Irish National Chapel in Lisieux, France – the final resting place of St Thérèse – and informed those that funded the initiative that Pope Pius XI would bless them for doing so.[58] The organisation's journal published a piece which suggested that

Jesus My Patient
A PRAYER FOR THOSE WHO NURSE THE SICK

Dearest Lord, may I see Thee to-day and every day, in the person of Thy sick, and whilst nursing them, minister unto Thee. Though Thou hidest Thyself behind the unattractive disguise of the irritable, the exacting, the unreasonable, may I still recognise Thee and say, "Jesus my Patient, how sweet it is to serve Thee.' Lord, give me this seeing faith, then my work will never be monotonous. I will ever find a new joy in humouring the fancies and gratifying the wishes of all poor patients. Oh! beloved sick, how doubly dear you are to me when you personify Christ, and what a privilege is mine to be allowed to nurse you. Sweetest Lord, make me appreciate the dignity of my high vocation and its many responsibilities. Never permit me to disgrace it by giving way to coldness, unkindness or impatience; and my God, while Thou art Jesus, my Patient, deign also to be my patient Jesus, bearing with my many faults, looking only with my intention, which is always to love and serve Thee in the person of each and every one of Thy sick. Lord, increase my faith, bless my efforts, sanctify my work now and forever. Amen.

A prayer from the *Irish Nurses' Magazine* in 1953. Digital content created, published and reproduced courtesy of Digital Library, UCD.

nursing nuns' 'sacrifice and service' was of a 'more truly noble' nature than that of lay nurses in 1937.[59] The organisation's Annual Council meeting was preceded by mass in the 1940s and, in the 1950s, Pope Pius XII bestowed a blessing on the INO which was framed and displayed at its office.[60]

Analysis of the official journal of the Irish Guild of Catholic Nurses, the *Irish Nursing News*, shows that although the guild also advocated vocationalism and frowned upon excessive state involvement in healthcare provision, the INO's publication did so more frequently and forcefully. The Secretary of the INO, Eleanor Grogan, even appealed to nurses to join the Catholic Nurses' Guild, owing to the importance of 'Catholic standards and Catholic moral law' and in light of 'pagan standards and immoral practices' in other countries.[61] A public health nurse who was a member of the organisation also suggested that the INO and the Irish Guild of Catholic Nurses affiliate and that one fee confer membership of both organisations.[62]

In light of all of this, there is an obvious contradiction in the INO's description of itself as a 'non-sectarian' organisation.[63] How can this be explained? From the 1920s, Ireland became 'a Catholic state for a Catholic people' in which Catholics comprised almost 95 per cent of the population.[64] Irish Catholics were extremely devout, particularly Irish women,[65] and this helps explain the INO's high level of Catholicism. Advertisements in Irish nursing journals for nursing positions in British hospitals reassured prospective applicants of the close proximity of local churches and of monthly masses at the hospital. This was essential, as some parents had reservations about their

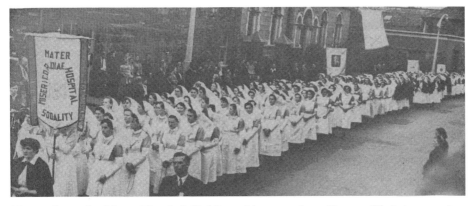

Nurses from the Mater Hospital, Dublin, taking part in a Corpus Christi procession in 1954. Digital content created, published and reproduced courtesy of Digital Library, UCD/Courtesy *Irish Press*.

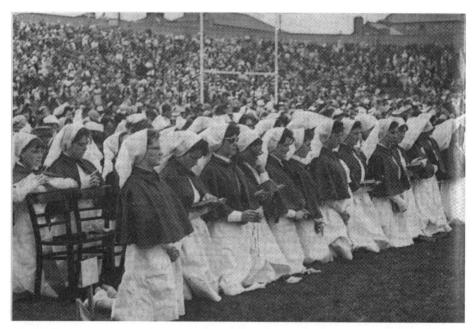

Nurses praying at the Patrician Congress Pontifical High Mass at Croke Park in 1961. Digital content created, published and reproduced courtesy of Digital Library, UCD/ Courtesy *Irish Independent*.

daughters emigrating to Britain to become nurses; one recalled her mother giving her £20 and a rosary, crucifix and prayer book before she departed for 'that evil, black Protestant Godforsaken country' in 1952.[66]

The devoutness of the Irish appeared unusual to some. Miss Goodall, Educational Supervisor at the Central Midwives Board in England, visited Ireland to survey the system of midwife training in 1953. In a letter to her employer, she wrote: 'Religious issues are rife here – it seems the peoples' lives are completely ruled by them – I've heard some queer things.'[67] Catholicism was an innate aspect of Irish life to such an extent that its influence was 'not even felt or noticed'.[68] The INO's endorsement of and adherence to Catholic teaching was consequently not regarded as breaching its supposedly non-sectarian position because Catholicism was essentially and de facto 'Irish'. If the INO's deference to the Catholic Church and to Catholic teaching was a manifestation of a broader societal adherence to Catholicism, then this could be expected to change if Irish society reappraised its relationship with Catholicism. An analysis of two divisive social issues and the extent to which these issues were infused by Catholic teaching suggests that this is what happened.

II.I. Contraception, Abortion and the Rise of Pluralism

In 1938, the INO's journal reproduced an article entitled 'moral disease' from the *Catholic Herald*.[69] It appears that the article was written by a Catholic nurse working in Britain. The nurse alleged that a 'pagan atmosphere' permeated hospital life there and that nurses who found themselves 'without Catholic influence' could lose their religiosity.[70] The first birth control clinic opened in London in 1921 and Durex began manufacturing condoms in 1934. Developments of this nature were not to the nurse's liking and, referring to women who limited or spaced their pregnancies, she concluded: 'It is only too obvious that birth-control has been practised.'[71] The piece was the first to establish a link, albeit tenuous, between Catholicism and contraception in the INO's periodical. This link was reinforced in the years ahead. In 1956, the *Irish Nurses' Magazine* devoted two pages, reproduced from the *Catholic Herald*, to the Pope's endorsement of the 'psycho-prophylactic method' – a pain relief technique during childbirth.[72] The technique was based on the Pope's assertion that a pain-free birth may lessen 'inducement to commit immoral acts' among married couples.[73] These immoral acts invariably related to the use of contraceptives.

The following year, the *Irish Nurses' Magazine* reproduced a series of lectures on medical ethics by Catholic priest Edward Hegarty of the Guild of Catholic Nurses.[74] The lectures were largely informed by papal teaching and, in one, the cleric remarked that 'contraceptive surgery [is] always sinful even when a future pregnancy would be dangerous.'[75] Readers, 'aware of [their] responsibility before God', were urged to refuse to assist during surgical sterilisations and were reminded that 'any attempt to impede the procreation of a new life ... is intrinsically immoral.'[76] The Catholic hierarchy's disapproval of artificial contraception was reaffirmed in the Papal Encyclical *Humanae Vitae* in 1968.[77] At the request of a number of nurses who had solicited her opinion on the topic, a doctor wrote to the INO, expressing her views, and the organisation published her correspondence: '[The Encyclical] sets forth perfect principles for people to attain holiness and happiness in their marriages ... Contraceptives diminish femininity and happiness by obstructing motherhood.'[78]

Two years later, a group of feminist activists laden with contraceptives purchased in Belfast, Northern Ireland, arrived into Dublin by train. The women, in bringing contraceptives into the Republic, flouted a ban that had been in force since 1935. Their actions triggered a national debate on the topic, which was featured in the INO's journal. The organisation published a

World Greets Papal Decision on Painless Childbirth

WORLD-WIDE interest and satisfaction has greeted the Holy Father's declaration in an address to some 700 doctors and midwives in the Vatican on January 8th that there is no moral or scriptural objection to a new technique to render childbirth painless to the mother.

His Holiness pointed out that " it is a question here of natural, painless childbirth, in which no artificial means are used, but the natural forces of the mother alone are called into action."

It is called the psycho-prophylactic method. Hypnosis is not involved : the mother is fully conscious throughout.

Pain is avoided through the absence of fear and the mother's own trained physical responses, including relaxation of tension, with the help and constant supervision of trained medical attendants.

His Holiness analysed the theory and practice of the Russian researchers, and said :

" For his part the Englishman, Grantly Dick Read, has perfected a theory and technique which are analogous in a certain number of points. In his philosophical and metaphysical postulates, however, he differs substantially, because his are not based, like theirs, on a materialistic concept."

The Holy Father remarked that if the method can avoid or diminish pain, it " can lead to positive moral achievements."

" If pain and fear are successfully eliminated from childbirth, that very fact," said His Holiness, " frequently diminishes an inducement to commit immoral acts in the use of marriage rights."

IRREPROACHABLE?

The Holy Father made it clear that he was passing judgment on the psycho-prophylactic method from the moral and religious point of view.

" The method," said His Holiness, " unquestionably has elements that must be considered as scientifically established; others that have only a high probability, and still others which remain as yet (at least for the present) of a problematic nature."

The Pope turned to the moral aspects and said : " Is this method morally irreproachable?

" The answer, which must take into account the object, end and motive of the method, is enunciated briefly :

" ' Considered in itself, it contains nothing that can be criticised from the moral point of view.' . . .

" The method is a natural elevating influence, protecting the mother from superficiality and levity; it influences her personality in a positive manner, so that at the very important moment of childbirth she may manifest the firmness and solidity of her character."

MORALLY NEUTRAL.

Having made it clear that the methods are in themselves morally neutral, the Holy Father explained that they should be undertaken with the highest purposes in mind. He listed three such purposes :

1. " **The interest presented by a purely scientific fact.**

2. " **The natural and noble sentiment which creates esteem and love for the human person of the mother, wishing to do her good and to help her.**

3. "**A deep religious and Christian feeling, inspired by the ideals of a living Christianity.**"

If, said the Pope, the methods are undertaken with intentions that are immoral, then it is the personal action of the agent which is to be judged wrong.

" The immoral motive does not change something that is good into something that is bad, at any rate as far as its objective nature is concerned, any more than the goodness of a thing in itself can justify a bad motive or furnish a proof of its goodness."

IDEOLOGY.

His Holiness next dealt with the theological evaluation, saying :

" The new method is often presented in the context of a materialistic philosophy and culture and in opposition to Holy Scripture and Christianity . . .

" The ideology of a researcher and of a scholar is not in itself a proof of the truth and the value of what he has discovered and expounded . . .

The Pope delivers his advice on childbirth. Digital content created, published and reproduced courtesy of Digital Library, UCD.

lengthy article written by Sister Mary Corona of Portiuncula Hospital, County Galway, in 1974.[79] Sister Corona aimed to put forward the 'true position of the Catholic' and advised that 'no contraceptive device is morally permissible'.[80]

MEDICAL ETHICS

The organisation's journal did not publish the counter position of those seeking a more liberal approach to contraception. Neither did it publish educational articles related to artificial contraception, and it is small wonder that, in 1974, some Irish nurses admitted to not knowing what the oral contraceptive pill actually was.[81] Soon the so-called 'Irish solution to an Irish problem' was arrived at when the *Health (Family Planning) Act* of 1979 permitted the sale of contraceptives on prescription.[82]

While the act was being drafted, the INO indicated to the Minister for Health, Charles Haughey, that it condemned devices and medications, including oral progesterone, that may have an abortifacient effect.[83] The

CONTRACEPTION   SR. MARY CORONA, F.M.D.M., S.R.N., S.S.M.

It is doubtful if any subject has caused such verbal and literary outpourings in recent years as contraception. Everything has been said, yet people behave as if nothing has been settled. An abundance of conscience-soothing articles have been written but still consciences go their unquieted ways. Theologians, priests, doctors and midwives (Religious and Lay) have all at one time or another mounted the rostrum to inform us why we need not cling too tenaciously to the teachings of Our Holy Father the Pope, and yet for so many the barque of Peter, though tossing on a sea of confusion remains the only hope of achieving stability, sanity and true conformity to what is right. On the other hand many Catholics in their efforts to defend good Catholic principles over-simplify the whole issue, ignore obvious difficulties, add many inaccuracies and end by convincing few.

The result? Confusion, division and serious anxiety. Into this sea of confusion I intend to throw my small pebble. Small it doubtless is but perhaps it will prove to be a tiny rock of hope for those who at times feel that they are all but drowning.

I intend to try to state the true position of the Catholic as I see it while at the same time not ignoring obvious difficulties and situations for which at present there is simply no answer.

I appeal to that growing number of theologians priests, doctors and midwives and others (who are I believe, betraying the trust inherent in their positions by interpreting Humanae Vitae in their own highly individual way) to stop sowing confusion; stop telling us that the Church should keep quiet on such personal matters (presumably so that they themselves can be better heard) stop telling us that the Pope is only one (to which we can answer 'so is God'). I ask these advisers in all earnestness to use the knowledge, talents, intelligence, ability and authority which they doubtless have to sow peace in souls not unrest; to encourage loyalty to the Holy Father and not division. If they cannot, 'in conscience', (a very over-worked phrase these days) then in the name of christian charity and truth will they not keep quiet. I make this appeal not for myself obviously, but for that silent majority whom I am convinced exist and who wish above all else to remain loyal to the Church: people who crave the truth and not a pale reflection of it; people who want only what is right and yet are in danger of being stirred around in the muddy pool of persuasive arguments and soothing noises to the extent that their vision will become dulled and they will no longer to able to appreciate the clear light of God's truth.

HISTORY OF CONTRACEPTION

As I have already indicated there are many inaccuracies on both sides. For example we are often told by those who are opposed to contraception that it is of modern origin — it is not. We have instances of it in the Old Testament and I myself have met it many times during the sixteen years I spent practising midwifery in the remote rural areas of Zambia. The methods used had been handed down to the present generation through many centuries.

When pregnancy was to be avoided there were two main systems available.

1. A contraceptive method of intercourse;
2. Abstinence as far as the lawful partner was concerned, with the man employing the services of another for the time being.

From this latter practice grew the establishment of concubinages which still exist today as an accepted system in many parts of the world. This is used fairly extensively when the wife is unavailable by reason of advanced pregnancy, illness, taboos or when pregnancy is to be avoided. However, since contraceptive methods of intercourse are notoriously unreliable and since the concubines are usually highly fertile, babies in great abundance result from these two systems. However, a high infant mortality rate takes care of this and maintains a balance. Should a woman die in childbirth the tragedy is short-lived and there is always another willing and ready to take her place.

As Christianity permeates an area this system is seen to be unacceptable. A husband is taught that his wife is not a mere instrument to be used for child-bearing, drawing water, cooking food or amusement, but a partner. She must therefore be accorded the respect and affection of an equal, which will at times be manifest only on the dimension of concern for her welfare and deep caring for the family already established. From this development comes the introduction of a way of life in which self-restraint, sacrifice, generosity, calendars, temperature charts and mucous tests come into play.

TWO MAIN GROUPS

All this of course is excellent for those who can accept it, but for those who cannot there is a problem. Those who cannot fall into two main groups.

1. Those married people who, because of one or more difficulties, find it almost impossible to follow this way.

These difficulties include:-

a) One or other partner unwilling to adopt any method requiring restraint;
b) Partner with alcoholic, mental or drug problem to whom any method would appear to imply rejection and cause untold misery;
c) Unreasonable partner;
d) Husband with erratic work pattern (always home at the wrong time);
e) Husband with 'wandering tendencies' and always more inclined to wander when wife not available;
f) Heavy drinking on part of husband.
   (On this latter problem one can say that in a country where we have a drink problem, we obviously have a high percentage of heavy drinking husbands — not necessarily drunkards, but heavy drinkers. It seems fair to say that if a man cannot control his drinking habit, there is small chance of convincing him to control his more urgent needs. Indeed even if he could be convinced of the necessity, a mind soaked in alcohol every evening will hardly be in a state to remember which values were accepted as sound earlier in the day).

2. Those married people who because of an almost complete breakdown in communication between them, except on the physical level, look on any method as unthinkable.

Group 2 requires no explanation, to state it is sufficient, but together with Group 1 poses the burning question 'What does one advise?'

DIFFICULT CASES

Many theologians, priests, doctors and midwives and others have no hesitation in these difficult cases in reading into Humanae Vitae—meanings that are not there, and also finding there that for individual cases contraception would be permissible. I have read and studied Humanae Vitae until I know it almost by heart, but I fail to find in it anything that inclines me even slightly to think that the Holy Father was leaving this loop-hole. For those then who are interpreting this document loosely one can only say that to advise something as an individual is one thing (though even this need not necessarily be morally defensible) — the person seeking advice can either take it or leave it depending on the esteem in which the adviser is held but it is quite another thing, to abuse authority in this manner, for those seeking advice usually see authority in those they approach for advice and to give advice as **coming from the Church** when there seems to be **no justification whatever** for doing so, is obviously wrong.

Perhaps a short digression would be useful here. I have used the word 'Church' in the time honoured sense of legitimate authority coming down from Christ through his Vicar on earth. It seems regrettably necessary to state this clearly for I have in recent times heard the Church defined as (a) The whole people of God (b) The Bishops' Conferences, and in several other way which seem to be employed to serve the purpose of those using the term. We know, of course, that the people of God are the Church in one sense, but NOT and NEVER in a teaching capacity. We also accept that the Bishops' Conferences have duties to instruct the faithful, but when the issue is one which requires the voice of Peter we then know that " . . . Some Bishops are not Episcopates, which together with the Pope — **and never without him** and under his authority and guidance have the complete and universal magisterium" (Osservatore Romano—October, 1968).

This statement in the Vatican's official newspaper makes nonsense out of a heading which appeared in a recent edition of an Irish Medical paper which ran "Cases when the Church can approve Contraception" then went on to explain " . . . most theologians and Bishops would approve contraception . . ."

It is very important that the Catholic laity be informed that theologians and Bishops' Conferences **do not** and **cannot** constitute 'The Church' in the sense in which we are using the term.

WHAT IS THE ANSWER?

So we go back to the question 'What is the answer?' There is none. That is, there is no answer which anyone can give **in the name of the Church** which will solve the problem. Those concerned may themselves settle for a course of action for which the Church has not legislated, they may for their own reasons side-step the Church's teaching. Such actions cannot be condoned, though on the other hand, **no one, no one at all,** has the right to judge of their motives, intentions,

guilt or anything else. Realising what God's love requires of them, let them make their decisions before God in the light of their own individual consciences and circumstances and, happily, God and not us will be their judge, just as he will be judge of the lack of charity that so often manifests itself in attitudes adopted towards these people by those who have not taken the same way.

Some of course will declare themselves shocked at the hardness of a Church that can cause such misery to people. This attitude (and we find it in the highly intelligent as well as in those of more limited mental means) would be absurd if the issue were not so serious.

The Church cannot bend the truth nor tamper with what she knows to be God's will for any reason whatsoever. Once she has decided that a particular practice is against God's law she is **in conscience** bound to speak in the plainest possible terms. (One could remark here that in these days of so much talk of freedom of conscience it seems that the only persons deprived of this privilege are those holding authority). Even if her decisions cause distress, which the Church would greatly desire to avoid, she cannot change what she knows to be right. She cannot say black is white when she knows it is not. Casti Conubii, the encyclical of Pope Pius XI, puts this very clearly ' . . . no alleged need or indication can convert an intrinsically immoral act into a moral and lawful one'.

We said above that people caught in these situations sometimes resort to means outside the moral law as taught by the Church. Two examples of instances occurring outside the context of contraception may help to illustrate this point.

a) In a polygamous society a Christian may heroically resist tribal pressures to take on extra wives. Eventually after many years his courage fails and to obtain peace he surrenders his monogamous state and becomes polygamous.

b) A much tried husband comes home one evening and finds his constantly faithless wife in the arms of another man. He shoots and kills her.

No one in his heart can condemn such men, though one does condemn the action. We admire the constancy of years. We regret deeply the steps they took. We support them as much as we can through the crises that inevitably follow. However — and this is the real issue — had either man consulted us prior to taking his drastic action **we would not have advised it, condoned it, nor co-operated with him in achieving it,** rather we would have **condemned any suggestion of it** as positively as possible.

Applying this to the contraceptives issue we see that it is right and lawful that we sympathise if, and when, steps are taken that are not morally right; we admire the years of faithfulness that have led up to the present. we continue to support the person without condoning what has been or still is being done, BUT — and this is the point — had we been consulted beforehand, we **would not, could not** have advised the action that was subsequently taken.

CONTRIBUTION OF SCIENCE

Being a true mother and therefore very concerned for the lives and welfare of her children the Church has through the lips of the Holy Father, urged that research will go on and that a way morally acceptable will be found to ease the stress of parents in these dilemmas. (Humanae Vitae) We should perhaps remember that the Church is not a science laboratory nor a medical research unit. However, such establishments do exist, and it is surely **their** work to find the answers to these perplexities, to **find a solution acceptable to Catholics.** Science has sent men to walk on the face of the moon, has found a way to detect a blighted ova as early as 32 days from conception, has made missiles, the principles of which the ordinary person and indeed even the more than ordinary person cannot even begin to understand. Human brains have thought out the workings of computers, jet flying, atom bombs and an almost inexhaustible range of commodities. Is it then too much to hope that soon science will find something that will satisfy two conditions, i. e.

1) Safety from pregnancy;
2) Moral acceptability, plus an auxiliary condition, that of satisfying the ego of the adviser.

For in my opinion our distress at not being able to help the woman confronted with the 'baby' problem is more sorrow for ourselves than for her, in a great number of cases. If we solve a problem, we no longer have to worry about it, we can forget it. If we cannot solve it, we have to live with our feeling of inadequacy — which is uncomfortable — or, if we are really heart-involved with the person concerned we will have to suffer, sometimes intensely so, in our efforts to relieve some of the loneliness and tension of that afflicted person. This is the rub — we do not like to suffer.

So in taking the position that contraception is not the answer to any of our difficulties I am not unaware of almost well nigh desperate problems. I have had twenty two years of active midwifery work, and as I mentioned earlier, almost sixteen were spent in the remote areas of Zambia where without doctor or fellow midwife I faced (and solved or failed to solve) the type of cases that in the obstetrical books do not even merit a pencilled note in the margin! Situations that cannot occur, occurred. Complications that cannot happen, happened.

Difficulties that are never met with these days were fairly frequently met. Examples of these would be the ruptured uterus following a five day obstructed 2nd stage of labour; the child-wife, underdeveloped to the extent of not being able to carry her frequent pregnancies for more than three months; the malnutrioned mother who produces premature infants who die within a month or so of birth; the locked twins that one somehow manages to deliver alive; the sloughed off cervix and vaginal wall following a full week of pressure from impacted shoulders; the massive 'three-in-one' fistula; the incurable uterine infection caused by such foreign bodies as grass, twigs, omens, pieces of rag, dung and leaves; the prolapsed cervix protruding for more than six inches from the vagina. In almost all these cases it would seem common sense to advise the avoidance of any more pregnancies by **whatever method.** However, one does not do this and when the woman again becomes pregnant as she invariably does, one is almost always able to see her through safely provided she presents herself for the necessary care. So I can say that in the circumstances in which I have worked I have helped many, though I have failed others and from it all I have learned that I am not God. I have now come back to the developed side of the globe to find that we have those in our midst who would usurp God's authority and set themselves up as masters of life and death, an attitude

which leads to a depressing lowering of values, a very definite decline in desiring to adhere to what is right, a frightening disregard for authority — all of which leads to a babelic confusion which makes the standards in the newly-developing countries by contrast appear half a century ahead.

LONG TERM
But although there is no ready-made answer to these problems, the long term view could be considerably improved if other values were seen for what they really are. Recently I was discussing the problem of now to avoid another pregnancy with a Catholic mother of five who told me that any method requiring restraint would be out of the question as far as her husband was concerned. At that moment the door opened and three of her young sons ran in. One tore open a completely new box of chocolates with absolutely no permission, threw no less than three into his mouth and then strewed the remainder around the room. The second boy jumped onto his mother's lay and banged her in the face yelling that she had spoiled his game by losing his football — and the reaction to this? The mother simply laughed! An uncontrolled child today will be an uncontrolled adult tomorrow, nothing is more sure. A boy who can hit his mother for spoiling his game will do likewise later on in life, when his wife appears to be doing the same thing. And yet the mother just laughed. She failed to see that she was creating for another the same problem that she herself was finding it so difficult to cope with, that of living with an unreasonable partner — a spoilt child grown to adulthood.

However, the long term view is far ahead and the problem is with us here and now. This problem, as we have already said, is not helped by giving answers that are no answers at all because they are based on false principles. Neither is it helped by ignoring it or getting hysterical about it. It is only helped by making an honest attempt to live with it. This is a lonely road and a weary one, but it should be said that many have similarly hard roads to walk — as is the case with those who suffer the degradation of unemployment, homelessness, poverty, hunger. Few sufferings could be more heart-breaking than young widowhood, mental breakdown, terminal illness in youth and drug addiction.

The difference is, of course, that in most of these cases, there is simply no answer, whereas with the issue we are discussing there is an answer **albeit a sinful one.** So it seems to me that we who are in the capacity of advisers have a serious responsibility to be brave enough to tell those who look to us for help that there is no easy solution this side of sin; the only answer is to accept the challenge and walk the hard way. Perhaps this is where the real trouble is — we have lost our courage; we cannot face the risk of losing our popularity, we cannot accept the hurt of being told that we are hard or lacking in understanding and compassion. Yet, if we do stand firmly on the side of truth, we will in the long run do more, much more for the afflicted than those who hand out ready-made solutions which are no solution at all. For we will show a willingness to suffer with the sufferer; we will walk at least a little of the way on the road with them; we will give of our time and energy, patience and friendship to make the way seem less lonely and long for them, and we will win their gratitude in the end for they will have kept their peace of mind knowing that they have not transgressed God's laws.

OTHER ASPECTS
There are, of course, other aspects of this contraception issue which I have not mentioned. There is the problem as it relates to the single girl. I do not of course refer to the normal girl living in normal circumstances, the answer for her is of course obvious. I refer mainly to the mentally retarded teenager who can only giggle and cannot say 'no', as also to other single women who through no fault of their own are in abnormally vulnerable circumstances. These situations beg a solution, but it must be a solution that is in complete conformity with moral law, otherwise it is no solution at all, rather an additional problem.

OPERATIONAL PRINCIPLES
The operational principles then as I see them are:-
Either contraception is
a) INTRINSICALLY WRONG and therefore NOTHING can justify it
   or
b) It is MERELY UNDESIRABLE in most cases and can therefore be left to the mature judgement of the individual who may or may not seek advice from competent people.
We are plagued by those who take the latter principle as their guide. They go even further, they seek to justify their position by reading into Humanae Vitae what is not there. Quite why they trouble to do this remains an obscure issue, for if it is not intrinsically wrong, i.e. according to the first principle, then the road is surely wide open and they can go right ahead without any reference to encyclicals or any other documents. My suspicion is, however, that the majority are not as sure of their position as they would like to be. There is still that feeling that Papal backing would spell security and they seek for it even when stating a principle that by its very wording does not require it.

THE MEDIA
One could hardly write on this subject without mentioning the media. One might be forgiven for having the impression that the Press publish what the majority desire whether this constitutes a healthy diet or otherwise. This is obvious in the contraceptive issue. We have been subjected to large scale coverage of speeches and meetings where unworthy ideas have been put forward, ideas that are already succeeding in brain-washing the public minds. The Press could do so much in the cause of truth. As it is, it is difficult to see how it could do less. What the media does not tell the public is that only a minority of those who are pressurising us to accept contraception are really interested in the individual woman, the family or the problem. The majority are simply interested in furthering their business projects, by securing employment, or increasing sales and production. We are encouraged to sell out our previous Christian heritage and to hand over the proceeds to line pockets already well filled. It will only be when it is too late that we will realise the value of what we have traded, and when that moment of enlightenment comes, let us then seek the aid of those who are so anxious to 'help' us at present and we will see where their interests lie. Wherever that interest is, one thing is certain — it will not be

with the woman, the family or the problem. Her 'problem' has been used to achieve a certain purpose for the business firms, clinics and shops — they will have no further use for her.

ANTI-CHURCH GROUPS
Perhaps we should also remember that this particular issue, because it touches on the vital principles of our religious beliefs as well as on a very fundamentally important aspect of individual lives, is being used to its fullest potential by those who are out of sympathy with the Catholic Church. If they can win over a goodly section of the Church's members (and their subtlety is that they offer an answer to a problem which is both deeply personal and urgent) this will indeed be a substantial victory for them and give them encouragement to take the next step.

CONTRACEPTIVE DEVICES AND ABORTION
These I mention simply to condemn. Since I hold that no contraceptive device is morally permissible there seems to be no point in discussing the merits of one type over another.
In regard to abortion, I am on the opinion that it is a serious mistake to link it with contraception, even in writing or speaking, for to do so creates a similar link in the mind and the result is only too obvious as we have seen in other countries. They are in my opinion completely separate entities.

GOVERNMENT LEGISLATION
I have reserved the proposed Government legislation for my final word. It should make no difference at all to the **committed** Catholic what a Government legislates — we should be strong enough to know and live our principles regardless of laws or absence of laws. Unfortunately, this is not always the case. So many of us founder under a persuasive speaker, sway with the breeze. We live our lives on shifting sands and as a result our balance is unsteady, and all this after centuries of Christianity, our grasp of which we would do well to question.

CONCLUSION
I am here somewhat sadly yet gloriously reminded of what a young Ugandan boy of only recent conversion said when he was told that he would be slowly burned to death if he did not agree to perform an immoral practice. He said: "But I am a Christian, how could I face God if I were to do that?", and then as an after-thought he added "And what would other Christians think", and with that he went to his martyr's death. It is a sad reflection on our present day society that his after-thought was wasted. It has to be said that many Christians on the so-called developed side of the globe would have thought precisely nothing — nothing at all.

Sister Corona is a member of the nursing staff of Portiuncula Hospital, Ballinasloe.

An article written by Sr Corona of Portiuncula Hospital, Ballinasloe, that appeared in the *World of Irish Nursing* in 1974. The piece was a reflection of the Church's thinking at the time. Courtesy INMO. With thanks to the Franciscan Missionaries of the Divine Motherhood.

organisation issued a policy document on family planning at the time: 'Married couples have the right to plan the size of their families ... We recommend the methods of family planning which are based on the natural cycle of fertility and infertility of the wife.'[84] It is arguable that the INO formulated its policy on family planning from a moral rather than religious stance, but accepting this would be ahistorical when one considers the frequent references to Catholic teaching by Catholic commentators in the organisation's periodical – after all, medical ethics and sectarianism were one and the same thing.[85] Some years later, the organisation's stance on abortion, another divisive issue in Irish society, suggested a more secular position.

One of Fr Edward Hegarty's lectures on medical ethics, reproduced in the INO's journal in 1957, noted: 'All moral duties come from the fact that *there is* a God ... He *rules* all and must receive honour and obedience from His creatures' [original emphasis].[86] The priest's lectures suggested that clinicians follow the teachings of the Holy See regarding the 'morality' of certain clinical practices,[87] and he likened abortion to 'plain murder'.[88] By the 1980s, the narrative in the organisation's journal was similar, but its inspiration had changed. Abortion was illegal in Ireland in the 1980s, but concerns were growing that court rulings might one day legalise the practice. Following the visit of Pope John Paul II to Ireland in 1979, an umbrella group, known as the Pro-Life Amendment Campaign (PLAC), organised. The group campaigned to hold a referendum to amend the constitution in order to safeguard the right to life of the unborn. The INO was among the groups that initiated the campaign for the PLAC, and commentary in its journal, the *World of Irish Nursing*, was unequivocal: 'Any deliberate interruption of human life is murder, whether it be before or after birth.'[89] The organisation's position on abortion was a reflection of the personal position of many Irish nurses and one nurse, Mary Hazard, recalled witnessing the delivery of a child who had been conceived as a result of rape. Hazard was stationed at a London hospital at the time:

The poor woman was given a Caesarean Section as the baby was nearly at term ... the most disturbing and shocking part was yet to come, and it would challenge me, in particular, as a good Catholic girl from rural, pious Ireland. The baby, once delivered, was utterly perfect ... I could see a perfect little face ... a little button nose and tiny fingers ... However, I was told to put 'it' on the draining board ... Surely someone was going to tend the baby? Surely, it could go to someone who wanted one? The baby was alive, for goodness' sake ... I felt like I had been party to committing the most terrible of all mortal sins –

murder. I could not find it in myself to forgive either myself, or the surgeons, for leaving this poor little mite to die.[90]

Delegates at the organisation's Annual Meeting in 1982 endorsed a motion that INO members support the PLAC.[91] The referendum was held in 1983, and the PLAC's position was endorsed by the majority of those who voted.[92] As it did in relation to contraception, the INO never disseminated or attempted to articulate the views of pro-choice groups; however, in contrast to its historical opposition to contraception, the INO's stance in opposing abortion was explicitly secular. Commentary in the INO's journal noted: 'Human rights arise from the nature of the human person, and they transcend questions of religion … The right to life is the same for the unbeliever or the agnostic as for members of all creeds and races.'[93] This more earthly position may have belied members' implicit religious views; after all, 2,000 nurses converged at Knock Shrine, County Mayo, in the early 1980s to 'pray that legal abortion will never be introduced' to Ireland.[94]

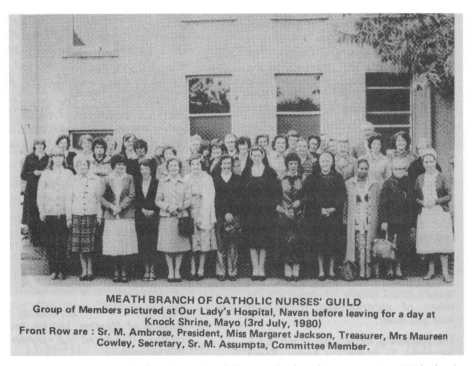

MEATH BRANCH OF CATHOLIC NURSES' GUILD
Group of Members pictured at Our Lady's Hospital, Navan before leaving for a day at Knock Shrine, Mayo (3rd July, 1980)
Front Row are : Sr. M. Ambrose, President, Miss Margaret Jackson, Treasurer, Mrs Maureen Cowley, Secretary, Sr. M. Assumpta, Committee Member.

An image from the Catholic Nurses' Guild's periodical *Irish Nursing News*. With thanks to the Catholic Nurses Guild of Ireland. Image courtesy of the National Library of Ireland.

Overall, the organisation's tone reflected the rise of pluralism and agnosticism in Irish society, evident in declining vocations and in the removal of the 'special position' of the Catholic Church from the constitution in 1972. The INO's position on abortion was also an expression of nursing and midwifery mores, as opposed to religious mores. In light of the crucial role that nurses and midwives were to play in the expanding health services, it became apparent in the 1950s that the *Midwives (Ireland) Act* of 1918 and *Nurses Registration (Ireland) Act* of 1919 needed to be revised. This resulted in the passage of the *Nurses Act* of 1950, which provided for the replacement of the Midwives' Board and Nursing Council with a joint regulatory body known as An Bord Altranais.[95] An Bord Altranais published its first *Code for Nurses* some years later which noted that nurses 'must at all times maintain the principle that every effort should be made to preserve human life, both born and unborn'.[96]

The rise in pluralism saw the beginning of the demise of Irish society's 'legalistic–orthodox' deference to the Catholic Church's teaching and signalled a shift toward individually principled ethics in which people increasingly decided for themselves what constituted moral and immoral behaviour.[97] This shift is evident in subsequent policies issued by the INO. The organisation's policy on tubal ligation was non-directional: 'A nurse who, on grounds of conscience, objects to assisting with this procedure is entitled to have his/her objection respected'.[98] The change in approach was also evident in various articles in the INO's journal: a 2001 article on contraception referred to the oral contraceptive pill, condoms, male and female sterilisation, spermicide, post-coital methods and natural methods.[99] In 2010, the journal contained a report of an event in Dublin at which the fiftieth anniversary of the contraceptive pill, a medical development that conferred women all over the world with 'reproductive freedom', was 'celebrated'.[100] INO conferences often opened with a recital of the Prayer of St Francis – a prayer that has at its core a willingness to embrace suffering and self-sacrifice – familiar themes in nursing and midwifery history.[101] By 2012, motions regarding the removal of 'all religious references' from addresses to the organisation's Annual Delegate Conference were being debated.[102]

III. From Spiritual to Temporal: Money, Militancy and Membership

What of the more temporal effects of the INO playing lickspittle to the Catholic Church and Catholic teaching? In *The Death of Religious Life*, Tony Flannery, a Catholic priest, writes of self-denial and 'a willingness to put the other person first' as hallmarks of the religious life.[103] The religious authorities sought to infuse nurses/midwives with this same sense of selflessness. A lecture by Rev Peter McKevitt, Chair of Sociology and Catholic Action at St Patrick's College, Maynooth, County Kildare, was reprinted on the front page of the INO's *Irish Nurses' Magazine* in 1948. McKevitt doubted whether the philosophy underpinning trade unionism was compatible with that underpinning nursing: 'The habit of self-sacrifice which puts the interest and well-being of the patient first [was at odds with workers'] personal comfort ... rights or privileges'; the cleric referred to this as the 'cheerful ... acceptance of privation'.[104] Some years later, in 1962, the front page of the *Magazine* carried an address by the Archbishop of Liverpool, Most Rev Dr John Heenan. The Archbishop advocated a salary increase for nurses but noted that 'Any profession is degraded ... when money becomes the incentive. The good nurse ... must be inspired by compassion for those she serves, so no woman should choose nursing as a career in order to make money.'[105] The INO's decision to publish McKevitt's and Heenan's pieces suggests partial agreement with the sentiments the clerics expressed and may have been partly responsible for the ambivalence its members expressed in relation to financial matters such as pensions.

The influence of nursing nuns is also notable. In 1978, the father of a student nurse at a Dublin voluntary hospital wrote to the Chief Executive Officer of An Bord Altranais, suggesting that the nuns in charge of his daughter's training hospital treated the lay student nurses as though they too wanted to become nuns: 'The real trouble, as I see it, is a confusion as [*sic*] the nuns' minds between novices in the order, who aim to rid themselves of all outside

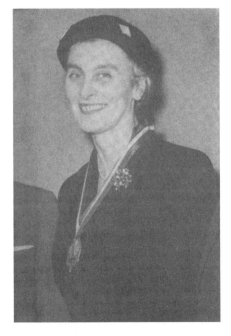

Mary Prunty, INO President, 1957–9. Prunty was unusually forthright for a nurse of her day. She hailed from Belturbet, Co. Cavan, and trained at the Charitable Infirmary, Jervis Street, Dublin. She graduated to a position as Ward Sister at Hume Street Hospital, Dublin, before becoming Assistant Matron, and latterly, Matron at Jervis Street. In later years she served as Matron at the Eye and Ear Hospital, Dublin. Courtesy INMO.

thinking and become only part of the Order, and lay girls who want to become first class nurses but to remain themselves.'[106] Whether or not aspirations to become a nun occupied the minds of most student nurses is unclear, but nuns undoubtedly had an effect on the lay nurses in their charge. Lenore Mrkwicka trained at the Charitable Infirmary, Jervis Street, Dublin in the early 1960s and recalled: 'The majority of training schools were run by religious orders and the ethos was … to serve.'[107] Another nurse elaborated:

> Being trained by a religious order really made you feel that you were there to do almost God's work … It was very much a vocation … There was none of this clocking in, clocking out … It wasn't a matter of just saying, 'I am done', and out you go … They made it seem like you had to work to the bitter end no matter what … Great demands were made of you, you stayed late and you came in early … the nuns did it and therefore you were expected to. They treated us like mini-novices [and] they made us do things like say prayers for patients … When I used to tell my friends that I did this they said it was ridiculous. And people in those [hospitals not run by religious orders] would say 'Why don't you just say no?' But you couldn't because it was part of the package, it was what was expected of you … Maybe there was a bit of Catholic guilt thrown in on top of us, good old Catholic guilt is a good motivator.[108]

The service-obligation of lay nurses who trained in hospitals run by religious orders was infused with and heightened by a pious vocational ideal – an ideal that appears to have tempered their militancy. In the already mentioned threatened mass resignation of nurses at Limerick County Infirmary in 1950, the only nurses who did not partake were those who trained at hospitals run by religious congregations.[109]

The large number of nursing nuns in Ireland may have also exerted a depressant effect on the INO's claims. Nuns were an alternative labour force whose 'philosophical indifference to money',[110] and seeming indifference to austere living conditions, endeared them to employers in times of economic austerity. In 1930, Annie Smithson attended a county Board of Health meeting[111] and protested that nurses' sleeping quarters were adjacent to the 'imbecile' ward, which was noisy and prevented nurses from sleeping.[112] Smithson requested a purpose-built nurses' home, but her talents and celebrity could only carry her so far. A board member took her apart:

> We have gone to an expense of £400 to provide apartments for [the nurses], and we are coolly asked by Miss Smithson to abandon them and put up a

nurses' home. We are asked to tax the people to accommodate those ladies ... if the nurses are not satisfied let them take their departure ... and then I will move that we have all nuns as nurses. I was anxious to have more nuns, and if those ladies resign we will get more nuns.[113]

The only defence Smithson could muster was wryly amusing: 'Will you excuse me if I ask who then will do night ... work? The nuns will not do it.'[114] The religious also had the potential to temper how INO members achieved their industrial demands. Drawing explicitly on the fifth of the Ten Commandments, 'Thou Shalt Not Kill', Fr Edward Hegarty set forth his opinion on strikes in an article in the *Irish Nurses' Magazine* in 1957: 'Any widespread *strike* by nurses or doctors – if it left patients without necessary attention, or the public accident services without sufficient personnel – would be nothing short of murderous' [original emphasis].[115]

The proliferation of religious articles in the organisation's journal may have had a more self-serving purpose by encouraging nursing nuns to join. Religious articles may also have been a strategy to induce lay nurses into membership. Pope Leo XIII's 1891 Encyclical, *Rerum Novarum*, put forward a stern defence of workers' rights.[116] In 1944, the Editor of the *Irish Nurses' Magazine* drew its readers' attention to a piece by 'Clericus', which reminded nurses that the Pope advocated workers' organisations and that Pope Pius XI and Pope Pius XII did likewise.[117] Clericus concluded that nurses remaining 'aloof' from the INO were on a 'Black List' and were 'false to the advice given by three Supreme Pontiffs'; this was a potent call to membership among a largely Catholic workforce who believed in the infallibility of papal teaching.[118]

IV. From Secular to Sectional

'Sections' are member subgroups in which nurses and midwives working in particular disciplines meet to address issues of common importance. They are a prominent feature of today's INMO. The organisation describes these sections as evolving out of a desire to address professional development issues and to provide social and personal support. Issues of a more pressing nature were also instrumental in the formation of sections. Trends in healthcare provision, including the proposed reorganisation of the health services touted in the late 1940s, had important consequences for INO members – particularly those engaged in the 'outdoor services', namely, public health nurses, Jubilee nurses and dispensary midwives. Social and statutory change affecting each of

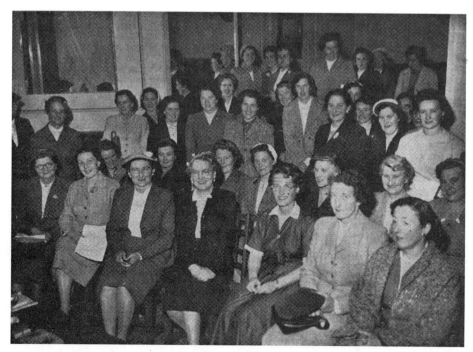

A meeting of the INO's Public Health Nurses' Section in the Hibernian Hotel, Dublin, in 1956. Digital content created, published and reproduced courtesy of Digital Library, UCD.

these groups threatened their roles and livelihoods, and each formed their own individual section within the organisation in response.

Public health nurses, who were dually qualified as nurses and midwives, formed the first section within the INO in 1951.[119] These practitioners were aggrieved that their salaries had not risen in line with the extra workload that the national campaign against tuberculosis and polio entailed. They were particularly unimpressed at hearing that the application of a new salary scale was dependent on their already onerous duties being extended to include home nursing and midwifery, which, up to that point, were the remit of district nurses and dispensary or private midwives. The role of the public health nurse, in contrast, was that of health promotion and disease prevention or, as the INO put it, 'to carry the gospel of health into the homes of the people'.[120]

The organisation's new Public Health Nurses' Section protested and refused to undertake the proposed extra duties, and the INO sought the employment of more district nurses in order to undertake home nursing. A compromise was reached whereby existing public health nurses could circumvent the

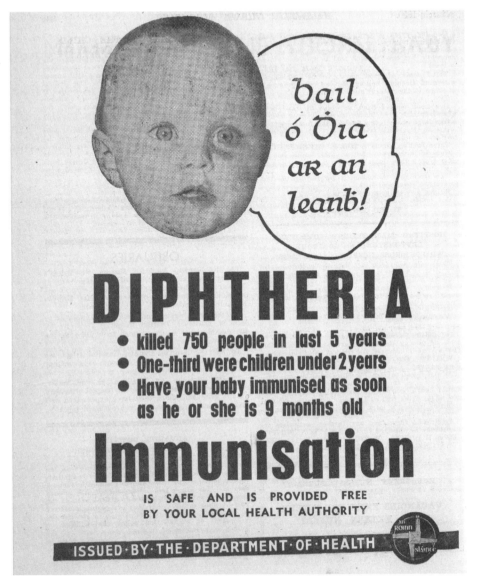

Immunisations comprised a large part of public health nurses' heavy workload. Digital content created, published and reproduced courtesy of Digital Library, UCD/ Courtesy the Department of Health.

additional duties, while newly appointed public health nurses would assume them.[121] This arrangement did not last long, however: by 1956, the office of the public health nurse was almost abolished in favour of a multifunctional district nurse. Tensions between the INO's Public Health Nurses' Section and the Department of Health continued for the rest of the decade before a final compromise was reached in 1959. Developments that year witnessed the retention of the public health nurse grade, along with the retention of home nursing and midwifery duties.[122]

Jubilee nurses formed the second section within the INO in 1952. These community nurses' salaries were partly funded by charity and, amid recession and increasing state involvement in healthcare provision, they feared for their incomes and their jobs. On behalf of their respective section, the INO requested that Jubilee nurses be absorbed into the local authority public health services as a means to safeguard their salaries and pensions.[123] That Jubilee nurses were clamouring to be subsumed into the state-run health services demonstrates a contradiction in the INO's opposition to statism at the time and suggests that, in its kowtowing to the Catholic Church, the organisation's stance was not always in members' best interests. It was finally decided that Jubilee nurses may apply for vacancies in the public health services as they arose. The last of the outdoor services to form a section within the organisation were dispensary midwives, who did so in 1953.

The hospitalisation of childbirth in Ireland intensified in the 1950s. Expectant mothers in urban areas increasingly attended metropolitan maternity hospitals in Dublin, Cork and Limerick, and mothers-to-be in rural areas increasingly attended district hospitals to have their babies. This trend threatened the livelihood of dispensary midwives, some of whom faced redundancy. The INO responded by seeking greater utilisation of their skills.

Up to then, the 'lying-in period' in uncomplicated childbirth comprised the labour and no less than ten days after the labour.[124] However, the 1953 *Health Act* provided for free nursing services for certain children up to the age of six weeks.[125] This was seized upon by the INO, which pointed out that the midwife was 'no

PRELIMINARY - MEETING -

TO DISCUSS

Formation of Dispensary Midwives' Section

WILL BE HELD AT

20, LOWER LEESON ST., DUBLIN

ON

TUESDAY, 27th JANUARY

at 3 p.m.

mere "delivery woman'" and was well suited to this role.[126] The organisation's protests were largely in vain, however: not only was hospital confinement for childbirth a largely unassailable trend, but public health nurses' increased involvement in midwifery (albeit under protest) likely infringed on dispensary midwives' dwindling caseloads – as did the fact that an increasing number of nurses appointed to dispensary districts were also midwives. The Minister for Health ultimately agreed to absorb dispensary midwives into the district nursing service and to subsume the remainder into other state-run health services.

INO sections conducted their own affairs, each having a president and chain of command and holding its own meetings to discuss topics of interest and concern. When pressing matters arose at section level they were brought to the attention of the organisation's Executive Council, who raised them with representatives of the state or employers. This mode of operation ensured that each section was dependant on the organisation as a whole, and this reduced the risk of a section leaving the INO altogether. The advent of sections was

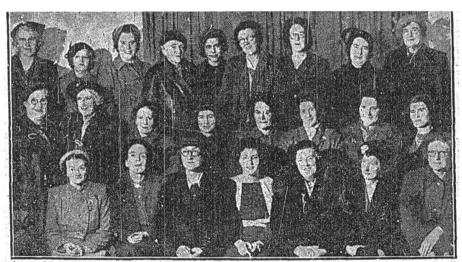

State Certified Midwives who attended the formation of the Dispensary Midwives' Section of The Irish Nurses' Organisation, Lower Leeson St., Dublin. Front row (from left)—Miss Porter, hon. secretary, Midwives' Section; Miss Fagan, Regional Organiser; Miss N. Healy, president, I.N.O.; Miss Meehan, assistant secretary, I.N.O.; Miss McDonnell, president, Midwives' Section; Mrs. Hickey, Kilkenny; Miss Brennan, Kildare. Second row — Mrs. A. Clarke, vice-president, Midwives' Section; Miss M. Whelan, Mrs. A. Stenson, Mrs. K. Mansfield, Mrs. S. Moore, Mrs. T. Foley, Mrs. M. Costello, Mrs. M. O'Connor. Third row— Mrs. D. Greene, Mrs. M. Byrne, Mrs. J. Kavanagh, Miss J. Brophy, Miss M. Ring, Miss M. Sherlock, Miss A. Boyle, Mrs. M. M. Roberts, Mrs. M. Fleming

The founding members of the INO's Dispensary Midwives' Section in 1953. With thanks to Irish Newspaper Archives and the *Irish Independent*.

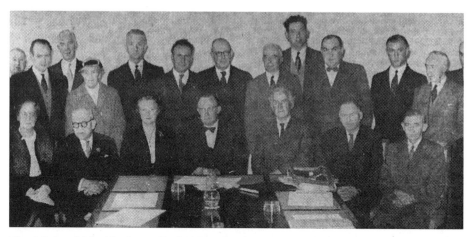

The National Health Council of 1956. Eleanor Grogan of the INO is pictured on the far left in the front row. Digital content created, published and reproduced courtesy of Digital Library, UCD/Courtesy the *Irish Press*.

wise; nurses and midwives were a fairly disparate bunch and some, such as psychiatric nurses, had never joined the INO in large numbers. The increasing specialisation that would take place in nursing in the 1960s had potential to further delineate one group from another, and sections offered a distinct identity, albeit under the INO's umbrella and control. Sections complemented the often ailing branch structure in which nurses and midwives from a motley array of clinical areas convened on a purely geographic basis. The establishment of sections attracted more members to the INO, the roll books of which swelled from 4,863 in 1948 to 5,840 in 1951.[127]

The *Health Acts* of 1947 and 1953 made provisions for the establishment of a National Health Council tasked with offering the Minister for Health advice on matters related to the nation's wellbeing.[128] Three nurses were appointed to the council in the late 1950s, including the INO's General Secretary, Eleanor Grogan. Grogan was an outspoken advocate for nurses and midwives and argued persuasively on a range of issues. Her efforts witnessed the council adopting a number of important resolutions in 1957: midwives should provide care for infants up to six weeks; the Minister should investigate, for infection-control reasons, if it was in the public's best interest to combine nursing and midwifery services by multifunctional district nurses; and that the public health nurse grade should not be done away with.[129] Grogan's arguments show that sections within the INO were capable of informing and influencing the organisation's policy as a whole. Her activities on the council also challenge

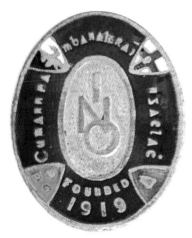

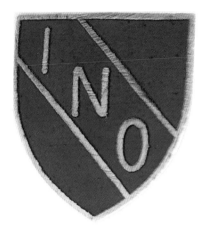

An early INO badge minted *c*.1945.
Courtesy Lisa Moyles/INMO.

New badge, new approach. The 1980s
were to herald a more trenchant and
combative INO and this was reflected
in a new shield-like badge. Courtesy
Lisa Moyles/INMO.

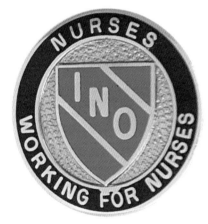

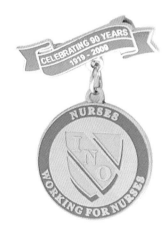

A slightly embellished take on the 1980s
badge which was rolled out in the mid–
1990s. Note that the shield remains as the
centrepiece. Courtesy Lisa Moyles/INMO.

The Organisation's ninetieth-birthday
badge. Courtesy Lisa Moyles/INMO.

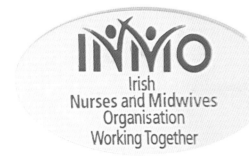

The INMO's current badge, which
came into being in 2010. Courtesy
Lisa Moyles/INMO.

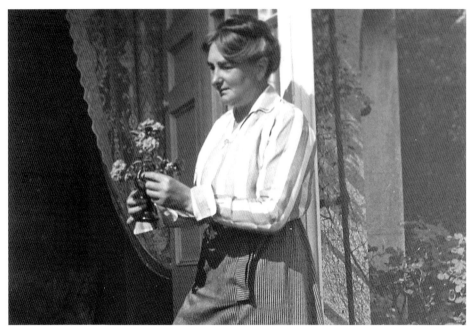

Louie Bennett in the period c.1915–20. Bennett would become the first President of the Irish Nurses' Union. Courtesy Rosemary Cullen Owens.

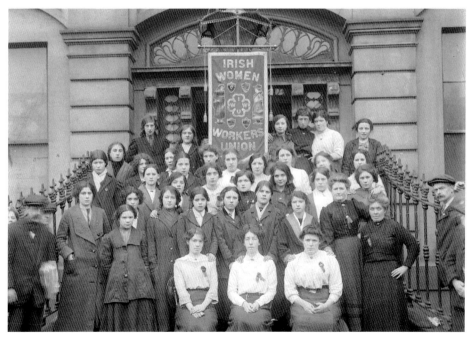

Members of the Irish Women Workers' Union on the steps of Liberty Hall at around the time the Irish Nurses' Union came into being. Delia Larkin is seated in the front row. This image is reproduced courtesy of the National Library of Ireland (Ke 203 Keogh Photographic Collection).

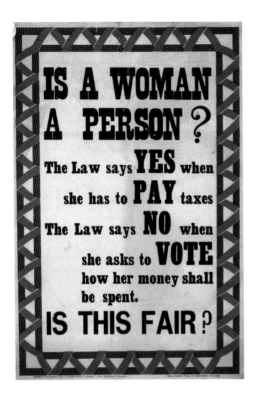

A poster used in the women's suffrage campaign in the years 1911–17. Image reproduced courtesy of the Women's Library Collection, LSE Library, UK.

The first-ever copy of the *Irish Nurses' Union Gazette*. Digital content created, published and reproduced courtesy of Digital Library, UCD.

Irish Nurses' Union Gazette

Telephone: 4994 Dublin.
20 SOUTH ANNE STREET, DUBLIN.

No. 13.   MAY, 1925.   Price 2d.

WE must begin by apologising for the long delay this time in the appearance of our Circular, but the Union work grows and grows to such an extent that the Secretary has little time to be editor and journalist as well as attend to the needs of members.

THE YEAR'S WORK.

The Report presented at the Annual Meeting last February showed a good record of work done for members.

Organising.

Organising tours were undertaken by Miss Gloster (who, unfortunately, is no longer with us) in Donegal, Galway, Dundalk, Armagh, Newry, Maryboro', Roscommon, etc. A splendid Branch is now in existence in Donegal, its success being largely due to the energy and enthusiasm of Miss McFadden, the local Secretary.

Every general trained nurse on the Register was circularised in November last in reference to a proposal of the Irish Matrons to revive the Irish Nurses' Association. We pointed out the actual improvements already gained for nurses by this Union, and the advantages of joining it. There was, unfortunately, a very poor response. Nurses have not yet waked up to the need of organisation, which is the real reason why conditions are still so bad in this country for the nursing profession. If even half the number of trained nurses on the Register (about 3,000) were loyal members of this Union, our strength would be enormously increased.

SEE THAT EVERY NURSE WITH WHOM YOU COME IN CONTACT JOINS THE UNION, and DO IT NOW.

Offaly.

Representations were made to the L.G.D. and the Commissioner on behalf of the nurses of Offaly County Hospital, and some improvements secured. This Commissioner has recently made a very harsh decision re sick leave, limiting it to four weeks in the year. We have sent in a protest to the L.G.D. against this decision.

THIS IS YOUR QUARTERLY REMINDER.

"Don't let your subscription fall into arrears." You never know when *you* may want the Union's help. *Foster its strength against the day of your need.*

Rates of Payment for Tuberculosis.

We successfully fought the attempt of the L.G.D. to force the Dublin County Council to employ a temporary nurse at lower fees than the standard rate for tuberculosis. After being forced by the L.G.D. to keep the patients without any nurse to visit them for over six weeks, the County Council at length employed one of our members and paid her at the full rate of salary, in spite of the refusal of the L.G.D. to sanction it. Miss Michie, of the Jubilee Institute, attempted to supply a retired Jubilee nurse at the lower salary, but the Co. Council declined to employ a nurse who was not a Trade Unionist. All members are asked to see that no nurse they know accepts a fee of less than £2 12s. 6d. per week, plus allowances, for tuberculosis work. The Nurses' Homes have all given us an undertaking that they will not supply a nurse at a lower rate, and we look to all private nurses to keep up the fees also. The fight will have to begin again for this year's holidays. In this connection Miss McCallum, Secretary to the English "Professional Union of Trained Nurses," writes that over three Private Nurses' Co-operative Homes charge 3½ guineas a week for general work and 4 guineas for tuberculosis, plus board, lodgings, etc., and that there are very few nurses who would take two guineas a week for anything.

Lectures.

A series of Lectures were again organised this winter, held in 5 Leinster Street. The following doctors very kindly gave lectures: Dr. Walter Stevenson, X-Ray and Radium Treatment; Dr. Davidson, Puerperal Sepsis; Dr. Bethel Solomons, Menstrual Complaints;

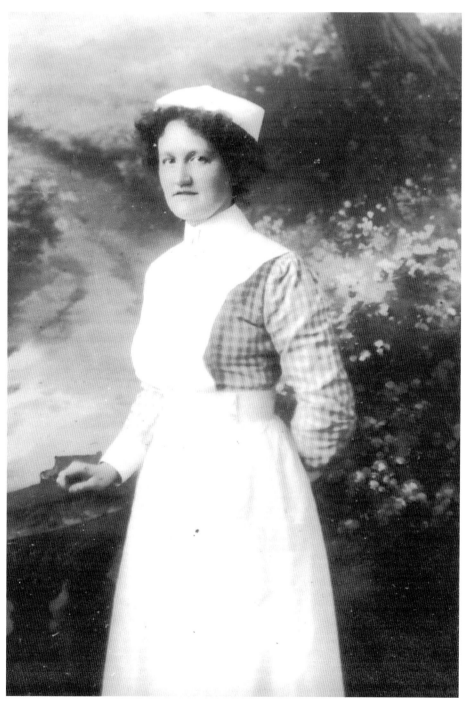

Marie Mortished during her days as a nurse. There is a suggestion that she trained at Crumpsall Infirmary in Manchester before returning to work in Dublin. This image is reproduced courtesy of Tony Cotton and John Vanek.

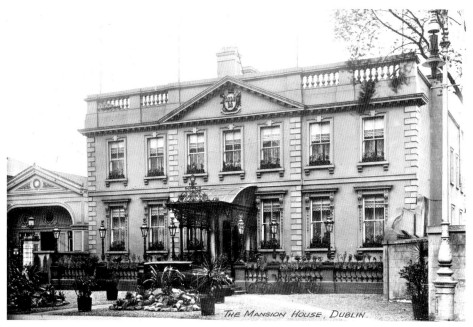

The Mansion House, Dublin, site of the INU's first public meeting, as it appeared when the Union was established. This image is reproduced courtesy of the National Library of Ireland (Eas 1705 Eason Photographic Collection).

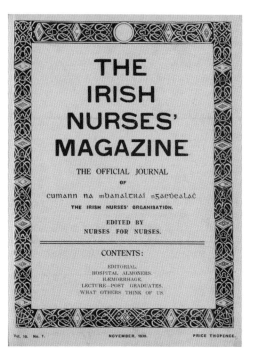

Irish Nurses' Magazine. Digital content created, published and reproduced courtesy of Digital Library, UCD.

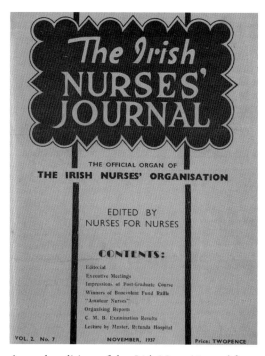

An early edition of the *Irish Nurses' Journal* from 1937. Digital content created, published and reproduced courtesy of Digital Library, UCD.

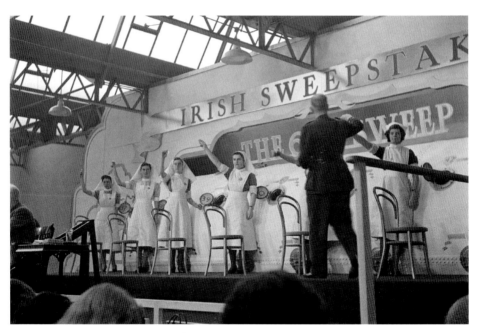

Nurses show the public the Irish Hospitals Sweepstake lottery tickets that they have taken from the drum in a draw in Dublin in the 1940s. This image is reproduced courtesy of The National Archives, The Hague, Netherlands. Photo: Willem Van de Poll – Glass Negative, Access Number: 2.24.14.02, File Number: 191-0888.

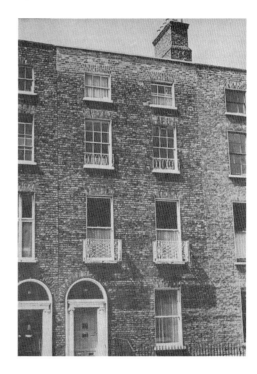

20 Lower Leeson Street, Dublin. Home of the INO, 1951–87. Courtesy INMO.

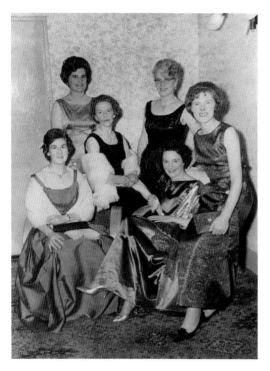

All dressed up! A dinner dance organised by the INO's Cavan Branch in 1965. From left seated: R. Meehan; A. Kelly; M. Quinn; K. O'Reilly. Standing from left: J. Osborne, INO Assistant Secretary and Ena Meehan, INO General Secretary. Courtesy INMO.

A Public Health Nurse making her daily rounds. The image appears staged and possibly comprised part of a recruitment or information campaign for Public Health Nursing. Courtesy Lensmen/Irish Photo Archive.

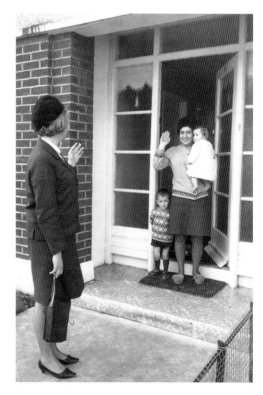

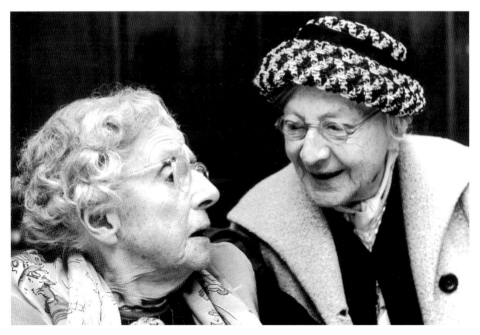

Retired nurses Sue O'Looney and Annie Donnellan in happy mood at the Christmas dinner organised by the INO's Dublin Branch Social Committee in December 1966. Copyright Mellifont Press.

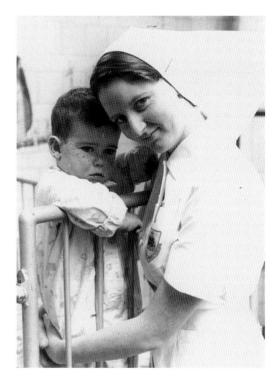

An image of a sick child and a nurse possibly taken as part of a recruitment or information campaign for paediatric nursing as a specialty. Courtesy INMO.

assertions that the INO was non-political; the organisation readily used political process to exert an influence. Grogan was careful to frame her representations to the National Health Council from a professional stance, drawing attention to optimum infection-control practices, for instance, but it seems that the industrial undercurrents to her arguments were viewed as a breach of Section 41 of the 1953 *Health Act*, which stipulated that conditions of employment were outside the council's remit.[130] Perhaps this was the reason for the Minister for Health, Seán MacEntee's decision, made 'with reluctance' in 1958, not to reappoint Grogan to the body.[131] Instead, he appointed representatives from An Bord Altranais to the council.

Changes to the system of public health provision in Ireland in the late 1940s coloured the INO's constitution and complexion. A range of sections was formed to lobby on sector-specific concerns, and these sections remain a vibrant part of the organisation to this day. The late 1940s also drew attention to the INO's yielding to two powerful lobbies: the medical profession and the Catholic Church. The organisation's journal became a sounding board through which the arguments of both factions were transmitted. The INO's support for the Church owed to the rising Catholic social movement. Its support for the medical profession possibly owed to traditionally gendered power relations between medicine and nursing. The organisation may also have been concerned at losing a powerful ally by not supporting the Irish Medical Association. The INO's support of vocationalism, which infused its opposition to the Mother and Child Health Scheme, somewhat conflicted with the organisation's early track record in campaigning on public health issues. When maternal and infant welfare were deemed to be threatened, as in the case of the

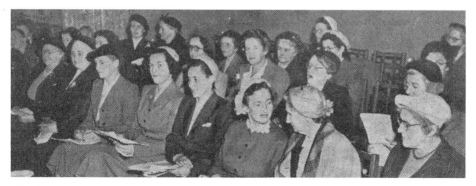

The INO's Annual Meeting in 1953. Digital content created, published and reproduced courtesy of Digital Library, UCD.

handywoman, the organisation launched a vigorous campaign of opposition and implored state intervention. By contrast, in the 1940s, the INO lamented efforts by the state to extend its reach into matters of public health. The organisation's opposition to statism conflicted with the socialist leanings of its early leaders; indeed, Louie Bennett endorsed the Mother and Child Health Scheme on behalf of the INO's former parent, the IWWU.[132]

Up to now, nurses' and midwives' service-obligation and aversion to striking have been portrayed as a humanitarian concern for patient welfare, but religious sentiment is also notable. Clerical teaching in the INO's journal equated nursing with self-sacrifice and service and referred to the murderous potential of a nurses' strike. Ulterior motives may have been at play here, as the religious were major employers of nurses/midwives in Ireland, and the voluntary hospitals they managed often encountered financial difficulties. It was arguably in the best interest of the religious to not only attenuate nurses'/midwives' demands by reminding them of the self-sacrifice that characterised their roles, but also to moderate their militancy in pursuit of what may transpire to be costly improvements in their working conditions, should a strike occur.

This was never acknowledged by the INO, even though nurses'/midwives' working conditions could reasonably be regarded as conflicting with the spirit of *Rerum Novarum*, which urged employers to pay employees a just wage. This realisation prompted one doctor to write a strongly worded letter to Archbishop Byrne in 1930, deploring nurses' working conditions at the nursing homes attached to St Vincent's Hospital, Dublin. The doctor finished his correspondence: 'As a Catholic, I think it particularly deplorable that such a system should survive in an Institution sufficiently wealthy to be a model in everything appertaining to the welfare of the nursing profession.'[133]

CHAPTER 7

Promise and Progress, 1960–9

In the shadow of the famous 'Hollywood' sign lies the sprawling and world-renowned Forest Lawn, Hollywood Hills Cemetery. On any given day there is a steady stream of both mourners and tourists to the cemetery, but the place is, nonetheless, an oasis of calm and serenity. There, under the hot Californian sun, in lot number 866, lies a discrete concrete slab with a simple inscription: 'Marie G. Mortished, Born in Dublin 1884, Died in Hollywood 1961'.[1] The brevity of the caption conceals what was an eventful life. With her family reared and having left her post as the INU's first General Secretary many years prior, a steady stream of fans, seeking an autograph from Marie's brother, Barry Fitzgerald, was a feature of Mortished's life in Dublin in later years. She decided to move to California to join him and her other brother, Arthur, in the 1940s. Fitzgerald was, by then, one of Hollywood's most sought-after actors. He died on a trip home to Dublin in early 1961, never making it back to Hollywood where he had intended to live out the rest of his days in convalescence with Marie, who died shortly afterwards. Mortished's demise had a broader relevance: it heralded the demise of the old INO and the emergence of the organisation that we know

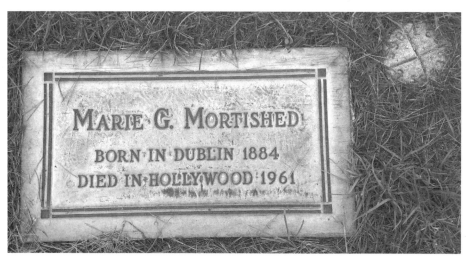

Marie Mortished's grave in Hollywood, California. Courtesy the author.

today – one that would begin to carve out a much more sizable professional and educational remit, driving change in the field of nurse education and training whilst all the while trying to improve its members' economic lot. Mortished had helped plant a garden that she never got to see grow.

The 1960s were a time of opportunity and advancement in Ireland. The state's previous economic policy of protectionism and self-sufficiency was replaced by one of free trade and foreign investment: annual growth rates quadrupled between 1959 and 1973.[2] Wages increased by 4 per cent annually from 1958 onwards.[3] Unemployment and emigration fell; trade union membership rose,[4] and the newly flourishing economy witnessed a rash of industrial disputes by workers keen to gain improvements in their conditions. The INO's long-time General Secretary, Eleanor Grogan resigned just as things were picking up. The end of her time at the organisation's helm was marked

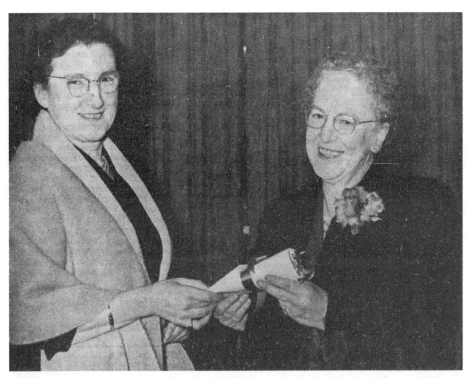

INO President Eileen O'Sullivan (left) making a presentation to Eleanor Grogan on the occasion of her retirement from the organisation in 1960. O'Sullivan was formerly a Ward Sister at Crooksling Sanatorium and later became a public health nurse at the tuberculosis services at Charles Street Clinic, Dublin. Digital content created, published and reproduced courtesy of Digital Library, UCD.

by a farewell do and sherry party at which she was presented with a piece of Waterford Glass.

Grogan was replaced by Christina (Ena) Meehan. One of thirteen children, Meehan was the daughter of two teachers. She had performed a number of roles at the INO since 1943, starting out as the organisation's Social Secretary and, by 1948, becoming the Assistant General Secretary. Outside of work, she is remembered as humorous, of having a love of children, meditation, art and books, particularly those by Roald Dahl – her education was in library studies, not nursing or midwifery. At work, Meehan, answering to Miss Meehan, displayed a more formal and formidable side. Her father died at a young age and her mother, a woman of 'strong personality', would reportedly 'not tolerate failure'.[5] Meehan had little time to waste in putting her considerable talents to use. If INO members were to achieve substantial improvements in their working conditions, then now was the time.

I. The *Employment and Conditions of Work of Nurses Report* and the Quest for Conciliation and Arbitration Machinery

The ILO published a seminal report entitled *Employment and Conditions of Work of Nurses* in 1960.[6] The report showed that, in Ireland, nurses at the starting point of the salary scale were paid less per hour than unskilled male labourers and significantly less than male carpenters and construction workers; nurses received 3.15 shillings per hour, in comparison to unskilled labourers, who received 3.38 shillings per hour and carpenters and construction workers, who received 4.29 shillings per hour.[7] INO President, Eileen O'Sullivan described the report as of 'the utmost significance to the nursing world', and the INO was forced to redouble its efforts in order to seek redress.[8] Action took the form of the attempted establishment of conciliation and arbitration machinery, but like the pension debacle, it would not be easy.

A conciliation service of sorts was already in operation for many employees. The Labour Court was established under the provisions of the *Industrial Relations Act* of 1946 in order to deal with the expected surge in wage claims that was anticipated when the Second World War ended.[9] The court acted as a mediator and resolved disputes between employers and employees.[10] Ronald Mortished, husband of Marie, was appointed first Chairman of the Court, but the INO could not hope to curry any favour as most nurses and midwives,[11] like many other state employees, did not have access to the court. This was due to the belief that such access would create a hostile relationship between them and their employer, the government.[12] INO members were at a disadvantage in

relation to certain other occupational groups who, although not having access
to the Labour Court, had access to conciliation and arbitration schemes. Civil
servants had access to such a scheme after 1950; primary school teachers after
1954 and secondary school teachers after 1955.[13] The state's fear in granting
access to nurses and midwives, to either the Labour Court or to conciliation and
arbitration machinery, was economic. In spite of the rise in Ireland's economic
fortunes, between the mid-1950s and early-1960s there was a 'disturbing rate
of increase' in health service costs in Ireland, and spending in the health sector
accounted for a significant amount of local taxation.[14] In an address to the
INO's Annual Council Meeting in 1961, the Tánaiste and Minister for Health,
Seán MacEntee, remarked:

> Your President ... has referred to the natural desire of the members of the
> Organisation to better their economic status ... With many of the sentiments
> contained in that address I am in complete agreement. [However] Nursing is
> a vocation in the sense that industrial or commercial employment can never
> be and the application to nursing of procedures now considered appropriate
> to industrial employment might well destroy its vocational character ... Can
> the community, can the tax-payers and rate-payers, afford it?[15]

MacEntee's remarks were echoed in the everyday lives of nurses. Kathleen
(Kay) Craughwell commenced her training at Galway Regional Hospital

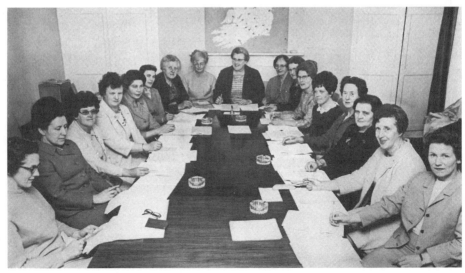

A meeting of the INO's Executive Council in 1969. Courtesy INMO.

in 1963. Craughwell recalled receiving reminders that the running of the hospital cost 10 shillings a minute, so she should make economies wherever possible; she also recounted how nurses had to pay for any items such as thermometers that they accidentally broke. Indeed, she remarked that nurses were docked an hour or so of their time off-duty if a baby in their charge lost weight.[16]

I.I. Acquiescence and Acceptance: The Realities of Aversion to Militancy

The INO rejected a new pay scale proposed by the County and City Managers' Association in 1961. The association recommended a salary of £430–£520 per year for a nurse, with two long service increments bringing the uppermost salary to £540 per year.[17] The organisation believed that the salary was not sufficient to attract nurses to the profession and to alleviate the nursing shortage, the effects of which were becoming increasingly evident considering the expansion of hospital services at the time. The organisation also believed that the proposed salary was low in relation to the salaries of other workers, such as teachers. The County and City Managers' Association then advanced an improved pay scale. This incorporated a salary of £450–£540 per year, with two long service increments bringing the uppermost salary to £560 per year. It also incorporated a 90-hour fortnight 'as soon as it can be arranged by each individual local authority'.[18] The INO again rejected the offer, as it still did not offer nurses parity with other equivalent occupations. Made wary by past experience, the organisation was also aggrieved at the failure to stipulate a definite implementation date for a 90-hour fortnight and was doubtful if the proposed salary would attract the number of nurses warranted to institute these reduced working hours.

The INO was right to be dubious. The 96-hour fortnight, recommended fifteen years earlier, was only just being implemented in some regions and the noise coming from the government did little to inspire confidence. The Minister for Health, Seán MacEntee outlined his position on a reduction in nurses' working hours: 'My functions in relation to this matter are secondary to those of the hospital authority concerned.'[19] Anger over members' working conditions grew, and the organisation's Dublin branch convened a meeting and resolved to deliver a petition of protest to the Dublin City Manager upon his return from a trip to France.[20] Some 920 INO members from Dublin signed the petition and members in Limerick and Clare followed suit. Up to that point in time, nurses'/midwives' protest strategies were quite insipid, with one recalling a planned act of rebellion at her hospital in the 1960s: 'We were going to wear brown stockings instead of black.'[21] Change was clearly afoot, and the petition represented the most vocal mass expression of discontent among INO members in the organisation's history.

The following month, after intensive negotiations, the INO accepted 'under protest' an offer of a salary of £465–£600 per year.[22] The organisation described the crux of the issue in an editorial in the *Irish Nurses' Magazine*: in the absence of conciliation and arbitration machinery, the rejection of the offer would result in a 'deadlock', meaning that the INO was obliged to accept it.[23] The organisation's acceptance of the offer demonstrated a marked contrast between it and the trade unions that represented nurses at the time. Nurses at St Kevin's Hospital, Dublin, who were members of James Larkin Junior's Workers' Union of Ireland (WUI), threatened mass resignation from their positions in 1961 in pursuit of an 80-hour fortnight and a salary increase. Similar to INO members, nurse members of the WUI had also recently rejected the offer of a revised salary scale which they perceived as inadequate. Larkin remarked that in the absence of conciliation and arbitration machinery, a 'position of impasse had been reached ... that in other circumstances ... would have resulted in a complete withdrawal of services'.[24] Indeed, nurse members of the WUI later upgraded their threat of mass resignation and voted in favour of strike action.[25]

For the WUI, deadlock resulted in threatened militancy; for the INO, it resulted in acceptance of a substandard improvement in members' conditions. This permitted the state to exploit it because, in realising that it would not take strike action, it could not bring sufficient leverage to negotiations to effect significant improvements in members' conditions. True, the INO did win some significant concessions in the 1960s, including a valuable allowance for members undertaking night duty, but its acceptance of suboptimal pay increases for members was the first in a salvo of disappointing outcomes. New salary scales for matrons and public health nurses were also soon accepted by the INO under protest. This trend did not go unnoticed by one commentator, T.P. Kilfeather, whose account in the *Sunday Independent* in 1969 summarised the situation:

> Bureaucracy tends to inaction when a situation contains no danger of crisis ...
> When a dispute threatened a shut-down of E.S.B. stations,[26] the Government,
> backed by public opinion, acted with all the resources of the State ... What's
> the difference between a claim for shorter hours by E.S.B. workers and a
> similar claim by nurses? The difference is that the Government knows the
> nurses will not strike.[27]

It would be another twenty years before the INO came around to the same way of thinking.

I.II. Salaries and Status: Achieving a Conciliation and Arbitration Scheme

In correspondence to the Hospitals' Commission in 1963, Ena Meehan, INO General Secretary, declared: 'The existing structure of salary scales do not bear reasonable comparison with the structure of scales applicable to other professions as a result of which the status of the nurse is inevitably diminished.'[28] A plan to pursue the establishment of conciliation and arbitration machinery received unanimous support at the INO's Annual Council Meeting in 1960, but the government refused to entertain the matter. However, the organisation was not deterred. Negotiating machinery for nurses, referred to as Whitley Councils, had been in operation in the UK since the establishment of the NHS

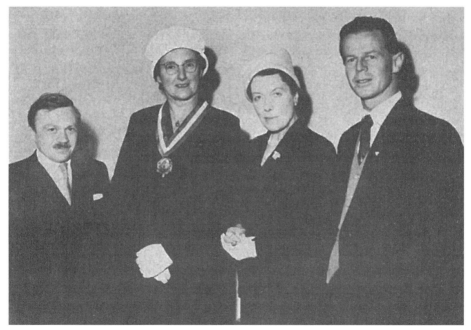

'The Staff-Side' from left: General Secretary of Cumann na nGairm Mhúinteoirí Charles McCarthy; INO President Eileen O'Sullivan; Chair of the Nurses' and Midwives' Whitley Council Frances Goodall; and representative of the Irish Conference of Professional and Service Associations J.C. Horgan. Pictured following Goodall's lecture on Whitley Councils in 1960. Courtesy INMO.

in 1948, and the INO invited Frances Goodall to address the Annual Council Meeting in 1960. Goodall was a former General Secretary of the Royal College of Nursing (RCN) and had negotiated nurses' working conditions under the Whitley Councils.

The INO also affiliated to the Irish Conference of Professional and Service Associations (ICPSA) in 1960. This was a federation founded in 1946 to represent the interests of 40,000 employees in the 'salaried and professional classes' who were not affiliated to the Irish Congress of Trade Unions (ICTU),[29] but were seeking improvements in their working conditions. The INO found like-minded company among the other professional groups who prized 'industrial and social harmony' and looked favourably on conciliation and arbitration machinery as a mechanism to avoid industrial action, which was not in 'the public good'.[30] The ICPSA declared that 'strikes, or threatened strikes' were not its policy.[31] The organisation, with the support of the conference, succeeded in having the conciliation and arbitration machinery issue for nurses raised in Dáil Éireann in 1962. Both bodies were informed that the matter was under investigation. The results of this investigation came to fruition later that year when the County and City Managers' Association submitted a proposal for a conciliation and arbitration scheme for local authority officers to the INO. The organisation considered the scheme unsatisfactory as it excluded nurses working in voluntary hospitals and omitted detailed analysis of the 'principles' that should decide nurses' salaries.[32] In essence, the INO feared that the scheme would not take into account members' professional status and that the improvements in conditions it might award would merely perpetuate their relatively low standing compared to other occupations. The proposed scheme also excluded deliberations regarding working hours at the arbitration stage.

The INO rejected the proposal and, along with ten of its fellow affiliates to the ICPSA, wrote to Jack Lynch, Minister for Industry and Commerce, imploring him to establish a revised Conciliation and Arbitration Scheme. The letter did not have the intended effect, and the INO's President, Miss O'Sullivan, informed members who gathered at its 1963 Annual Council Meeting that the Minister 'holds out no hope of being able to concede … national Arbitration [*sic*] machinery for professional bodies whose charters do not allow them to direct strike action'.[33]

Nurses and midwives were not alone in the manner in which they were treated. Civil servants did not resort to strike action and, as a result, they 'not uncommonly found themselves treated in a summary and very casual fashion' by the state.[34] Members of An Garda Síochána were another occupational sector that did not engage in strike action. Gardaí were precluded by statute

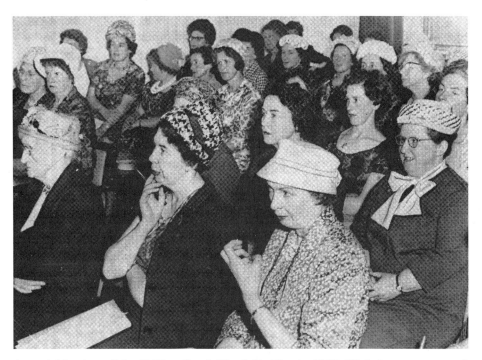

Annual Meeting of the INO at Jury's Hotel, Dublin, in 1963. Digital content created, published and reproduced courtesy of Digital Library, UCD/Courtesy the *Evening Herald*.

from taking strike action. The *Garda Síochána Act* of 1924 proscribed trade union membership for gardaí[35] and provided for imprisonment 'with or without hard labour' for anybody convicted of organising a withdrawal of labour in the national police force.[36] Revealingly, gardaí were not granted a conciliation and arbitration mechanism until 1962, some ten years after civil servants and seven years after teachers.

In 1963, the INO invited the ICN's Sheila Quinn to address its Annual Meeting on the subject of arbitration. Quinn crystallised what the INO had found out to its detriment when salary negotiations had reached a deadlock two years previously: the absence of conciliation and arbitration machinery meant that employers had the 'final word' in deciding nurses' employment conditions.[37] She continued:

> [Nurses] have a tendency to regard [themselves] as a special group ... this is perhaps not a good thing. We have much to gain, and nothing to lose, by comparison with other groups of workers ... If we give up the right to strike

or are deprived of it, it means we have lost our greatest weapon … it is highly possible that employers may make use of this fact, knowing that however many times they may refuse reasonable demands … the nurses will carry on with their work.[38]

In 1964, the INO, along with a number of other professional associations and trade unions, decided to take part in a newly proposed conciliation and arbitration scheme for local authority officers. The change in the organisation's tune owed to an assurance that any improvements secured for members employed by the state would also be applicable to members working in voluntary hospitals. The INO had five representatives on the staff panel of the scheme, to which it submitted two claims for conciliation: one was successful in its entirety and the other, following disagreement, went to arbitration. In February 1965, the INO accepted the arbitration award and correctly heralded it as historic; the award represented a significant salary increase and brought members' salaries from £465–£600 per year in 1961 to £525–£750 per year in 1965.[39] Other challenges remained. The *Employment and Conditions of Work of Nurses Report* recommended a 40-hour week.[40] It was not within the remit of conciliation and arbitration to address working hours, and the organisation continued to lobby local authorities and the Minister for Health in this regard. The INO achieved a partial victory when Donogh O'Malley, Minister for Health, issued a circular to health authorities recommending the introduction of an 85-hour fortnight by January 1967.[41] O'Malley even agreed to sanction the employment of any extra nurses that the introduction of a shorter working week would necessitate.

The organisation's successes were finally beginning to stack up: an allowance for night duty, a significant salary increase, a reduction in members' working week and, in 1969, an allowance for nurses working in specialist areas such as intensive care. Why the sudden change in fortunes? At the time, the United Kingdom lacked over 7,500 nurses and midwives, and the USA had a shortage of almost ten times that figure – in spite of better working conditions in those countries.[42] The INO's *Irish Nurses' Magazine* carried the story of three Irish nurses who accepted jobs in Texas, USA in 1963. The nurses were met on their arrival at the airport and given bouquets, honorary citizenship of the state and a police escort to their workplace.[43] Another emigrant penned an article that same year, having settled in Boston, Massachusetts. She described good promotional prospects, a 36-hour working week, fully funded opportunities to pursue bachelor's and master's degrees and last, but by no means least, the freedom to wear her hair in any style she chose.[44] In contrast, the addition of chicken to the nurses' Sunday dinners at Baltinglass District Hospital, County

Wicklow, was a sufficiently significant development to warrant mention (and an exclamation mark) in the *Irish Nurses' Magazine*.[45] If Ireland was not to experience, again, its own shortage of nurses, then further improvements in conditions were clearly necessary.

II. The Pension Campaign Concludes

Although more and more voluntary hospitals were adopting the Federated Superannuation Scheme for Nurses, the INO remained concerned with the lack of pension reciprocity between voluntary and state-administered hospitals. This hindered nurse mobility, and Ena Meehan wrote to the Hospitals' Commission in 1962, noting that 'local authorities do not recognise permanent service given in voluntary hospitals, for the purposes of salary increments [or] pension rights'.[46] The Department of Health wrote to the INO in 1964 indicating that a Special Committee on Superannuation had been established to investigate the matter further. The INO made representation to this committee and, drawing on research published by the Economic Research Institute, and adding a hefty dose of persuasion, directed the committee's attention to the fact that nursing

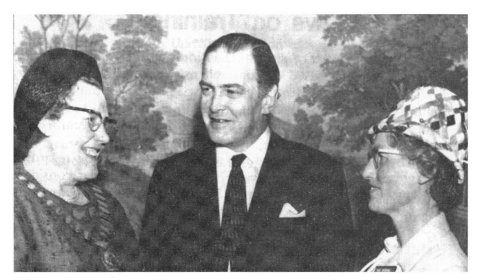

Minister for Health Donogh O'Malley with INO President Maureen McCabe (left) and General Secretary Ena Meehan (right) in 1966. McCabe was a tutor at Dublin's Coombe Hospital and, to this day the Maureen McCabe lecture is delivered in her memory on International Day of the Midwife at the hospital. Digital content created, published and reproduced courtesy of Digital Library, UCD.

was largely a profession for single women and that 'loneliness' among single people was an 'increasingly grave social problem' in later life.[47] The INO continued that older singletons' 'known vulnerability to illness cannot but be a source of anxiety which is further emphasised by a lack of security about their future'.[48] The ploy was somewhat successful. Donogh O'Malley took an acute interest in the long-standing issue of providing an adequate nurses' pension scheme. Addressing public health nurses in 1965, he remarked:

> The time is past when nurses can be treated differently ... according to whether they are providing health services in the employment of a local authority or of a voluntary agency ... When I get [the *Report of the Special Committee on Superannuation*], if there is any delay in introducing a scheme, it will not be for lack of will on my part.[49]

Shortly after making these remarks, O'Malley was assigned to the government's Education portfolio and a new Minister for Health, Seán Flanagan, was appointed. Nurses inundated the INO's headquarters with letters of commiseration: such was the measure of the esteem in which they had held O'Malley. The sentiments expressed in a satirical commentary piece in the *Irish Times* came very close to the mark. Its author, writing under the pen name 'Backbencher', pondered who would be most 'disconcerted' by O'Malley's sudden transfer: 'The weeping nurses' went the conclusion.[50] Progress on establishing a satisfactory pension scheme suddenly stalled, and INO members' fears over the cabinet reshuffle were being realised. A petition containing 4,000 nurse signatories was sent to Flanagan in 1968, imploring him to establish a reciprocal pension scheme without further delay. Help was to come the INO's way from a touted overhaul of how the health services operated. Plans to rationalise the health services, in particular to prevent their duplication and to ensure concord between state-run and voluntary institutions, accelerated in the 1960s with the seminal 1966 White Paper *The Health Services and their Further Development*, which recommended closer coordination between state-run and voluntary services and the replacement of the existing twenty-seven local Health Authorities with a smaller number of Health Boards.[51]

The White Paper also suggested that the central exchequer, and not local rates, should fund the ever-increasing cost of the service.[52] Further plans to rationalise the health services continued in 1968. That year, eighteen prominent doctors, comprising a consultative council charged with recommending changes to the system of hospital organisation, delivered their *Outline of the Future Hospital System: Report of the Consultative Council on the General*

Hospital Services to the Minister for Health.[53] The report, often referred to as the *Fitzgerald Report*, concerned itself with the rationalisation and standardisation of the health services and recommended that every nursing post should be pensionable and that employment conditions in the profession should be standardised.[54] The recommendations resonated and, shortly afterwards, the INO received correspondence from the Department of Health in which a new pension scheme for the staff of voluntary hospitals was touted. The scheme became operational in January 1969, and virtually all voluntary hospitals subscribed to it. The proposed scheme incorporated reciprocity between state-operated and voluntary services, meaning that INO members could transfer their employment between different employers without interruptions to their pensions. The pension saga had finally come to an end.

III. Professional and Educational Issues Assume Greater Significance

The nursing reformation that commenced in the 1800s is widely attributed to two developments: the selection of middle-class women of 'good character' for entry to nurse training and the establishment of systematic schemes of nurse training within hospitals. Trainees, known as probationers (sometimes called pros), endured dire working conditions, and prospective nurses were chosen partly on account of whether or not they were envisaged to be able to cope with the onerous workload. One application form for a position as a probationer inquired: 'Are you strong and well?'[55] One-time General Secretary of the INO, Eleanor Grogan, penned a poem in which she reminisced about her time as a probationer. Its title, 'The Pro's Lament', left little to the imagination: 'Tell me not in penny numbers, Nursing is a lovely dream! I am dead for want of slumbers, Things are harder than they seem. Doctors, Matrons, Sisters, Patients, Though my heart is strong and brave, With their trying ways will drive me very shortly to my grave.'[56]

Marie Mortished, for the INU, protested at the conditions endured by probationers in 1919, which included working for: '14 hours a day, seven days a week, learning her profession by the exhausting practice of it, as well as by attending lectures, and also doing in very many cases an enormous amount of emptying pans, polishing brasses, scrubbing, and other sheer manual labour [whilst] frequently subjected to ... intolerable bullying.'[57] Mortished's concerns were warranted, but the fledgling union's concern at probationers' plight was fleeting, as very few were members of the union in its early days – possibly owing to matronly disapproval. The move away from trade unionism and the evolution of the INU into the INO in the late 1930s brought with it a greater focus on educational issues.

III.I. Pre-Registration Apprenticeship Nurse Training

Pre-registration apprenticeship nurse training entailed working on hospital wards as paid employees and, at the same time, fitting in lectures at one's hospital or at a centralised training school between, before or after shifts or on one's days off. This resulted in constant conflict between the probationer's role as an employee and her role as a trainee. The 1940s witnessed an important modification to the system of apprenticeship nurse training with the introduction of preliminary training schools to some hospitals. These schools provided a number of weeks of dedicated instruction to probationers before they commenced work on hospital wards. They also helped to ameliorate the conflict between the trainee's dual role as labourer and learner. It was at this time that the term 'student nurse' entered parlance. Preliminary training schools were badly needed, as some students were clearly unprepared for the tasks that awaited them. One student, Anna Hennigan, who trained at Cork's North Infirmary in the late 1950s, recalled:

> We were put into wards the first day we arrived with our uniform, suddenly we were called nurse [but with] no experience whatsoever ... I remember being put into the boys' ward [and] there was ten boys in the ward and one of them said to me 'Could I have a bottle please nurse?' ... I said 'A bottle of what?' ... 'Ha, ha, ha, she doesn't know what the bottle means' ... I reddened up to the two ears and soon learned, of course, what the bottle was.[58]

The INO lobbied that all nurse apprentices should commence their training with a three- to four-month period in a preliminary training school studying anatomy and physiology, hygiene, nursing theory and practice and science and ethics. The organisation eventually got its way and such schools became a requirement in all schools of nursing in Ireland by 1960.

In 1955, the World Health Organisation convened a study group that recommended the establishment of an experimental school of nursing in each country. Each school was to provide education to nursing students, where the focus was on learning as opposed to labour. One such school was established in Glasgow, Scotland in 1956. A theoretical syllabus was taught in years one and two alongside ward-based work that was specially chosen for its educational

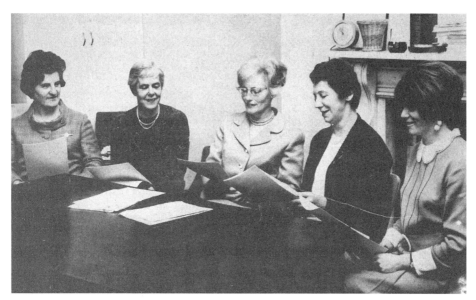

The INO's staff at the organisation's headquarters in 1969. From left: J. Osborne, Regional Organiser; M. Brophy, Information Officer; Ena Meehan, General Secretary; M. Watson, Assistant Secretary and T. Brangan, Receptionist. Courtesy INMO.

merit; a third year of clinical practice preceded the granting of registration.[59] The INO took great interest in the development and lobbied An Bord Altranais to establish an experimental school of nursing, in the form of a university-based school of nursing, in Ireland. The results of the Scottish experiment brought precisely what the INO desired and understood by 'student status' into closer focus and laid the basis for much of the organisation's educational endeavours for the next thirty years. A lecture delivered by Margaret Lamb, Education Officer at the RCN, to INO members in 1963 was unambiguous, and she remarked that advances in medicine and surgery demanded increased technical understanding by nurses. Nonetheless, the students that undertook the Scottish experiment were dissatisfied and complained: 'You couldn't possibly … learn how to *do* things in the school' [emphasis added].[60]

The Scottish students' experience pointed to an enduring tension between nursing as a practical pursuit versus nursing as a theoretical pursuit. The criticism of the course resulted in Lamb revising her opinion that full student status was desirable for trainee nurses, and she reverted to a view that protected study time within an apprenticeship style model was superior, provided '*we do not sacrifice* [the student] *to the needs of the wards*' [original emphasis].[61] The INO seemingly took its lead from Lamb and, thereafter, turned its attention to optimising the living and learning experience of student nurses within the existing apprenticeship model. There are a number of reasons why the organisation adopted this less radical stance. Firstly, some nurse educators in Ireland in the 1960s prized the practical bent of apprenticeship nurse training: 'Graduates of a degree programme in nursing would not be good *practical* nurses' [emphasis added].[62] Commentary in the *Sunday Independent* in 1969 also rubbished any suggestions of university education for nurses and advanced a practical as opposed to theoretical view of nursing: 'A university degree, after all, is a poor substitute for a needed drink or a cool hand on a hot brow.'[63] Secondly, many of the INO's Executive Council were also senior nurse managers who were possibly averse to the staffing difficulties that dismantling the apprenticeship model would incur; after all, student nurses were an indispensable part of the nursing workforce. Last, and by no means least, the apprenticeship model was a cheap form of labour.

Improvements in student nurse education were dependant on increasing the number and educational preparation of nurse teachers, known as tutor sisters. In Ireland, some tutors did not have any formal teaching qualification and such a course of study was only available in Britain. When An Bord Altranais established its first course for tutor sisters at University College Dublin in 1960, the INO awarded a scholarship of £25 to members who

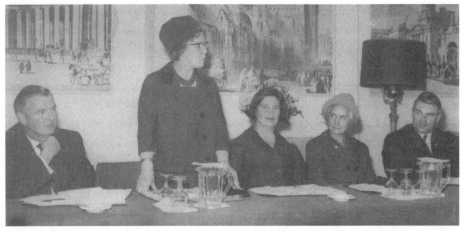

A meeting of the INO's Nurse Tutors' Section in 1965. From left: Dr N Reilly of the Irish Medical Association; B.N. Fawkes of the General Nursing Council for England and Wales; T. Barrett of St Laurence's Hospital, Dublin, and Chair of the Section; A. Young, Matron of St Kevin's Hospital, Dublin, and E. Hannon, Longford County Secretary. Courtesy INMO.

undertook it. Lobbying by the INO was also responsible for the establishment of refresher courses for tutors two years later. The advent of the tutors' course was followed by the establishment of a Tutors' Section within the INO in 1961. This vocal, energetic and well organised sector led the organisation's drive to effect improvements in nurse education from that point on. Yet, some of the most effective catalysts to change came from unexpected sources.

III.II. A Wake-Up Call

In autumn 1965, four student nurses at Galway Regional Hospital were reportedly asked to resign for failing to attend a house examination which, as a result, they were adjudged as having failed.[64] In a vivid illustration of the conflict between student nurses' dual role as labourer and learner, it was claimed that the students had finished night duty, retired to bed and did not hear a call for them to rise at midday in order to take the exam.[65] Ordinarily, student nurses were a fairly acquiescent bunch. Many had secured a training place through an opaque and inequitable system that smacked of 'pull' wherein, it was who you knew, not what you knew that dictated your success at interview. Many students possibly felt obliged not to rock the boat as a result. Students were also browbeaten by a multitude of rules and regulations as well as an ever-present system of surveillance of both their working and personal lives. Nevertheless, and continuing the trend of slowly evolving militancy witnessed in the conciliation and arbitration campaign, 200 of the Galway students' colleagues protested to local politicians, complaining about 'how unfair it is to expect nurses to sit for an examination after spending twelve hours on night duty'.[66]

The INO attempted to intervene and argued that the students had never been given any official written notification that the quality of their work was in question or that failure in a house examination would result in dismissal which, the organisation maintained, was custom and practice for civil servants.[67] The organisation also advised the students not to sign resignation letters and they were discharged from their posts on 1 October 1965 following a disciplinary meeting.[68] A request by the INO to attend the meeting was reportedly ignored. The Galway Trades Council, which represented thousands of trade union members in the region, then became involved and requested that Donogh O'Malley, with all his known sympathies toward nurses, investigate. Three days after the students were discharged, O'Malley addressed nurses at an INO refresher course in Dublin: 'In some hospitals there is authoritarian approach towards the nurse, and personal disciplines are imposed which would not be tolerated by workers in other fields. Change in hospital nursing practices and attitudes is [*sic*] sometimes not considered, because time has made them sacrosanct. Let me say firmly I am against sacred cows.'[69] O'Malley's utterance was not merely more of the same rhetoric that characterised politicians' remarks on nurses' working conditions.

Within weeks of the incident, O'Malley had visited Galway Regional Hospital and issued a diktat regarding student nurse training: that a block system be introduced; that student nurses' hours be reduced to ninety per fortnight; that split shifts and night duty be minimised; that the ratio of students nurses to nurse tutors be 30:1; that petty restrictions on students' freedom be lifted and that periods of night duty not be scheduled within one month of a student sitting an examination.[70] These stipulations mirrored many of the recommendations that the INO had made to the Minister during the drafting of the White Paper, *The Health Services and their Further Development*, in 1966. Once again, external forces were playing a role in the INO's success. O'Malley also dismantled what was known as 'fourth year'. Many nurses who completed their three-year training period were expected to provide a further year of service to their training institution. During this year, nurses were not paid the salary of a registered nurse to which they were entitled. Rather, they were paid little more than a third-year student: 'You gave the year to the hospital and you got £5 a month ... Talk about cheap labour' recounted one nurse.[71] Nurses that declined to undertake fourth year were not given their hospital training badge – a coveted asset. Lenore Mrkwicka, who resigned from her training hospital during her fourth year, recalled:

> I didn't get this lovely badge until about twelve years later I was working in a hospital and I was looking after a patient whose relative was a nun from the same community that I had trained in and [we] got chatting and [she asked] 'Why aren't you wearing your badge?' I said, 'I didn't get it because ...' So I had it a week later ... Now when it is shined up it looks great – the Jervis Street Hospital badge.[72]

The INO disagreed with fourth year and, up until events in Galway, argued, without success, that it be abolished in order to permit newly qualified nurses to gain experience in diverse clinical areas in other institutions.

The enthusiasm to bring about change to student nurse education can partly be explained by a need to reconsider old approaches. The 1960s brought about a slowly expanding range of professional and educational opportunities for women. If nursing was to remain a popular career option, then this necessitated lifting some of the petty pinpricks that training entailed. Developments in Galway were just the beginning. The *Fitzgerald Report* suggested a possible future need for nurses to undertake training in hospitals with at least 300 beds in order to gain a greater range of clinical experience.[73] This recommendation mirrored a view long-held by the INO. In 1925, Kathleen Nora Price for the INU, gave evidence to the Commission on the Relief of the Poor and Insane and suggested that some hospitals persisted in training nurses in spite of not being able to offer them a comprehensive clinical experience.[74]

The INO was, however, concerned that the imposition of a bed quota on training hospitals may result in the closure of some schools of nursing attached to smaller hospitals. The organisation successfully argued that schools work together in order to increase their available bed complement to at least 300; the interchange of students from smaller to larger institutions, known as transfer schemes, was underway by 1971. There was a particular impetus behind this campaign, as 1968 witnessed criticism and concerns that students who trained in Irish hospitals with less than 300 beds would no longer be eligible to register as nurses in Britain. One nurse wrote a letter to the *Irish Independent*, noting: 'If I go to Britain I shall have to do a further training of six months before I can register … We have been all used obviously as just a pair of cheap useful hands, with no thought to our future career … May I appeal to the students and their parents to demand some action now [?]'[75]

As the 1960s drew to a close, the INO established a working party on nurse education and passed a number of key resolutions at its 1967 Annual Meeting. The organisation noted the 'general dissatisfaction' regarding pre-registration nurse training and urged An Bord Altranais to address a number of issues: adequate staffing at training schools in order to ensure an optimal ratio of tutors to students, adequate numbers of qualified nurse tutors, the provision of the best available library and lecture room facilities and regular inspection of schools and hospitals in order to optimise students' theoretical and clinical experience.[76] The frequency with which the INO made the same or similar requests to An Bord Altranais underscores the slow pace of progress in the area of nurse education. It also highlighted what would become a sometimes strained and fractious relationship between both bodies that would simmer for the time being but would, at a future date, boil over.

III.III. Post-Registration Education

The INO's endeavours and successes in the field of post-registration education eclipsed those of its endeavours on behalf of would-be nurses. The organisation's

THE PATIENT

By Frances Condell

ILLNESS is a calamity which strikes all of us at some time or another and which e q u a t e s us at the common denominator as patients. Hospitals, to you, may be an home from home, or the environment in which you choose to work; while an hospital to me is a place I frequent only as a visitor, os as a voluntary social worker or, more often than not, as a place of refuge from pain.

Illness usually comes as a shock to the normally healthy and, unless it be of a dangerous type, the sick person tries to cope with it himself; or, perhaps, his family or friends help him until the responsibility becomes too great and then—usually days later and at a late hour at night !—he G.P. is called in and if, upon consultation, conditions no longer lend themselves to home care, the hospital takes over. That is one way of becoming a patient.

Another person may have a complaint for which he has already been treated at home or in hospital, then ignoring or distorting to his own likes and whims the doctor's instructions, his acute condition gradually becomes chronic. Invariably, such a patient ends up paying calls at frequent intervals at the doctor's consulting rooms, or he attends at a Dispensary or at an Out Patients' Department for "the bit of a note" which enables him to acquire medications or drugs. Finally, of course, the time comes when he, too, ends up in hospital—but before he gets that far, let us try to see his position as it may appear to him.

From my own experience in dealing with sufferers of this, that and the other complaint in the social welfare field, if a person has a complaint, no matter how chronic, a visit to the doctor is based on apprehension. He may be an old-stager at the game, like myself; nevertheless, the fear is there. The fear, for instance, that a common complaint, or one to which he has become accustomed, has now reached an alarming extent, or is at the stage of becoming a potential danger.

I know that you doctors are very busy people. I know that you have your exasperations; but, please, try to put yourselves in our place and be patient with your patients.

Whether you like the elevation or not, or whether you bask in the pleasure of it, however unadmitted, every grateful patient has a secret idolatry of his doctor. How distressing, therefore, is for any patient to discover that the faith he has had in his doctor's concern for him is somewhat shaken by being rushed through a consultation, given the "bit of a note" for medicines, a pat on the back and led to the door with the rapidity of an usherette showing a late-comer or patron to his seat in a crowded cinema or theatre; or quietly, but firmly dismissed with : **"Ah, you'll be all right. Repeat the tablets and come back in a month !"** . . .

You in your busy lives may not realise that a visit to the doctor is a very important happening in the day of a patient. You may not realise that the day, however repetitive, may be the one red-letter day in a dreary month for a despairing, troubled and chronic patient. A visit, no doubt, which that patient will recall and discuss at length with anyone who will listen to him. What you

say to that patient may be magnified beyond all your diagnostic or prognostic capabilities. In fact, that patient could become your best—or your worst !—public relations officer. It's up to you.

Occasionally, of course, if you fail to diagnose what a patient thinks you should diagnose and which he may hope or expect you to diagnose (provided it's not too serious), especially if he is a bit of a malingerer, his disappointment may cause him to state quite openly in company that, as a doctor, you are no so-and-so good. He may refer to you disparagingly as: **"That fellow ! I know more about medicine myself than that 'quack' !"** . . .

Generally speaking, however, most patients to-day are intelligently capable of probing a doctor's diagnosis, due perhaps to the availability of a better educational system than in my young days and to the communication media and public discussions and, perhaps, the reading of a certain digest of information.

Patients, on the whole, like to be treated as intelligent beings, capable of understanding the implications of a treatment and what is being done to their bodies in that treatment.

The apprehensiveness of patients scheduled for surgery, for instance, cannot be exaggerated. Most of us are terrified of the experience which is so commonplace to the hospital team concerned that their familiarity with, initially, even the pre-surgery procedure, may cloud their understanding of the patient's fears. Unless we patients are spoken to as intelligent adults and told otherwise, we, on the beds, can visualise that the area of skin being prepared will conform to the area to be cut open by the largest and sharpest scalpels possible. The mere rattle of the drums on the trolley is nothing to the fearful pounding hearts of those prone on the beds !! We may recall films of a surgical team surrounding an inert form on the operating table, plus the silent tension of dramatisation programmed for our entertainment or interest, and so familiar to us now on television. Such a medium of communication re-suggests itself to the mind of a patient scheduled for surgery, so can you really blame him if the drama which he has witnessed on the screen so many times suggests to his apprehensive mind, now that he is the one "for the table", that he will be the one whose body will be opened up, that he will be the one whose innards will be probed and that, maybe, each of you green-gowned, booted and masked "terrorists" will "have a go", once you have him semi-drugged and hijacked from his hospital bed where he was surrounded by understanding allies in pain and discomfort. He visualises himself, perhaps, waking up, untimely, in the middle of all the probing and stitching, an island of suffering in the sea of his own blood ! Yes,

You In The Know could well laugh at his fears—but fears there are, nevertheless, in your strange world of having to cause pain in order to ensure recovery.

Matter-of-fact attitudes by hospital staffs to patients can be reassuring to some but downright terrifying to others and especially, strangely enough, during the ordinary procedure and non-medical formalities of admission to hospital.

May I stress that a simple understanding and kindness which recognises a patient's individuality at this time greatly relieves his feeling of inadequacy and so reduces the impersonal and unintentional bureaucratic element which all of us can develop in our everyday work through familiarity and practice. All of us patients complain at some time or another of the lack of privacy and of the long waiting to be picked out of the "assembly" line in a doctor's consulting room, or in the Out Patients' Department. We may crib at the incessant form-filling and not understand that details of our personal and medical history are essential for hospital records and all because their importance is not explained to us, however briefly—and how we hate to be regarded as mere ciphers or numbers in the compiling of those records !! . . .

Proficiency at one's job, in or out of hospital, is an essential in these times; but if proficiency is bounded only by the carrying out of the immediate requirements of a job, to the exclusion of the human element and human feelings, especially in an area involving possible undesirable human reactions to such super-efficiency, then it is high time for all of us to have a good hard look at its limited boundaries of the overall effect

What I personally expect from such desirable co-operation and co-ordination is progression and not regression. I feel, too, that it must be so easy for you of the medical profession to become the prisoners of your own legend. Legends may have gone out with the beloved Fairy Tales of my own youth; nevertheless, tread softly, because you tread on my dreams . . .

To my way of thinking, a "physically-minded" doctor (for want of a better term) can be very off-putting to a patient. He may have the reputation amongst his colleagues of having no time at all for any of this reassuring and necessary "psychological nonsense". Such a doctor is usually described by us patients as being "very abrupt", and indeed in other terms not so complimentary. He may be accused of not permitting the patient to "tell him anything"—you know the type of comment and reaction by the patient, like : "I couldn5t get a word in edgeways, even to tell him what was wrong with me !" . . .

I say "accused", for this type of comment is an accusation and is not conducive to the relief of anxiety. I may be wrong, but I feel that disregard for the feelings, apprehensions, actual fears and fantasies—within reason, of course—of a patient can aggravate physical conditions and, often, indeed, distort the whole physical picture. Unfortunately, too, this attitude is "catching", especially with very young, impressionable and ambitious young colleagues on the medical team, and has contributed more to the term—however undeserved !—!of **"The Medical Mafia"** than anything else I know.

With all due respects to the doctors, those who typify hospital care are the nurses. They are the nearest, constantly, to the patient and they, above all others, can prevent the hospital service from becoming too impersonal. Therefore, it is very encouraging that our student nurses' curriculum now includes courses in psychology, sociology and allied areas of knowledge added to terms of work in psychiatric hospitals, thus giving them a greater insight into patient involvement.

The present trend in encouraging nurses, upon qualification, to "stream" into administration or teaching in hospitals may cause some of us to cry out in the future: "Where have all our nurses gone ?". However, I think that most of us would agree that any professional in any profession should feel free to "stream" God-given talents. Nevertheless, for all our sakes, it is desirable that those who opt for hospital nursing, as we know it, be given the opportunity and the **time** to **nurse** their patients without having their work schedules cluttered up with ancillary jobs, however necessary, that could well be done by non-professionals.

Of course I am aware that nurses have a daily routine to fulfil. I am aware that wards must be kept tidy and as spotlessly clean as possible and that we "mummified" patients in our horizontal tombstones of beds are expected not to let the nurses down until the daily "Processionals" are over—but all of us patients are not in plaster ! We like to move our lower limbs if we can and to lift the weight of restrictive bed-clothes without fear of reprimand! Also, we like the doors or apertures of our lockers to be facing us at a convenient get-at-able angle, and not positioned where, admittedly, they look better, as if they were on display in a furniture stores. We like to have our waste-paper bins within comfortable reach and not placed over in a far corner, just because they have always been kept there ! We hate being left sitting enthroned on a bed-pan, just because the poor nurse is run off her feet or is called away to perform another duty before she has the time to remember our predicament ! I remember receiving Holy Communion one morning so enthroned ! Never was the prayer : **"Remember me, O Lord, in the hour of my adversity"**, so fervently uttered . . .

We female patients hate having to ring the bell when some sudden upset or call of nature catches us unawares and, if regarded as ambulatory, have to dash for the bath-room or toilet, barefooted and conscious of our "see-through" nighties, like a half-hearted Godiva, and all because our slippers and dressing-gowns must be—and repeat **must be** !—kept in that press in the far corner of the ward and not readily accessible to our beds where they should be !

Thank you for listening and, in conclusion, may I ask you of the medical and nursing world to remember that we patients depend our lives on you; that we admire and are grateful for your dedication in looking after our bodies—but, in your care of us, please do not forget that with every body goes a mind and feelings, fears and apprehensions and, in order to equate us as human beings on your planet, do remember that most of us have the power of hearing, and speech and eyes to see and that we are not beings apart or merely pieces of anatomy held together by the rigid sides of an hospital bed. I ask you to remember, too, that the long night is very long indeed when one is suffering and that the early morning welcome sleep is often more beneficial to us, as patients, than being roused to be washed and to have our temperatures taken at some very early hour, or to be fed with a breakfast which we cannot see, at times, because we, like you of the medical world, are exhausted from our efforts to get well and to aid our own recovery—and which, after all, is your whole aim in life, too, isn't it ? . . .

(Above is text of address given at IMA Conference in Killarney, April, 1972).

An insightful article by Frances Condell that appeared in the *World of Irish Nursing* in 1972 and detailed the travails of patients in the healthcare system. Courtesy INMO. With thanks to Jeff Condell.

refresher courses for midwives and nurses, the only such courses in the country, had been in operation since 1928 and 1938, respectively. The esteem in which the organisation's educational remit was held can be judged by the fact that, in 1948, the Department of Health requested that the INO organise a course of training for public health nurses. But a change to the power brokers in nursing education was looming. Minister for Health, Noël Browne, addressed the Senate in 1949 and indicated some of the changes that the touted *Nurses Act* of 1950 was to incur. Browne made provision for An Bord Altranais to arrange post-registration courses for nurses, such as public health nurses. The act also stipulated that An Bord Altranais could provide nurses with scholarships and with accommodation when attending courses.[77] Part of the INO's utility lay in its educational remit, and education was a conduit to membership of the INO. Any change to this arrangement posed a threat to the organisation's raison d'être, and the INO redoubled its efforts at effecting change in post-registration education thereafter.

The INO remained especially keen to establish university links to post-registration education and prized the comprehensive and varied theoretical instruction that such an education could offer. The move toward a more liberal education was one that was emerging from the USA at the time, but it was not long before the organisation's requests were tempered. The continual refusal of universities to establish post-registration courses resulted in the INO setting its sights on a college of nursing. Such an institution would deliver lectures, circumventing the lack of resources cited by the universities, but a university would issue diplomas to nurse graduates. Correspondence from Ena Meehan to An Bord Altranais in the late 1960s shows that the INO viewed the college as an interim measure until such time that a university faculty of nursing was established.[78] It was esteem and standing that endeared some nurses to university education: 'Such a scheme is a definite step forward in raising the status of the nurse' said one correspondent to the INO.[79] Nurses' standing, as a result of some of the tasks they were expected to do, was indeed questionable. Kathleen Craughwell recalls what was expected of students at the Galway Regional Hospital, where she trained, in the 1960s:

> The sister on the medical floor ... always brought a student nurse around [who] had to turn the patients' heads away so they wouldn't breathe on the doctor [and] there was another ward sister ... [who] used to get us to cut the corners off the soap for [a particular consultant] ...and if we were giving him a towel we had to hold it a certain way, a bit like a server at Mass.[80]

Craughwell also recalls that, even when she became a ward sister, one particular doctor anticipated that she would take charge of having a clean white coat laundered for him each day, until she set him straight on the matter.[81] It is little wonder that some newspapers posted advertisements for 'nurses and maids' under the same heading – a phenomenon that resulted in an incandescent Eleanor Grogan, for the INO, penning a letter to the Rathdown Board of Assistance in 1951 in which she stressed that nurses were professionals, in a separate category to maids.[82]

For all of the talk, the term 'status' was applied inconsistently and arbitrarily: for some it referred to prestige, for others it was the route to better financial reward. The term was most often understood by the INO in a relational manner, and the organisation's efforts to effect university education waxed and waned in line with developments in other occupations. The organisation's efforts to establish a college of nursing intensified in 1969 when it was touted that primary school teachers were to be awarded university-accredited degrees through the national teacher training colleges. Status aside, university education was necessary, as ongoing advances in medicine necessitated corollary advances in nursing. Nursing had always been an exacting profession that required great skill. Community Jubilee nurses, for instance, needed to be well versed in emergency tracheotomies in order to treat the large number of children who succumbed to diphtheria in Ireland up to the 1930s.[83] Treatment modalities continued to change apace mid-century. A case study published in the *Irish Nurses' Magazine* in 1958 described the meticulous nursing techniques employed at St Finbarr's Hospital, Cork, to cool an anaesthetised patient to 31°C in an ice bath prior to open-heart surgery for repair of an atrial septal defect.[84] The range of new treatment options at the time was bewildering to some, and one onlooker in 1963 recalled:

> I went into a hospital the other day and could not find anybody in the ward, but there were screens around a bed, and when I put my head around the screen I realised that everybody in the ward was at work on a patient; on the floor … I went back to see Sister and I said to her 'what on earth is going on there?' 'Oh,' she said, 'that man had just died and you know you are not allowed to die now if you are under eighty … [we do] this famous "kiss of life" and you have just got to get this man living again.' I said 'Well Sister, when I come in to you, will you please let me die in peace [?]'[85]

Nurses noted some of the tests they carried out on hospital wards in the 1960s: supine and standing blood pressure readings, glucose tolerance tests and

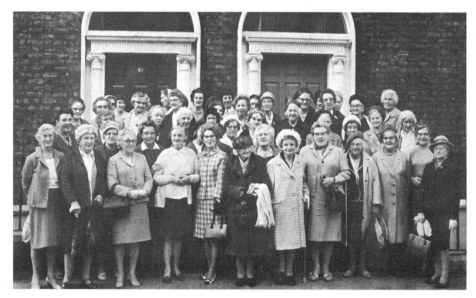

Members of the INO's Retired Members' Section gather at the organisation's headquarters in preparation for a day trip in 1969. Courtesy INMO.

phlebotomies. This contrasted sharply with the range of tests they performed some years earlier, when urinalysis was reportedly 'the sum total'.[86] Midwives also undertook novel roles, such as the administration of intravenous injections for the first time in the 1960s.[87] The lack of post-registration education options rendered INO members poorly prepared to meet the demands of the evolving clinical arena, as Ellen Broe, Director of the Florence Nightingale International Foundation, pointed out to assembled nurses in Dublin in 1955: 'The complexity in duties, which nurses in later years have had to undertake, has been rather frustrating … I do not think that any other profession has tried to do so many tasks for which they were not prepared, as nurses.'[88]

More specialist areas were also emerging. The INO foretold this and soon incorporated specialist components into its refresher courses. Subsequent refresher courses for nurses incorporated visits to specialised institutions and clinical areas including paediatrics, dermatology, oncology, geriatrics and mental health and, for midwives, incorporated specialised teaching in institutional and domiciliary midwifery at the three Dublin maternity hospitals. The growth in specialisation was also evident in the organisation's periodical. The Sister at the Intensive Care Unit of St Laurence's Hospital, Dublin contributed an illuminating piece to the *Irish Nurse* in 1967 related to intensive care nursing.[89] Members attending the INO's refresher course in 1967 received a lecture on enteral and parenteral feeding and care of patients with tracheostomies.[90]

Another specialist area that the INO concerned itself with was that of nurse management. The 1960s saw the establishment of a working group to investigate and make recommendations on senior nurse staffing in Britain. The group's report, the *Report of the Committee on Senior Nursing Staff Structures*, more commonly referred to as the *Salmon Report*, was published in 1966 and recommended an increase in the number of managerial strata in nursing.[91] Any similar recommendation remained a long way off in Ireland, where managerial positions were grossly underdeveloped: some institutions employed no ward sisters at all, necessitating nurses to 'act-up' without extra remuneration. In 1961, at the County Hospital, Bantry, County Cork, the only ward sister post was that of theatre sister. The INO inquired as to when the hospital intended to fill its other ward sister vacancies but received 'no definite assurance' from the institution.[92]

The *Salmon Report* provided reason for optimism if nothing more, and the INO took notice. The organisation incorporated lectures on management and administration as part of the syllabus for its refresher course from 1960 onwards. A Ward Sisters' Section was formed within the INO in 1961, and the new section made progress by initiating classes in management at the Catholic Workers' College, Dublin in 1962.[93] INO General Secretary, Ena Meehan, wrote to the Minister for Health and to An Bord Altranais in 1968 and requested that a qualification in administration be obligatory for all ward sisters and that, in the absence of courses in administration for nurses in Ireland, that prospective ward sisters be seconded to take such courses in Britain.[94] The organisation had some success, and An Bord Altranais established a course in administration for ward sisters in 1970.[95]

IV. The Nurse Wants to Nurse

The INO received a letter from the Engine Drivers' Union in 1937, complaining that the boiler-man at the National Hospital for Children, Dublin had been laid-off and that a nurse now attended to boiler maintenance tasks when necessary. The organisation's Executive responded that they did not approve of nurses attending to boilers and assured the engine drivers that the nurse in question was not a member of the INO.[96] The incident laid bare the vast and dubious range of roles and responsibilities that were expected of nurses, and the trend showed no signs of abating. In the 1960s, student nurses were expected to make surgical caps and masks on sewing machines when assigned

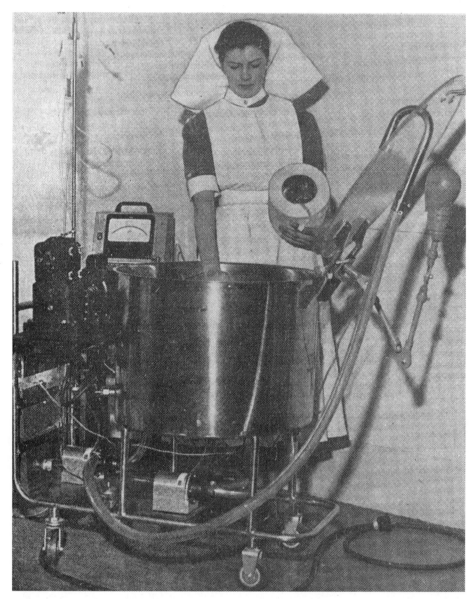

Nurse M. Fagan with the new artificial kidney at the Charitable Infirmary, Jervis Street, Dublin, in 1958. Digital content created, published and reproduced courtesy of Digital Library, UCD.

to their hospital's operating theatre,[97] and registered nurses were assigned to their hospital's catering department when the need arose.[98] The volume of clerical work was also cumbersome and much lamented by the INO. Whilst garment-making, catering and clerical duties could all be linked to patient care at some level, however tenuously, it was more difficult to consider other duties under the nursing rubric: revelations that nurses were expected to take care of the Matron's pet parrot, not to mention the patients, at a particular Dublin hospital exemplified the extent of the issue.[99] Attempts to delimit the nurse's role were stymied by the lack of clarity in defining that role. One definition described nursing as:

> An art and a science which involves the *whole* patient, – body, mind and spirit; promotes his spiritual, mental and physical health ... stresses health education and health preservation as well as ministration to the sick; involves the care of the patient's total environment – social and spiritual as well as physical; and gives health service to the family and the community as well as to the individual [original emphasis].[100]

To make matters worse, the ILO found that some nurses were not in receipt of an employment contract detailing their conditions of service.[101] The nursing role was, by contract and in practice, vague, sprawling and growing.

The INO harboured concerns over the limits of nurses' responsibilities for many years; after all, it was a member's refusal to compile lists of patients' belongings that resulted in the organisation's first withdrawal of labour in 1920. But it was amid increasing activity at ward level (owing to developments such as early patient ambulation) and the evolving global nursing shortage that renewed debate emerged about what exactly constituted nursing practice. Sheila Quinn, Director of the Economic and Social Welfare Division of the ICN, addressed the INO's Annual Council meeting in 1962: 'The profession should decide upon the proper function of the professional nurse. Is she doing what we want her to do? If not, are we quite sure what it is that we want her to do?'[102] Quinn continued 'the nurse wants to *nurse*, and not to spend time in unnecessary duties which take her away from the patient' [original emphasis].[103] Quinn's sentiments were echoed in the everyday lives of nurses in Ireland. Kathleen Craughwell again recalls her days as a student nurse: 'We were treated as domestics for the first year. We washed window sills, we cleaned windows, we washed skirting boards and at that time each of the wards had a day room with a fire place so we used to have to wash the fire place [too]'.[104] How was the situation to be remedied?

Ireland was somewhat unique in not employing auxiliary personnel. This militated against nurses' efforts to relinquish routine duties, as had been done elsewhere. In April 1966, Miss Conway, Assistant Matron at Belfast

City Hospital, indicated that the employment of auxiliary personnel at that institution was going some way toward absolving nurses of non-nursing duties.[105] The INO requested that auxiliary personnel be introduced on a national basis but with a number of stipulations: that candidates be carefully selected, that they be trained and that their duties be circumscribed to exclude nursing duties.[106] The organisation was involved in a delicate balancing act as, if lesser paid auxiliaries were to assume nursing duties, they might one day supplant registered nurses altogether. The INO lauded the Dublin Health Authority for employing trained auxiliary personnel in 1966, but progress on the establishment of a national auxiliary grade was protracted.

This resulted in the INO issuing a protest to the Minister for Health on the matter in 1967. Although the Minister announced a planned pilot project in the creation of the grade of Ward Assistant at the County Hospital, Letterkenny, County Donegal, the following year, and although the proposed scheme met the INO's demands, it was not replicated nationally. Local arrangements regarding the employment of support staff continued. The INO employed economic arguments in an effort to effect the introduction of auxiliary staff. It argued that nurses' time and the state's finances were being 'squandered on duties that could be performed by a less highly skilled person'.[107] The organisation was correct with regard to the squandering of nurses' time, but its concerns regarding the waste of state-monies were less so. As long as the apprentice model of nurse training existed, there was little impetus for the state to establish an auxiliary grade because trainee nurses were doing multiple nursing and non-nursing duties at a fraction of the cost of support personnel.

Furthermore, the trend toward multifunctional grades, as seen in the case of public health nurses in the 1950s, was one that the state encouraged. This flew in the face of the increasing demarcation of roles and responsibilities that the INO sought. Debate regarding the introduction of auxiliary staff was closely aligned with debate regarding the introduction of the State Enrolled Nurse (SEN) grade in Ireland. Enrolled nurses had their genesis in the nursing shortage that emerged in Britain following the Second World War. The grade was similar to that of a nursing auxiliary, and the focus of training was practical, with on-the-job assessments instead of written examinations. The INO's Matrons' Section urged formal recognition of the Enrolled Nurse grade in Ireland in 1969, but the Matrons' Section's enthusiasm was tempered by a number of INO Branch Secretaries who feared that enrolled nurses may one day replace registered nurses, as was allegedly happening in some parts of Britain.[108] They also feared that the grade may exert a depressant effect on salaries. An extraordinary General Meeting of the INO was held at the Montrose Hotel, Dublin in January 1970 and considered the topic.

The organisation's Matrons' Section put forward a motion calling on An Bord Altranais to establish a syllabus and training centres for such a grade but, the motion was defeated. Thereafter, the INO formally opposed any further attempts to introduce the grade. Matrons' keenness at establishing the Enrolled Nurse grade suggests that they were swayed by the necessities of staffing their institutions. Opposition by rank-and-file members was not likely down to protectionism alone; the proposed advent of the Enrolled Nurse grade came as the organisation was struggling to further nurses' professional legitimacy; a new occupational grade with a shorter training period, no written assessment and yet retaining the title 'nurse' stood to injure its endeavours. But did nurses and midwives have the right to lay claim to professional status?

V. Professional Status

The *Midwives* and *Nurses Acts* of 1918 and 1919, respectively, increased midwives' and nurses' professional standing, but their professional status was fragile. The *Local Government Act* of 1941 expressly stated that registration/certification as a nurse/midwife was not tantamount to professional status.[109] The INO's actions belied its own insecurities in its members' standing. As the 1961 *Nurses Act* was being drafted, the INO lobbied the Minister for Health to incorporate an amendment to the 1950 *Nurses Act* that would make explicit nurses' professional status, i.e., a reference to the 'profession of nursing' and not merely 'nursing'.[110] The Minister declined and noted that nurses' professional status 'has long been recognised'.[111]

Definitions as to what constituted professional status changed with time. An article in the *American Journal of Nursing* in 1959 referred to a number of determinants of professional status.[112] The piece suggested that professionals were driven by a service-obligation and not by 'personal gain'.[113] If this was the sole criterion of professional status, nurses went a long way toward measuring up. Indeed, while the *Nurses Act* of 1950 was still at the bill stage, one commentator, Dr Barniville, went as far as to suggest that student nurses should work for free – this being the conduit to becoming 'a professional woman'.[114] Yet nurses did not meet many of the other criteria referred to. For instance, professionals attended institutes of higher education and had a unique body of knowledge. Florence Nightingale envisaged nursing as a distinct profession and maintained that nurses were not merely 'ancillary doctors'; rather, they had their own unique role, much of which concerned the maintenance of good hygiene and sanitation: 'nursing and medicine ... must never be mixed up'.[115]

In spite of the Nightingale ideal, in practice, there was a broad cross-pollination between nursing and medical knowledge. A glance at the speakers at the organisation's first refresher course for midwives at the Rotunda Hospital, Dublin in 1928 shows that the vast majority of lectures were delivered by doctors. The same was true of the INO's refresher courses for nurses, with just three of the twenty-two lectures, in Mercer's Hospital, Dublin in 1939, delivered by nurses.[116] Considering that university courses for nurse tutors were only established in Ireland in 1960, the teaching of nurses and midwives by doctors continued for some time to come. Engagement in research was also a determinant of professional status. Sheila Quinn, in her address to INO members in 1962, noted that nursing knowledge was more the product of 'tradition and authority' than it was the product of critical scientific inquiry.[117]

The INO took note and, that same year, invited Kay Lynch of Belfast City Hospital to address a seminar titled 'Research into the Work We Do'. Shortly after, in 1966, on the fiftieth anniversary of the 1916 Rising, the INO collaborated in the establishment of the Elizabeth O'Farrell Foundation Committee. O'Farrell had once been an active member of the INU, and it was fitting that Ena Meehan acted as Honorary Secretary of the Committee, which aimed to fund nursing and midwifery research and post-graduate education.[118] But in spite of the organisation's best efforts, a research basis for many nursing/midwifery practices was slow to take-off, as Anne Cody, who trained as a nurse in the early 1970s, recalled: 'We did [things] because it was always done that way. We took temperatures in the morning, we took them in the afternoon, we took them in the evening, nobody knew why until somebody started doing research ... A lot of it was ritualistic and you never asked a question.'[119] Their exclusion from university, their lack of a distinct body of knowledge and the lack of research activity meant that nurses' and midwives' professional standing was questionable if judged in relation to the determinants of professional status that were in vogue at the time. This hampered INO members achieving, in greater measure, another of the determinants of professional status: financial security.

The 1960s was a time to take stock of how far the INO had come. The twenty pioneering visionaries that had founded the organisation in a one-room office could scarcely have guessed that it would grow to become Ireland's most authoritative voice on nursing and midwifery matters, with a membership of

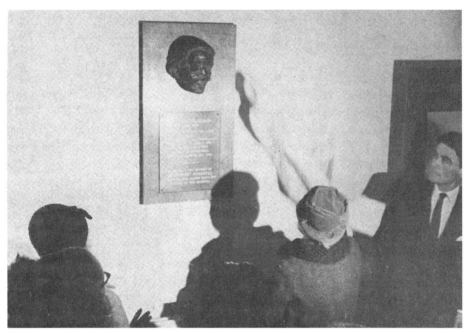

Unveiling a plaque to the memory of midwife Elizabeth O'Farrell at the National Maternity Hospital, Dublin, in 1967. The plaque still stands in the hospital's main foyer. Courtesy INMO.

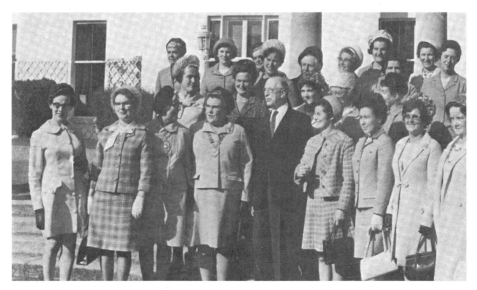

Golden Jubilee: members of the INO's Executive Council and staff meeting President of Ireland Éamon de Valera, at Áras an Uachtaráin on the occasion of the organisation's fiftieth birthday in September 1969. Courtesy INMO.

almost 4,000 by the end of the decade.[120] This was a cause for commemoration and, as the INO turned fifty, it marked the occasion with some fanfare. A fetching souvenir booklet was published and a Golden Jubilee mass was celebrated in St Andrew's Church, Westland Row, Dublin on 8 September 1969. A number of members embarked on a coach outing to County Wicklow and others took a cruise on the River Shannon. The organisation's personnel were also received by Éamon de Valera, the President of Ireland. Margrethe Kruse, President of the ICN, made an address to INO members in the auditorium of Dublin's Mater Hospital on 10 September, entitled 'The Next Fifty Years'. Kruse pined for a crystal ball to help her with her task and told assembled members how 'many unknown factors' made it difficult to predict the future.[121] One such factor, the second wave of the women's movement, was about to make its presence felt. Even a crystal ball could not have predicted the indelible mark that it would leave behind.

CHAPTER 8

Marriage, Money and (Moderate) Militancy, 1970–7

R eaders of the *World of Irish Nursing* in the early 1970s were bemused to find a photograph of an all-female, all-nurse rugby team among its pages. The nurses, who worked at St Vincent's Hospital, Dublin were photographed having just lost a charity match. Their opponents, also pictured, were consultants at the same hospital, and a piece beside the picture read: 'Women's Lib. suffered a marginal defeat [when] the consultants won 14-12.'[1] If taken in the light-hearted manner in which it was intended, the piece was a humorous one. On a more serious note, 'women's lib' was suffering far more than just a marginal defeat in Irish society. In 1971, over fifty years after the first public meeting of the INU in Dublin's Mansion House, some 1,000 women again assembled at the same venue on Dawson Street. On this occasion, women did not convene to debate the merits of a nurses'/midwives' trade union. A flyer circulated at the meeting made their intentions clear: 'Equal rights for Irish women – do you think it's just that for every 26p a women earns a male counterpart gets 47; do you think it's just that the civil service and state sponsored bodies … sack

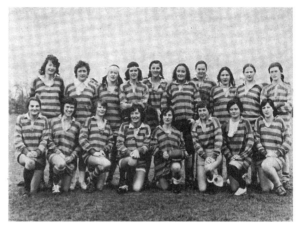

NURSES

RUGBY

Right, the vanquished, front row, from left : Geraldine Walsh, Angie Gilligan, Deirdre Reddin, Ann Meagher, Geraldine Deasy, Joanie Reddin, Flossie Ryan and Ronnie Owens. Back row, from left : Mary Byrne, Monica McGlew, Liz Clear, Marie Duffy, Esme McCann, Anne Murray, Captain, Marie Walsh, Sheila O'Beirne, Pat Fogarty and Marie Hearne.

Courtesy the *Irish Medical Times.*

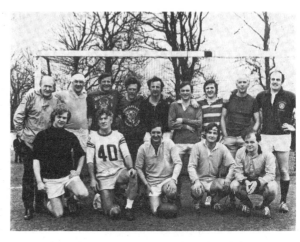

THE VICTORS

Women's Lib. suffered a marginal defeat when the nurses of St. Vincent's Hospital were defeated by the consultants in a rugby match at University College, Belfield recently. The consultants won 14-12 in the charity match which was in aid of a Dublin Welfare Centre. From left, front row : Dr. John Fitzpatrick; Prof. Don Hengarty, Mr. T. W. Keveny, Dr. Don Buckley, Dr. R. De Vere-White. Back row(from left : Dr. John Fleetwood, referee, Mr. Joe Cahill, Dr. D. Maher, Mr. Neil Galvin, Dr. Bhil Quinlan, Dr. Liam Byrne, Dr. D. Megihan, Mr. F. Fonovan and Dr. C. Ryan.

By courtesy of Irish Medical Times

Find out why they are all smiling .... on page76.

Courtesy the *Irish Medical Times.*

women upon marriage [?].'[2] The second wave of the Irish women's movement was under way.

I. The INO and the Women's Movement

The INO was comprised mainly of the fairer sex – indeed, its periodical was geared specifically toward them: Bronwyn Conroy, a beautician, wrote a regular column for the *Irish Nurse* on the topic of 'beauty culture'. Conroy noted: 'It is essential for a girl to cultivate everything that is 100 per cent. Feminine – good dress sense – make-up and hairstyle perfect.'[3] A subsequent article inquired: 'Have you by any chance looked in the mirror … and decided that you are not exactly thrilled with your reflection? … Have your skirts suddenly become a little too tight … These are all, in themselves, fatal signs that you are putting on weight.'[4] Aware that its constituents were, in the main, women, the INO was also aware of the gendered nature of the work that they carried out.

Caring was firmly rooted in womanhood, and the connection was one that was reinforced in the organisation's journal. An advertisement for a popular brand of baby formula appeared in the *Irish Nurse* in 1966 and pondered: 'Quite why fathers, who are normally sensible, competent men, should be reduced to a state of complete incompetence when faced with the necessity of making baby's feed is difficult to explain … But they'll have no difficulty in making S-M-A … *Yes, even fathers can make, and feed, S-M-A!'* [emphasis added][5] Yet the consequence of the gendered nature of nursing and midwifery work, in particular the view that such work was women's work and, therefore,

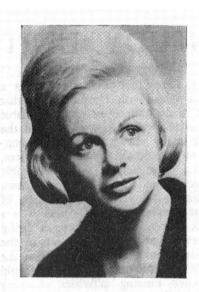

Bronwyn Conroy to write for IRISH NURSE!

Miss Bronwyn Conroy, Chief Consultant Revlon International Corporation, Television Beauty Consultant and Manicure Specialist.

We are pleased to announce that we have just concluded arrangements with Miss Bronwyn Conroy, the well-known beauty consultant, for an exclusive series of articles on beauty culture which will, we believe, be of particular interest to all readers of this journal. The first of Bronwyn's articles will appear in our November issue.

BOOK FOR EVERY ISSUE NOW!

not remunerated appropriately, did not seem to be in the organisation's consciousness. It took the second wave of the women's movement to raise the INO's awareness that its members' employment conditions were a manifestation of women's inequitable employment conditions in general. But this had not always been the case.

The INU derived valuable support from organisations such as Louie Bennett's Irish Women's Reform League in its infancy. It appears that some of the INU's early leaders were also imbued with greater aspirations for women than those that generally existed at the time. Fanny Ungerland, mother of the first General Secretary of the INU, Marie Mortished, failed to see why women should be restricted by prevailing gendered norms and left her German family to take up a position as a governess in Scotland. Ungerland may have inculcated Marie with a similar philosophy. Mortished became chairwoman of the Irish Housewives' Association (IHA) in 1947, over twenty

Look your best — 3

with

Bronwyn Conroy

HAVE you by any chance looked in the mirror during the last few weeks (just as I have done) and decided that you are not exactly thrilled with your reflection? During the long winter months when the weather is cold and you are definitely feeling miserable, naturally you tend to eat more of the fattening type of foods. Consequently, your figure, face and general appearance suffer as a result. Finally, when the weather becomes a little brighter and you have more time to take a good look at yourself you may find that "things aint what they used to be!"

Well, if you want to do something about it do join me in a four month plan for a more beautiful you. Should you decide this is not for you because, perhaps, you consider yourself plain-looking, put that idea right out of your head. Admittedly, despite what all the advertisements say, not every women can be beautiful, but all women can be attractive. That is a much better word. It is the key to a completely happy disposition. Don't think that this plan is going to take up lots of your time and energy. It is not, because not for one minute do I overestimate the length of time nurses and business girls have to spare for beauty routine and diets. If you decide to think of the potentials that lie within your reach rather than imagine the drawbacks you possess, you will be on the right road to success. This is the first initial step you will have to take completely unaided.

I suggest you begin by taking a really good look at yourself standing in front of a full length mirror. Try to look at yourself as somebody else would . First of all consider your hair. Does the colour suit you? Does the style suit you? If not, make a note to do something about it. Also, what about your skin? Are you wearing make-up? If so, does it look well? Are your nails long and elegant; or are they broken and your hands badly cared for? Now for your figure. Have a really good look at this, too, bearing in mind that you are not exactly thinking of entering for the next 'Miss World' Contest. Have your skirts suddenly become a little too tight around the waist? Don't just blame the cleaners. Have you suddenly decided that dark colours are definitely more suited to you than others? These are all, in themselves, fatal signs that you are putting on weight.

If this penetrating look in the mirror has depressed you a little, don't worry unduly. You are, after all, only starting out on your four-month trip to beauty, so take a notebook and pencil and mark down all the things that you consider need improving. First of all weigh yourself, then take your measurements, exactly what they are—not what you would like them to be. Now let us consider your 'diet', that dreadful word. However, this is something that must be faced. Remember, your ideal weight is the one at which you feel best and look your best. If your increase in weight is due to the fact that you very often eat between meals —you must stop this habit. Eating quickly is a very easily acquired habit and one I am sure that nurses very often are obliged to indulge in. This often causes overweight simply because you are inclined to eat more.

If by any chance your mirror shows no excess weight but, instead, salt-cellar collar bones, with arms and legs that are much too thin, then you have a different problem to deal with. You will have to put on weight and this as actually much more difficult than losing it. In this case there is, however, the joy of not having to watch what you eat and being able to indule in all of the fattening foods most people have to avoid. Incidentally, it is a good idea to have a medical check-up if you consider yourself overweight.

During your four months' course you should consistently take half a desertspoonful of lemon juice in half a glass of luke-warm water as a 'before breakfast pick-me-up'. This will help your complexion as well as your figure. Try to have three well balanced meals per day, cutting down on the high calorie foods such as bread, potatoes, cakes and pastries, sweets, chocolates, tinned fruits and, of course, alcohol.

Don't say after reading this list of 'musts' that life is no longer worth living! It really will be, when you look in the mirror in four month's time and see the transformation that has taken place.

With thanks to Bronwyn Conroy. Digital content created, published and reproduced courtesy of Digital Library, UCD.

years after she left the INU.[6] The IHA was a feminist organisation that aimed to 'unite housewives, so that they may realise, and get recognition for, their right to play an active part in all spheres of planning for the community'.[7] Similar to her concerns for nurses and midwives, Mortished's concerns for housewives were also of a material nature, and prior to relocating to Hollywood, she remarked: 'We are all housewives doing the daily round … Some of us may have ambitions and real talent for other things but – perish the thought. Can I stretch the butter until Friday?'[8]

Some years after Mortished resigned as General Secretary, the INU, while in the process of transitioning to the INO, broke ties with its parent, the IWWU. The IWWU wrote to the INU and remarked that it had 'misunderstood' its status, which was that of a 'woman's organisation permanently attached to the I.W.W.U.'[9] The correspondence demonstrated an important distinction between both entities: the IWWU was a women's organisation, the aim of which was to 'improve the pay and conditions of Irish women workers'.[10] The INU, and more especially the emerging INO, was a nurses' and midwives' organisation, the aim of which was to improve nurses' and midwives' conditions, but the membership of which just happened to be women. There was little explicit acknowledgement by the INO that its members endured substandard

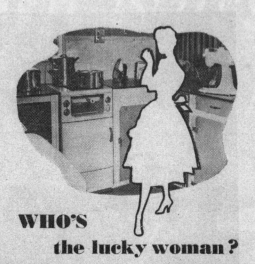

WHO'S the lucky woman?

And she is, indeed, a lucky woman, because she is admiring the new electric cooker which will make such a difference to her kitchen and her purse. From now on all her meals will be perfectly cooked and her kitchen will look smart and up-to-date. She'll have more time to spare, too, because her new electric cooker has two wonderful high speed hotplates to quicken her cooking. She has a family of five and from now on her cooking will cost less than 4s. 6d. a week by electricity. If your cooking costs you more, it will pay you to follow her example and switch over to electricity.

A new three-plate electric cooker complete with thermostatically controlled oven and two high-speed hotplates can be yours for only £1 12s. 7d. every two months. If you wish, installation charges may be spread over five years.

E.S.B. SHOWROOMS

Listen to Maura Laverty, famous cookery expert, author and playwright, from Radio Eireann every Tuesday at 2.15 p.m.

'A woman's place …': the old adage was reproduced time and again in the INO's journal. With thanks to © ESB Archives, esbarchives.ie, MK/PA/6/92. Digital content created, published and reproduced courtesy of Digital Library, UCD.

conditions because they were women, and there was little evidence that the INO espoused an active desire to change the position of women in society. Rather, the organisation's primary aim was to change the working conditions of nurses and midwives. The INO's core concern was labourism not feminism.

This began to change in the early 1970s. An article appeared in the *Sunday Independent*, following the precedent set when INO representatives became the first all-female team of negotiators at the Labour Court in 1972. The article declared: 'Although the [negotiators] are not Lib members they point out that they are all for Women's Lib. The reason, says Miss [Ena] Meehan, is that the majority of our members are women and this has affected their situation.'[11] In spite of its new-found feminist consciousness, progress proved to be protracted and problematic, not least because of some nurses' and midwives' ambivalence toward emerging redefinitions of women's roles.

I.I. The Marriage Bar

Many Irish women resigned from employment of their own volition after marriage, but from the 1920s onwards, the obligatory retirement of women was instituted with the advent of a marriage bar. The bar coalesced with other inequalities such as the tendency to alter a woman's employment status from permanent to temporary should she get married. By 1946, just 2.5 per cent of married women were categorised as employees.[12] The situation in nursing was not radically different. In 1936, just 5 per cent of female (working) nurses were married, and in the years 1946, 1951, 1961 and 1966, the number of female married nurses was 5 per cent, 8 per cent, 8 per cent and 9 per cent, respectively.[13] Of course it is a wonder that nurses got the opportunity to marry at all considering that their love lives were subject to the same surveillance that characterised their working lives. One student nurse recounted her predicament when a young male patient arrived at her room in the nurses' home in order to wish her well with an upcoming examination: 'I had to hide him in the wardrobe. I would have been excommunicated if they had seen him.'[14] Another, who failed to cover her tracks quite so well, was summoned to the Matron's office and lost her days off for striking up a relationship with a former patient:

> I got friendly with this guy in the male surgical ward, a very, very nice guy ... and I said: 'How would you like to go to [the hospital's annual] dress dance?' And he said: 'yes, sure'... The guys had to come to the nurses' home [before the dance] ... and the doorbell would ring and the Matron would answer the

doorbell and she would bring the guy into the room … and she could come in and say, 'Nurse so and so, whoever is here.' And [when] it came to me … she came in and she said, 'Nurse … bed number thirteen St Joseph's Ward, I will see you in the morning.'[15]

For better, for worse; for richer, for poorer; in sickness and in health, marriage and nursing were somewhat of an odd couple: mutually exclusive yet strangely synonymous too. In 1970, the INO's *Irish Nurses' Journal* published the names of members who had got engaged or married: 'Cupid [was] very busy' at the County Hospital, Bantry, County Cork, where seven nurses got engaged or married in a two-month period in 1970.[16] Additionally, in the popular Mills and Boon series of books, hospitals were sometimes the background or the setting for 'romantic drama' for nurse protagonists, and the profession was portrayed as a route to marriage.[17] The prospect of romance was also a subtle but recurring feature of nurse recruitment advertisements. In one advertisement for positions at the University Hospital of Wales, carried in the *Irish Nurses' Journal*, the accompanying picture was that of a demure woman, presumably a nurse, stepping off a train into the arms of a dapper man.[18]

In another advertisement for posts in a range of hospitals in New York City, the picture depicted a nurse walking arm in arm with a prospective suitor, both of whom were gazing into each other's eyes. The caption read: 'His name is Bob…we've been dating three months.'[19] There was even a financial incentive for those who married. In 1943, Wicklow County Council awarded a bonus of 5 shillings per week to married midwives and 3 shillings, 6 pence to single midwives. The incentive was not enough for one midwife, who quipped: 'Personally I would not take a husband on myself for the extra 1/6.'[20] In 1970, one nurse, so frustrated that she was planning to emigrate to Canada, commented: 'The big temptation to come into nursing used to be the marriage gratuity after five years. I've been qualified five years, but I have no man to marry. I'm penniless and nearly frigid.'[21]

Some married nurses, depending on whether they worked in state-run or voluntary institutions, did return to work following marriage, but they were entitled only to temporary positions and were paid at the minimum point of the salary scale, indefinitely. Over time, in response to the shortage of nurses, some employers, such as those in County Cork, relaxed their rules about non-payment of increments to temporary married nurses and, in spite of having to recommence employment at the bottom of the pay scale, began to pay them salary increments. The INO sought to capitalise on this and to have a national agreement on incremental credit implemented. The organisation wrote to the

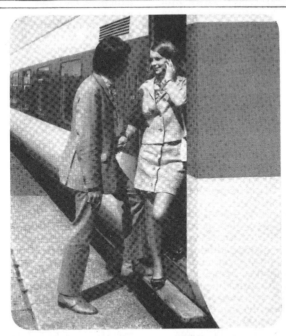

QUALIFIED NURSES
Come home to Wales!

THE NEW UNIVERSITY HOSPITAL OF WALES NEEDS YOU
Forget the trouble and expense of travelling home
—come and work in ideal conditions, with every
facility for modern nursing plus wonderful leisure
and recreational opportunities in the newest and
most superbly equipped hospital in Europe !

S.R.N's & S.E.N's
Write now to Matron: THE UNIVERSITY
HOSPITAL OF WALES
Heath Park, Cardiff CF4 4XW
Interviews to be arranged in Republic of Ireland

With thanks to University Hospital of Wales/Cardiff and Vale Health Trust. Digital
content created, published and reproduced courtesy of Digital Library, UCD.

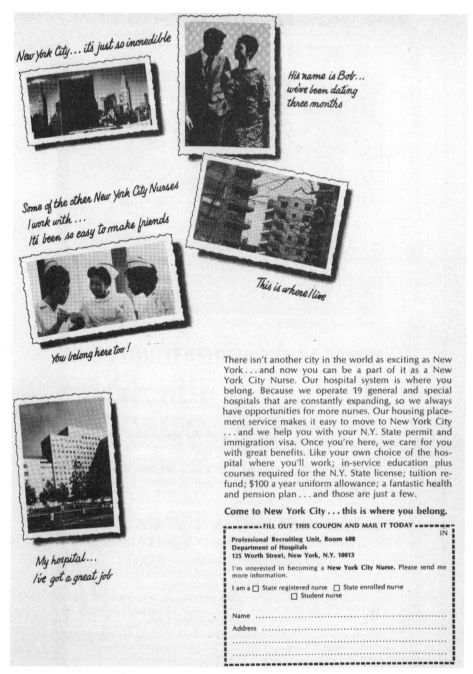

New York City... it's just so incredible

His name is Bob...
we've been dating
three months

Some of the other New York City Nurses
I work with ...
It's been so easy to make friends

This is where I live

You belong here too!

My hospital...
I've got a great job

There isn't another city in the world as exciting as New York... and now you can be a part of it as a New York City Nurse. Our hospital system is where you belong. Because we operate 19 general and special hospitals that are constantly expanding, so we always have opportunities for more nurses. Our housing placement service makes it easy to move to New York City ... and we help you with your N.Y. State permit and immigration visa. Once you're here, we care for you with great benefits. Like your own choice of the hospital where you'll work; in-service education plus courses required for the N.Y. State license; tuition refund; $100 a year uniform allowance; a fantastic health and pension plan... and those are just a few.

Come to New York City ... this is where you belong.

■■■■■■■■FILL OUT THIS COUPON AND MAIL IT TODAY ■■■■■■■■

IN

Professional Recruiting Unit, Room 608
Department of Hospitals
125 Worth Street, New York, N.Y. 10013

I'm interested in becoming a **New York City Nurse.** Please send me more information.

I am a ☐ State registered nurse   ☐ State enrolled nurse
                        ☐ Student nurse

Name ....

Address ....

....

....

With thanks to New York City Health and Hospitals. Digital content created, published and reproduced courtesy of Digital Library, UCD.

County and City Managers' Association, requesting that 'salary increments for married nurses in continuous temporary employment be allowed on a national basis'.[22] The Minister for Health acceded to the organisation's request by late 1969, and married nurses, although re-entering employment at the minimum increment of the salary scale, received increments similar to their unmarried counterparts thereafter.[23] This was another of the somewhat qualified successes that had become characteristic of the INO. The marriage bar in teaching was removed in 1958, largely due to a shortage of teachers in primary schools.[24] Considering the nursing shortage, the concession possibly owed as much to necessity as it did to equity or progressiveness on behalf of the state.

However, much work remained to be done. Incremental salary increases were in the bag, but those who returned to work following marriage were entitled only to temporary positions. This was soon to change. The Irish Housewives' Association, in conjunction with a number of other bodies, including the INO, formed the Committee on Women's Rights in 1968 and lobbied for the establishment of a Commission on the Status of Women. The campaign was successful, and a commission was established in 1970 that sought to recommend how women could participate on equal terms with men in Irish society.[25] The commission's 1972 *Report of the Commission on the Status of Women* was the most significant document to date affecting the rights of women in Ireland and recommended several measures aimed at eradicating sexual discrimination. The report recommended the abolition of the marriage bar, and its authors continued that they 'see no reason' why a woman's employment status should be altered from permanent to temporary following marriage.[26] One nurse who invariably endorsed this recommendation was Noreen Muldoon. Muldoon trained as a nurse in Birmingham, England in the late 1960s. She got married, became pregnant and returned to live and work in Ireland in the early 1970s. As a married woman, she was accorded temporary employment status on her return and, following the birth of her first child, she encountered difficulties getting rehired. She recalled:

> All I wanted to do was to go back to work … It was the actual status of employment that really bothered me … I ended up with no work, and I wasn't alone … It was a very, very difficult time and I found it extremely traumatic myself as a young mother and a young woman to think that we as women were treated so differently to single people or married men.[27]

The INO appears to have shared Muldoon's sentiments and, at its Annual General Meeting in 1971, one of the resolutions adopted endorsed the provision of permanent positions for married nurses.[28] However, it seems that this position ran contrary to the prevailing view among many members at the time, which suggested that they took issue with the provision of permanent posts for married nurses and midwives. Why was this so? The marriage bar created a labour throughput that favoured the employment and promotional prospects of younger nurses, and any changes to this discriminatory arrangement, including the provision of permanent posts to married nurses, caused 'considerable unease' among some members.[29] Dan Spring, a Labour Party politician, appeared incredulous in 1971 when he recounted how he could not secure a position for a singleton at a hospital in Kerry: 'Single nurses cannot get jobs because of the married women.'[30] Sensing members' ambivalence, the INO's Executive put it to a referendum of members. In all, 4,000 INO members were balloted on whether they favoured the provision of permanent posts for married nurses. Some 1,775 returned ballot papers. Representing just over half of those voting, 912 members voted in favour of the resolution and 863 voted against.[31] Speaking at the organisation's Annual General Meeting in 1972, Erskine Childers, Tánaiste and Minister for Health, remarked that he was 'a little surprised' by the narrow majority of INO members who supported the abolition of the marriage bar,[32] and notwithstanding many INO members' misgivings, the marriage bar was abolished in late 1973.

For years, the decision rankled with some nurses and witnessed the 'over worked [*sic*] Nurses' of Temple Street Children's Hospital, Dublin writing to the Chief Executive Officer of An Bord Altranais as late as 1977 grumbling about the number of 'Grannies' and 'married women with "key posts" [at the hospital] while their husbands earn a fine salary, and so many trained nurses (Single) looking for work'.[33] The increase in the number of married members brought with it new challenges for the INO. The organisation made a detailed submission on job-sharing to the Department of Health in 1984, but the Minister for Health, Barry Desmond, harboured qualms that job-sharing would interrupt the continuity of patient care.[34] The organisation persisted and won a major success with the establishment of job-sharing posts in 1986. The development was sorely needed considering the prevalence of the 'second shift' phenomenon in women's working lives; by 1993, nurses accounted for two-thirds of job-sharers in the health service.[35]

I.II. Equal Pay

The tenth wage round came into effect in 1966, and all employees whose salaries were decided by conciliation and arbitration received salary increases.

In employment sectors that were open to men and women, each employee received an increase of £1 or 20 shillings per week. Where positions were only open to women, the salary increase was set at 15 shillings.[36] This trend was both long-standing and stubborn: in 1960, women workers received 53 per cent of the rates accorded to their male colleagues; in 1969, they received 54 per cent and, by 1971, they received 59 per cent.[37]

The first challenge the INO encountered in redressing the trend related to men or, more precisely, a lack thereof. Historically, where men adopted traditionally female roles, the perceived value of the role increased. This suggested that if more men entered nursing, salaries would rise. The INO does not appear to have recognised this, and in 1967 it asked: 'Do all nursing posts have to be thrown open to men in order to prove that the individual nurse's responsibilities and performance is of equal significance to that of a man?'[38] This implied opposition to men in nursing was not new. In 1932, 'Disgusted' wrote to the *Irish Nursing and Hospital World*: 'Can men find no other more suitable work than attending by the sick bed? Are they to attend women as well as men? The whole thing is too silly for words.'[39] Men could not train to be general nurses in Ireland at that time and, as a result, the number of male general nurses in the Saorstát numbered between just three and five.[40] Discrimination also meant that it took seismic events for men to be invited to join nurses' associations. Male nurses were invited to join the Irish Guild of Catholic Nurses in 1939, but the invitation was extended more out of necessity than desire. In a letter to the Archbishop, the Guild's Secretary, Ruth Nicolls, noted that men were invited to join because a male nurse had recently failed to alert a priest to the death of a patient in his charge. The nurse was seemingly bemused when asked to explain himself and replied: 'But the man was dead … what was the use of calling a Priest [?]'[41] By the end of the 1960s, just nine male general nurses were employed in local authority hospitals in Dublin.[42] In 1967, just three schools of nursing accepted men as student general nurses: St Finbarr's Hospital in Cork, the Mater Hospital in Dublin and the City and County Infirmary in Waterford.

The promise of change was to come from Europe. Ireland's accession to the European Economic Community (EEC) in 1973 made it incumbent on the state to introduce equal pay measures, and the government instituted the *Anti-Discrimination (Pay) Act* in 1974. In principle, the act provided for equal pay between men and women. In practice, things were more complex. The provisions of the act meant that men and women should be paid the same rate 'if both are employed on like work', but the lack of men in general nursing and midwifery made comparisons challenging.[43] This was not the case in

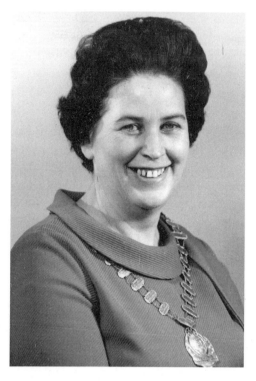

Maeve Keane: hailing from Co. Roscommon, Keane trained as a nurse at St Michael's Hospital, Dún Laoghaire, and later specialised in tuberculosis nursing and worked at St Kevin's Hospital, Dublin. She became a Ward Sister at James Connolly Memorial Hospital, Dublin, and was appointed as Assistant Matron of that institution in 1969. She later served as Matron of St Mary's Hospital, Phoenix Park, Dublin. She was President of the INO 1971–5 and 1979–81. Copyright Pat Sweeney Photography.

psychiatric nursing, where men were more plentiful and where equal pay was conceded and set for implementation in 1973. By contrast, the lack of men in general nursing and midwifery prompted INO President, Maeve Keane to rail: 'There are so few men in these services their existence is almost regarded as of no account.'[44] This, somewhat conveniently, gave the state the perfect excuse to drag its heels on the matter.

Women's socially ascribed roles as wives and mothers influenced the apathy of INO members in relation to the establishment of a pension scheme in the 1930s. In essence, nursing and midwifery were preludes to marriage, and there was little impetus for INO members to become involved in the long-term commitment that such a scheme necessitated. However, the abolition of the marriage bar represented the beginning of the demise of the male breadwinner model; this, in turn, refashioned nursing and midwifery into lifelong careers for women. Census returns for 1971, 1981 and 1986 reveal an ever-increasing number of married female nurses at work: 14 per cent, 35 per cent and 45 per cent, respectively.[45] As the number of married female nurses in the profession continued to rise, so too did their expectations for improved working conditions. They became less likely to acquiesce to substandard improvements in their employment conditions. A more vocal rank-and-file INO member began to emerge, compelling the organisation to redouble its efforts on their behalf.

WOMANS RIGHTS

Nuala Fennell

No debate or thesis on the subject of Woman's Rights if it were to be honest, would ignore the Woman's Liberation Movement. Not since the Suffragettes has their been such a female revolution. It all began when a group of discontented women burned their bras outside yet another presentation of that American national review, the Beauty Contest. We all know the repercussions to this, the women who did this unseemingly act were called shrews, harpies, lesbians, and the whole thing was written off as a dog-in-the-manger gesture by a group of females who never would qualify for a beauty contest in the first place.

Maybe now some years after we read those headlines most of us are a little more aware of why the women threw dignity to the wind and made their famous protest. Since then we have seen a radically changed situation in America. Women are seen to be active in politics, even being elected to high Government office; legislation has been passed to make it illegal to discriminate against women in job selection. That's America, and whether we like it or not it is the world laboratory. What is invented and tested there, eventually in some shape or form makes its appearance everywhere else.

But, American, German, English, Swedish or Chinese women are not Irishwomen, and their fight for equality as they see it in their own countries, would not be our fight for equality. Because the entire Women's Lib and attendant movements for female equality have in most cases made strong please for liberal abortion, contraception and divorce as a human right, we women in this country have tended to shy off the entire campaign as it has been publicised and have, if I may be so impertinent to suggest, preferred our totally unfair and discriminating system, to the alternative of getting involved with such radical sexual ideas. What a pity that our defenciveness about our moral standards has meant that we allowed the international trend for female equality to pass us by ? Why were we not able to handle it our way ? Why could we not have stated that as a nation we did not see abortion as an individual right to be enforced by law, or that we did not approve of easy divorce, while at the same time, continuing fiercely and relentlessly the fight for the deprived, deserted or mistreated wife, the need for contraception, equal pay, fair family law, and changed adoption legislation. All these areas affect our lives as women. We threw out the lot, and this country is a little the worse for it. Is it not strange then, that we have a tradition of women's organisations, clubs, society's all proudly boasting constitutions that are totally non-political. This is fact means that they will not operate in the political arena, no matter that the deserted wife has to live with one child on £6 a week. Meddling in that situation could be called political, so none of our often numerically powerful women's associations will get caught up in promoting justice for this woman. This is a luxury I think that we in Ireland just cannot afford.

At every vantage and on every level we should be pushing women toward the political field. We should be telling her that as a citizen it is her right to involve herself in active politics, instead of intimidating her and making her so uptight about politics that mostly she doesn't value her vote greater than her super-market checkout slip.

I would reject the idea of putting a woman into the post of President of Ireland, to be me it would be like putting icing on a particularly stale cake, and I would resist any suggestion that a woman should take this post until we have taken our place in every other area of public administration, the legal profession, national and local politics. Let me say emphatically that I am not anti-men. This is one of the areas where long ago I parted company with Women's Lib. Nothing can be achieved by entering into ideological conflict with men, and anyway it is unnecessary, as most men would support the justice of equality for women, and Women's Lib only anticipate antagonism by their attitudes.

The single greatest factor that I think has caused women to have accepted inferior status for so long is a lack of faith in their own abilities. We have been conditioned to believe that women couldn't do male jobs. Who ever heard 15 years ago of a woman judge, and now we have one, Justice Kennedy. Would our parents have approved of a female Cabinet Minister ? Or what would they have said about a woman Minister for Transport as capable as Barbara Castle ?

(The above is summary of address given by Miss Nuala Fennell, founder member of AIM at the February meeting of the Dublin Branch of the I.N.O.)

Summary of an insightful address given by Nuala Fennell to the INO's Dublin Branch in 1973. Pieces like these were indicative of a rising feminist consciousness within the organisation. With thanks to Garrett Fennell. Courtesy INMO.

II. 'Militant Mood': Frustration Reaches a Crescendo in 1970

Keen on gaining a salary increase and a 40-hour week, the INO entered the 1970s in a militant mood. Nurses in Britain had recently secured a salary increase through a publicity campaign, referred to as the 'Raise the Roof' campaign, organised by the Royal College of Nursing. The INO decided to emulate the college's campaign and to fund it with a 'Fighting Fund' it established.[46] Members contributed money to the fund and, in return, had their names mentioned in the organisation's periodical. The term 'Fighting

Fund' ultimately proved too inflammatory for some and, at the organisation's Annual General Meeting in 1977, a resolution to change the fund's name to the 'Action Fund', proposed by the INO's Meath branch, was adopted as a 'more appropriate' title.[47]

This was a critical time in the organisation's development. In the 1940s, the INO employed rhetoric in pursuit of its claims. In the 1960s, it rejected offers of salary increases, organised a protest meeting and sent petitions to employers. Now, in the 1970s, it threatened the 'token withdrawal' of services should its claims not be met.[48] Nurses employed by the Limerick Health Authority planned to boycott clerical duties should a raft of improvements in their conditions not be conceded.[49] Nurses in the INO's Athy/Baltinglass/Carlow branch, in the absence of a porter, refused to carry stretchers up the stairs at the Midwifery Unit of St Dympna's Hospital, County Carlow.[50] The INO also threatened the withdrawal of on-call nurses for ambulance duty in the District Hospital, Gorey, County Wexford, in 1972, as such nurses were not being paid an allowance for performing this duty.[51] (The necessity for nurses to leave their hospital wards to undertake ambulance duty, without replacement, was a recurring issue for the organisation and was brought into sharper focus following the bombings of Dublin City Centre, by paramilitaries, in the early 1970s.) These actions were radical for the INO and showed that members were slowly beginning to reappraise old approaches in pursuit of their goals.

The core of the INO's campaign was a series of nationwide protest marches. The first such march took place in Dublin on 25 February 1970, just three weeks after the establishment of the Commission on the Status of Women. Speaking in anticipation of the marches, INO President, Drogheda woman and Richmond and Coombe Hospital-trained Maureen McCabe remarked: 'I'm going to get myself a good pair of walking shoes.'[52] McCabe had her priorities right, as subsequent marches were held in Cork, Galway, Sligo, Waterford, Athlone, Kilkenny, Limerick and Dundalk. The marches were good-humoured affairs with a social element. One march held in Tralee, attended by the Rose of Tralee (a student nurse at Dublin's Mater Hospital), was followed by dinner at a local hotel and a cabaret with music provided by 'the ever popular Bunny Dalton'.[53] Yet the slogans on marchers' placards demanded action: 'We have been in labour long enough and need delivery now' went one, whilst another pondered 'What price a vocation [?]' A plethora of organisations supported the INO's protest march, and in Kerry, nurses were joined by the Kerry Medical Association, the Irish Countrywomen's Association and Macra na Feirme. The Estoria cinema cancelled a movie screening and allowed the INO to use its auditorium for a meeting in Galway. The Mayor of Galway, Fintan Coogan,

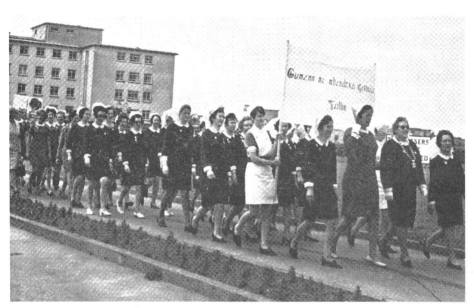

INO President Maureen McCabe leads the organisation's protest march in Galway in 1970. Also pictured are Áine Walsh, Maeve Keane and Mary Byrne, Chair of the INO's Galway Branch. Digital content created, published and reproduced courtesy of Digital Library, UCD.

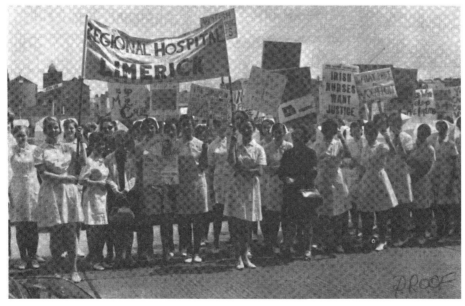

Protest marches spread to Limerick in 1970. Digital content created, published and reproduced courtesy of Digital Library, UCD.

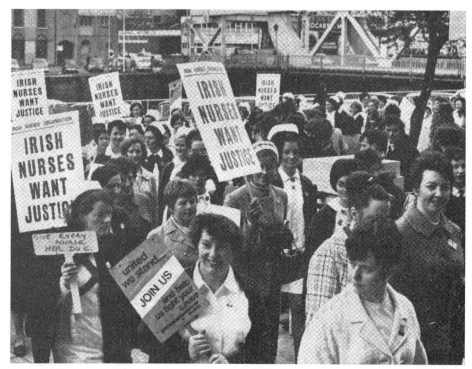

Protest marches spread to Cork where nurses marched to City Hall in order to meet with the Lord Mayor. Digital content created, published and reproduced courtesy of Digital Library, UCD.

was even ruled out of order when he produced a protest poster in support of nurses in Dáil Éireann.[54] It was clearly time for the state to make some concessions.

Tánaiste and Minister for Health Erskine Childers noted that he was 'unhappy' to see nurses marching and cited recent improvements in their conditions of employment, such as the establishment of an 85-hour fortnight and salary increases awarded under the wage rounds and conciliation and arbitration scheme.[55] Nonetheless, Childers acceded to the introduction of an 80-hour fortnight and, crucially, set a date for its implementation. This represented progress but was by no means a windfall. The Tánaiste was content to draw attention to salary increases gained under wage rounds but failed to mention that, in 1970, on foot of salary increases, the charges for nurses' rations and hospital accommodation were increased by 25 per cent. This rendered INO members' net 'pay rise' questionable, as hospitals effectively found a way to recoup their extra financial outlay; the rise in boarding costs at the National Maternity Hospital, Dublin resulted in midwives boycotting the hospital's dining hall.[56] In addition, Childers remarked how nurses' pay and conditions had not kept pace with their 'sisters in other occupations'.[57]

His choice of words provided a valuable insight into the state's mindset: nurses were women, and their salaries were to be benchmarked against the relatively diminutive salaries of other women, not men. A small but perceptive group of grassroots INO members were less than pleased with the outcome of the 1970 protest marches. The organisation's means and results were coming under increasing scrutiny, and a sense of disquiet was emerging. Some members were also reportedly leaving the organisation in favour of trade unions. The INO's modus operandi would soon face sustained questioning and criticism from both within and outside the organisation.

III. Digging its Heels in: Increasing Opposition to Trade Unionism and Striking

Maeve Keane, President of the INO, remarked in 1975: 'In conscience, a nurse is of the Florence Nightingale mentality she cannot forsake a patient in furtherance of any dispute.'[58] But Flo's reputation was laudable and lightning-rod alike and, at a protest march in Dublin, one nurse thundered: 'If we had Florence Nightingale here, we'd hang her. She's responsible for most of our bad conditions.'[59] Resolutions submitted to the organisation's Annual Meeting in 1974 by the INO's Meath and Clonmel branches, respectively, recommended that the INO affiliate to the ICTU and reconsider its no-strike policy.[60] Although neither of these resolutions were adopted, a change in attitude in relation to trade unionism and militancy among rank-and-file members was becoming apparent.

A key impetus in this change in attitude was external pressure. In 1969, an ITGWU official, Edmund Browne, launched an invective at the 'false prophets' who, out of 'stupid snobbery, have unsuccessfully masqueraded as unions for many years'.[61] Browne poured scorn on no-strike policies as a measure that 'utterly compromises' nurses' hands in bargaining and asserted his view that nurses 'have the same right to withdraw their services from their employers as any other group'.[62] He continued: 'It is time that general nurses realised that they must dispel the starry-eyed Florence Nightingale vision … Protests and demonstrations may be a useful part of a strategy aimed at focusing public attention on the plight of the general nurse [but they] are no substitute for effective trade union action.'[63] On that occasion, Browne never mentioned the INO. In 1975, in an interview with the *Irish Independent*, he was less circumspect. Explicitly referring to the INO, he noted: 'They have a naive approach to industrial relations ... you don't get into an economic argument and then strip yourself of your muscle power. Most nurses wouldn't strike – but why tell the employer that?'[64]

The INO was not (yet) for turning, however, and was willing to sacrifice members who dallied with trade unionism. In 1975, Carmel Taaffe, INO President and Matron at Dublin's Cherry Orchard Hospital, told members of the organisation who were also members of a trade union: 'Make up your minds – you cannot serve two masters, you cannot take leadership from 2 sources and remain loyal to both.'[65] Even the faintest whiff of trade unionism was enough to make the INO retch. The organisation minted a variation on its standard members' badge in the 1970s, emblazoned with the INO's acronym and the title 'steward'. The badges were intended for those INO members who acted as shop stewards in their workplaces. Members were not impressed, as recalled by Anne Cody: 'Not many of the members know this but we went ahead and we designed a lovely badge. They threw it out at the Annual [Meeting] so the badges never saw the light of day ... The members were very conservative, they didn't want [a] shop steward ... that was too uniony for them.'[66] Yet there was a recognised need for better representation of members at ward level, as the organisation was deemed to be somewhat aloof.

A compromise was arrived at in 1975, which witnessed the deployment of 'nurse representatives', essentially shop stewards by a different name, as a means to expedite and better address members' workplace issues. These representatives joined an expanding array of INO staff all geared toward making the organisation more receptive to members' needs: an Information Officer, an Organising Coordinator and a number of regional and promotional officers were all hired. Communication between rank-and-file members and the organisation was also augmented with the advent of the answering machine in the 1970s. The extra expense in financing these developments was met through a new system of deducting members' subscriptions from their salaries, as this helped ensure a more reliable income at head office and eased the burden on Branch Secretaries. Further efficiencies were achieved with the computerisation of the INO's headquarters in 1982.

The ill-fated Nurse Steward badge that never saw the light of day. Courtesy Lisa Moyles/INMO.

But for all the change taking place in the INO, its stance on strike action was unwavering. Addressing a protest march in Limerick, that city's former Mayor, Mrs Frances Condell, remarked:

> In comparing the work of nurses generally with the work of other people in other areas of employment, I am doing them an injustice ... I am reducing the nurses' status of dedication to work ... I am very proud that our nurses ... have not taken the easier and more common way out today, of leaving their work and going on strike ... Surely that decision in itself displays their mettle, their strength of purpose, their dedication ... in not exploiting the sick and the helpless.[67]

A short time later, Minister for Health, Brendan Corish, sang a similar tune: 'Your organisation's approach ... is the only rational one in this day and age ... no profession within our health services should lightly substitute direct action techniques for reasonable negotiation and discussion ... Your organisation's attitude in these matters has been exemplary.'[68]

The attempted gaelicisation of Irish society in the early years of the Saorstát, evident in attempts to have state-employees conduct their business through Irish, witnessed the INU holding Irish classes for members in the early 1930s. The INU's successor, the INO, also occasionally referred to itself in Irish as 'Cumann na nAltraí Gaelacha'. But the organisation's command of the *cúpla focail* seemingly did not extend to one commonly used term: *plámás*. Time and again, the INO fell for persuasive ploys (perhaps unintended) that manipulated and controlled nurses and midwives – ploys that reassured them of the moral legitimacy of not taking strike action in spite of the detrimental consequences on their employment conditions.

Carmel Taaffe, INO President, speaking at the organisation's 1975 Annual General Meeting in Galway, remarked that trade union officials 'will never fully understand nurses [sic] problems and attitudes'.[69] For Taaffe, chief among these attitudes was members' service to patients: 'How is it possible to talk at the same time of striking and seeing that the patients do not suffer? The two situations are totally incompatible ... It is the acceptance of this ethic or philosophy that distinguishes professional from non-professional groups.'[70] She also distilled INO members' position on strike action in one word: 'NEVER' [original emphasis].[71] Still reeling from members' tabled motions questioning the INO's position outside congress, in 1975, the organisation's Executive recommended that the INO should not join the ICTU.[72] Worried that members might defect to trade unions, and cognisant of the ever encroaching ITGWU, the Executive also recommended that no member be permitted to join any other nurse representative organisation while the INO possessed a negotiating licence under the 1941 *Trade Union Act*. Both motions were adopted.

In 1975, Ena Meehan remarked on the organisation's disinclination to take strike action in its early days and on its status as an excepted body, which was dependant on it not striking. Meehan commented on the 'tough women' of the INO's past and added 'We must pay them the courtesy of thinking that they knew what they were doing.'[73] Meehan's contribution is notable. After Louie Bennett's death in 1956, a park bench was erected in St Stephen's Green, Dublin in her memory. The bench is inscribed: 'In memory of Louie Bennett, 1870–1956, builder of the Irish Women Workers' Union, worker for social justice, world peace and the unity of Ireland, her sympathy and love for humanity knew no boundaries.' The INO penned a small biography of Bennett in its *Irish Nurses' Magazine*. The piece lauded Bennett but did not acknowledge her role as the organisation's first president and merely noted that she had taken 'a keen interest' in and was a 'source of encouragement to' its founding members.[74]

Bennett had led a fourteen-week-long strike of laundry workers in the 1940s. It is possible that her involvement in strike activity did not fit with the INO's contemporary image and, as a result, it distanced itself from her. The organisation's reasons for its aversion to strike action soon became tenuous. In December 1975, an editorial in the *World of Irish Nursing* recalled an address at the INO's Annual General Meeting that appealed for the release of Tiede Herrema, a Dutch businessman who was kidnapped and held hostage, as ransom, pending the release of republican prisoners from Limerick prison. Herrema was released unharmed two weeks later. The editorial remarked:

> The theme implicit in this appeal that the innocent should not be imprisoned or injured in order to barter for some other gain might well be examined in relation to many aspects of industrial relations. Where the nursing profession is concerned, the person who is seriously ill in hospital is imprisoned by illness and is not to be further imprisoned by a withdrawal ... of essential nursing services.[75]

In 1976, Carmel Taaffe remarked: 'Every nurse and indeed every employee has the right to strike but we have voluntarily rejected this right ... But having taken this decision it does not deter us from using other forms of direct action ... I can tell you now that embarrassment can come in many forms.'[76] In spite of Taaffe's protestations, nurses' and midwives' primary source of embarrassment remained their salaries. Buoyed by a feminist narrative, and under pressure

Kyran Lynch, the INO's first industrial relations officer in 1977. Courtesy Fennell Photography.

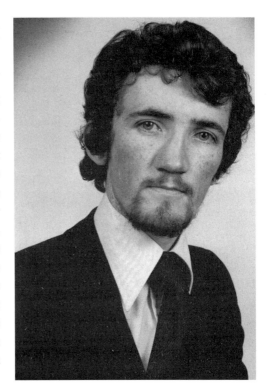

from trade unions, a belief among some rank-and-file INO members was growing that the organisation's leadership was ineffective and that its no-strike policy was injurious to members' interests. The organisation's decision to employ its first industrial relations officer, Kyran Lynch, in 1977, was a case of too little too late. Members had become impatient with the slow rate of progress, and this would soon find expression in the organisation's decision to return to the trade union fold, and, in a reappraisal of its no-strike policy.

IV. Marking Time

The 1970s was largely a period of marking time for the INO's educational endeavours. The organisation addressed a number of educational issues to An Bord Altranais in 1970, chief among which was that the board appoint an inspector of schools of nursing.[77] This was considered important because, as an example, there was just one qualified nurse tutor for 234 students at Galway Regional Hospital in 1971, a situation which students found to be lacking.[78] Hospitals also continued to charge student nurses a hefty fee in order to secure a training place. These fees all but excluded working-class applicants, and some candidates had to go to extraordinary lengths in order to meet the cost of training. The father of one would-be student at Cork's North Infirmary turned to gambling in order to secure his daughter a training place. She recalled:

> We had to pay sixty guineas as a down payment [to train] … My father was a bit of a gambler … He put £8 on [a horse] … He won at 8/1, so that was £64 … He said 'Here you are now Anna and if anyone ever asks you who made a nurse of you, you can say it was Vincent O'Brien', he was the horse trainer.[79]

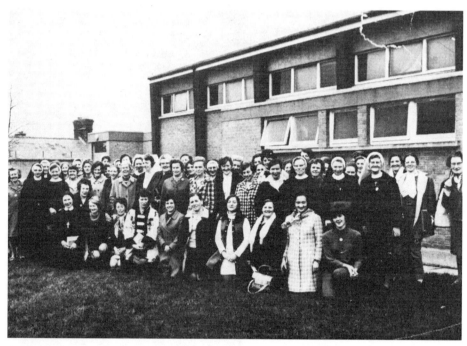

Attendees at the Midwives' Refresher Course at Dublin's Coombe Hospital in 1972. Courtesy INMO.

In 1970, the INO suggested that the fees payable by students be replaced by an educational grant payable by An Bord Altranais to individual schools of nursing, if the schools complied with certain obligations. The INO maintained that the board would then have at its disposal an 'effective weapon' in ensuring that high standards of training were met by each school.[80] The organisation also urged a revision in the reported ratio of 1:100 clinical instructors to student nurses, to 1:40, as it 'must be obvious that no teacher could possibly cover adequately the number of wards that the former figure implies'.[81] Carmel Taaffe also suggested the establishment of a course for clinical instructors in order to translate classroom teaching into clinical practice as, up till then, such courses only existed in Britain.[82] This campaign was sorely needed. One nurse who trained at the Charitable Infirmary, Jervis Street, Dublin in the 1970s recalled:

> One Sunday evening I was assigned to give a young chap two suppositories to secure a bowel motion before he went to Theatre the next day. I duly carried out the instruction [but] came to realise I had given him Aminophylline

suppositories which would aid breathing but certainly were not designed to urge bowel evacuation.[83]

Another nurse who trained in Dublin's Richmond Hospital in the same decade recalled:

> At that time we were learning from each other … it was students teaching each other … You were very responsible, very accountable and you did worry an awful lot about the patients … but your knowledge was limited … I think it was as good as they could give at that time … I don't know how they could have done it better because you didn't have the Clinical Tutors, you didn't have sufficient Tutors [and due to the marriage bar] you didn't have the senior staff either.[84]

The 1960s witnessed moves, long touted by the INO, to make students' clinical learning experience more comprehensive, and the organisation sought to build on this trend in the 1970s. The INO lobbied for the inclusion of geriatrics, psychiatry, public health and obstetrics in its efforts to broaden the general nursing curriculum.[85] Ireland's accession to the EEC, and the associated directives regarding nurse education that flowed thereafter, placed the wind at the organisation's back. Directive 77/453/EEC stipulated that students of general nursing gain clinical and theoretical instruction in maternity care, a longstanding goal of the INO.[86] An Bord Altranais allocated a minimum of forty hours of maternity care teaching in an approved hospital in order to meet this directive, but the INO regarded this as too little and successfully lobbied the board to increase students' maternity secondment to four weeks.[87] The same directive noted that student nurses' clinical experience 'should be selected for its training value [and] should be gained under the supervision of qualified nursing staff'.[88] The organisation's Tutors' Section responded by lobbying training hospitals to increase their complement of registered nurses. Student nurses were also frequently 'seconded' to hospitals other than their training hospital, in cases where their training institution could not provide an educational placement in a particular clinical area. For example, students training in hospitals with no children's ward spent time working in the children's ward of another hospital, or in a dedicated children's hospital, usually under a reciprocal agreement. The organisation warned against using seconded students to solve staffing issues at other institutions and argued that secondment sites be approved only if they could offer students a 'meaningful' clinical and theoretical experience.[89]

The rise in the INO's militancy on industrial issues found an echo in relation to professional and educational issues. A perceived breach of European guidelines on nurse education resulted, in 1979, in a proposal that the INO's nurse tutors and clinical teachers not participate in student nurse examinations in protest. That comparable European guidelines related to medical, dental and veterinary professionals were all being implemented,[90] suggests that nurse education remained low on the state's list of priorities. The INO continued to address the bulk of its concerns regarding nurse education to An Bord Altranais, but in 1972 the board indicated that it lacked the power to establish the INO's long-sought college of nursing and lacked the funds with which to make educational grants to schools of nursing. It was, however, about to commence a course for clinical instructors.[91] That the board was only in a position to deliver on one out of three of the INO's key requests typified the painstakingly slow rate of progress, and the INO's frustration with the board, which simmered in the 1960s, was beginning to bubble. Nor was there much impetus for change. Fifty-seven per cent of student nurses interviewed in 1969 were of the opinion that the existing system of nurse training was good or quite good; four out of five students training in hospitals with a block system wished for no alternative system to be introduced and less than one in ten believed that university education was a realistic alternative to the apprenticeship model.[92] The apprentice model, for all its shortcomings, was popular, and considering that 1,800 applications were received for just thirteen training places at Sligo General Hospital in 1975, the state was in no rush to change things.[93]

Progress regarding post-registration education for nurses was a little more tangible. Following lobbying by the INO, a course in management for nurses was established at the Regional Technical College, Dundalk, County Louth, in 1971. In 1971, Carmel Taaffe urged, unsuccessfully, that post-registration education be made mandatory for nurses and (proving herself ahead of her time) that An Bord Altranais maintain a record of nurses'/midwives' educational achievements. Dubious as to whether a college of nursing would ever materialise, the INO threw its weight behind a proposed Faculty of Nursing at the RCSI in 1971. The faculty was founded in 1974 to provide post-registration education for nurses, and the INO contributed £100 to the venture.[94] A sizeable 289 nurses registered for courses upon the faculty's inception and, by the end of the decade, 1,000 nurses were on the faculty's books. These nurses were undertaking short courses leading to a diploma or a number of courses leading to a fellowship.[95] Diploma courses at the faculty took their place alongside the INO's refresher courses, which ran throughout the 1970s, and the organisation employed an educational

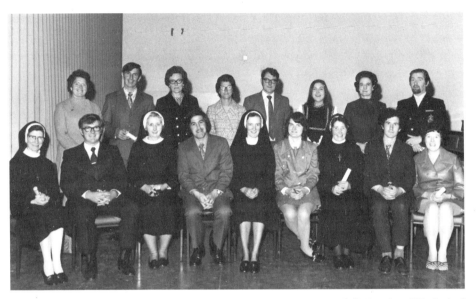

Successful candidates in the Middle Management course at Dundalk Regional Technical College. Courtesy INMO.

correspondent, from 1975 onwards, who wrote a monthly article concerning education in the INO's periodical.

Research activity remained intertwined with professional legitimacy, and the INO's enthusiasm to inculcate members with an awareness of the research process increased in the 1970s. This manifested in a series of articles in the *World of Irish Nursing* that outlined the importance of nursing research and attempted to equip members with the skills necessary to carry out their own scientific studies. A scientific basis for nursing work was also being forged through developments such as the nursing process. The nursing process originated out of General Systems Theory, and its influence spread to Ireland in the 1970s, where it was championed by the INO. The process replaced the former task orientation model of work in which nurses/midwives were allocated patient-related tasks such as medication administration and wound dressings by their ward sister; that system witnessed patients receiving disparate and sometimes arbitrary care in a disjointed manner. The gusto and fanfare with which the nursing process was greeted in Ireland spoke volumes as to the underdeveloped state of the scientific method in nursing work it was, after all, a simple algorithm. It was timely that research was the theme of a session at the INO's Annual Meeting in 1972; that same year, Miss McFarlane, Head of the Division of Nursing at Manchester University, told INO members:

'Only by research can we apply the basic sciences to nursing situations and identify a scientific basis for improved patient care; only by research can we gain the necessary facts on which to base enlightened action; only by research can we evaluate methods.'[96]

V. Policy and Politics

The 1966 White Paper *The Health Services and their Further Development* laid the basis for administrative changes governing the health services and for the replacement of the existing local health authorities with eight regional Health Boards charged with administering the services. Legislative provision for the creation of Health Boards was incorporated in the *Health Act* of 1970, and members of these boards were appointed by central or local government or were democratically elected by a range of health service professionals.[97] Nurses were, by far, the most numerous grades in the health service, and it may have been expected that the number of peers they could elect would reflect this. On the contrary, the proposed Southern Health Board was to have thirty-three members: eighteen were to be mayoral or County Council appointments, eight were to be elected by doctors, one was to be elected by dentists and pharmacists, respectively, three were to be appointed by the Minister for Health and two were to be elected by nurses.[98]

Nurses'/midwives' own apparent nonchalance in relation to policy, political and administrative matters was an issue that the INO tried hard to address. Carmel Taaffe attempted to raise members' political conscience in 1971, noting that nurses' 'inactivity in the past' was causative in the Minister for Health giving them such a 'weak voice' on Health Boards and implored graduating students at Dublin's Coombe Hospital to 'become vocal [because] it is too bad to hear medical men, unions and other disciplines speaking out while nursing remains silent'.[99] Some nurses were politically active, including Ward Sister at Galway Regional Hospital and member of the INO's Executive Council, Mary Byrne. Byrne was a member of Fianna Fáil and, in 1975, became the first woman to serve as Mayor of Galway.[100] Byrne is remembered fondly by her colleagues and recalled as both an inspiration and an able negotiator with a knack for bringing people around to her point of view.

Yet most nurses and midwives avoided policy, political and administrative matters: just 808 nurses out of an eligible 5,000 voted in elections to the board of An Bord Altranais in 1963.[101] In one election to the INO's Executive Council in the 1970s, just 800 out of approximately 8,000 members voted.[102] The reason behind their political detachment is not clear, but research carried out in 1970

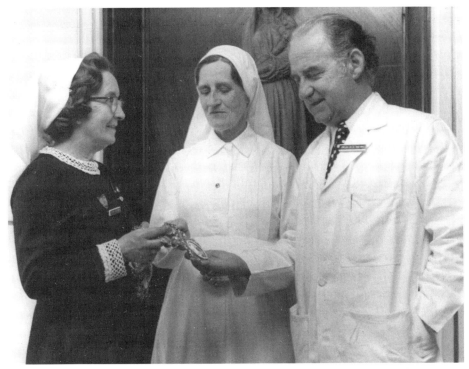

Mary Byrne, Mayor of Galway and member of the Executive Council of the INO, shows her chain of office to Sister Kieran, Matron, and Dr S. O'Beirn of Galway Regional Hospital in 1975. Courtesy INMO.

showed that women in Ireland were less interested in political matters than men, and among those who were members of a political party, very few held official positions.[103] Many nurses and midwives, particularly in the period following the marriage bar, had the added challenge of shift work, including that of the 'second-shift', which may have impeded involvement in political activities such as attending meetings and canvassing. The INO's ostensibly 'non-political' stance may also have been an issue as members of apolitical organisations were fearful of cross-contaminating their organisational activities with political activities and avoided active involvement in political process as a result.[104]

The INO persisted. It implored members to interest themselves in the election of nurses to their local Health Boards and a number of INO alumni did indeed assume Health Board positions.[105] In a stark illustration of the under-representation of women at policy level in Ireland, nurses were often the only women on Health Boards and, staggeringly, in the early 1970s, of the

243 people who sat on Health Boards, just fifteen were women.[106] The INO met with representatives of the Department of Health in 1970 to request nurse representation on Consultative Health Committees – the administrative strata below the level of Health Boards charged with acting in an advisory capacity to the boards. Although the Minister did not increase nurse representation on Health Boards to greater than two, he did accede to a further two nurse representatives on local Health Board Advisory Committees.[107] The state was clearly more amenable to situating nurses/midwives in the lower decision-making tiers than it was in the upper ones. The INO also sought nurse representation on the proposed Comhairle na nOspidéal, a body that offered advice to the Minister for Health on the operation of the hospital services. The organisation had limited success in its campaign and, of the twenty-three persons appointed to the first council, just one was a nurse.[108] The board elected to the new St Kevin's Hospital, Dublin had no nurse representatives in 1971, in spite of the INO's best efforts.[109]

The organisation could be forgiven for bemoaning as mere lip-service the consultation with nurses and midwives on issues affecting the health services; it grew tired of citing the evidence supporting the benefits of involving nurses and midwives at strategic planning level. The subsequent gaffes range from the blackly humorous to the downright feckless. To what extent has a lack of consultation with nurses/midwives been responsible for questionable hospital design and planning? Anecdotal evidence reveals a number of hospitals that warranted retrospective works in order that they be able to accommodate trolleys and store equipment. In one hospital, a bedpan washer was installed in the neonatal unit,[110] and at another, St Felim's Hospital, County Cavan, the installation of a bar (yes, a bar) was proposed. A piece in the *World of Irish Nursing* wryly remarked that St Felim's was overcrowded, lacked an elevator and concluded: 'Conditions ... do not it seems, lend themselves to the innovation of "bar" facilities.'[111] Furthermore, in spite of the INO's protests, the state rode roughshod over public health nurses' health promotion and prevention role in the 1950s, diluting it into that of a multifunctional practitioner. It is today paying the price, literally, for creating a system that, in the absence of relatively cheap health-promotion strategies, relies on much more expensive hospital-care alternatives.[112]

It was not until 1975, amid the second wave of the women's movement, that Ena Meehan inquired, with a feminist lens, as to the reason underlying her members' suboptimal representation at strategic levels in the health services. Meehan inquired: 'It is fair to ask, is this because nurses are nurses ro [*sic*] because so many of them are women [?]'[113] Analysis of women and public policy in Ireland shows that, from the advent of the second wave of the women's movement, women's representation at strategic level increased slowly.[114] This trend is evident, albeit tentatively, in the INO's successes from that point. In 1976, the organisation was successful in having a nominated member of its Executive Council appointed to Comhairle na nOspidéal, and in 1977, after lobbying the Minister for Heath, Charles Haughey, the organisation secured the addition of a nurse to the fourteen-strong male planning team charged with delivering a new hospital at Beaumont, Dublin.[115]

In tandem with its campaign to advance the nursing and midwifery perspective nationally, the INO waged a campaign to advance its own perspective among its peers. The INO disaffiliated from the National Council of Nurses of Ireland in 1949 in a spat over proportional representation. The organisation was aggrieved that, in spite of it being the council affiliate with the largest number of members and, therefore, paying the largest affiliation fee, the INO's voting strength was equal, not larger, to that of smaller affiliates: 'Voting strength, therefore, is not related to financial interest.'[116] The INO assumed that the council would capitulate on the issue of proportional representation or, in the absence of INO monies, dissolve altogether – opening up the possibility of the INO becoming the conduit body for affiliation to the ICN and, perhaps, increasing INO membership in the process. It was wrong on both assumptions. The impasse rumbled on for three years until, in 1952, the INO affiliated once again to the council.

The same issue arose in 1975, and the INO withheld its affiliation fees. The organisation was due to pay the National Council £1,000, four-fifths of the council's income, yet was only entitled to nominate one quarter of the council's delegates, with the rest being nominated by the council's other affiliates. These affiliates comprised the Irish Guild of Catholic Nurses, the National Florence Nightingale Committee of Ireland, the Adelaide Hospital Nurses' League and the Irish Matrons' Association. The Catholic Nurses' Guild's historian puts its membership at 1,051 and falling in 1965, suggesting that membership was less than 1,000 by the 1970s.[117] Membership of the Florence Nightingale Committee was fifteen; of the Adelaide Nurses' League was approximately 400; and of the Matrons' association was 200.[118] Membership numbers at the INO, in contrast, were approaching 8,000. The INO argued that its relatively large membership should afford it more delegates on the National Council. The council acquiesced, possibly fearing for its survival in the absence of INO funds, and the organisation was granted one extra delegate for each of its sections. The INO then had twenty-one delegates, and each other affiliate organisation had eight.[119] The INO's real goal was to subsume the council altogether, just as the

The immensely popular 'Nurse of the Year Competition' was co-sponsored by the INO and ran throughout the 1970s. Courtesy INMO/Reproduced with the permission of Lucozade Ribena Suntory Ltd. All rights reserved.

COULD YOU BE THE NURSE OF THE YEAR 1977?

The search for the Nurse of the Year 1977 is now under way. She (or he) will be the nurse who best reflects the correct image of the nursing profession in Ireland. The Lucozade Nurse of the Year Award, £1,000, could go a long way towards helping you achieve many of your ambitions. In addition, a special commemorative plaque will be presented to the hospital you represent.

All nurses who are professionally qualified or under training for a professional nursing qualification are eligible. There will be eight regional finals and a national final to be held early in April. Get full details from your matron now . . . you could be the 1977 Nurse of the Year.

Presented by

LUCOZADE

RCN had done in Britain in 1963. The organisation feared that the 'identity of the nursing profession' was injured by it being 'splintered' into multiple groups; elsewhere, the 'most representative nursing organisation has direct affiliation with the International Council of Nurses'.[120] The INO got its way in 1978 when it incorporated the National Council altogether. The new company was titled: 'The Irish Nurses' Organisation and the National Council of Nurses of Ireland'.[121]

The 1960s witnessed many protest meetings and petitions, the results of which were somewhat disappointing. Militancy increased in the 1970s and saw protest marches and works-to-rule. Further increases in the organisation's militancy were problematic, however. The INO's status as an excepted body and its no-strike policy precluded members from a withdrawal of labour. Frustrated by the narrow range of militant options available to them, some members began to ask questions of their own organisation. For the first time in the organisation's history, these questions were about to become deafening.

CHAPTER 9

Some Striking Developments, 1978–90

The INO entered the 1980s on what appeared to be a firm footing. Membership of the organisation had risen from 4,499 in 1968 to 8,055 in 1977.[1] But as the 1970s drew to a close, nurses and midwives had not benefitted to the same degree as other workers in relation to pay and conditions of work. Moreover, when National Wage Agreements became the standard manner for determining state employees' salaries in 1970, the INO's position outside the ICTU rendered it unable to influence the process. Feeling disenfranchised and disillusioned, INO members' demands for wage justice and their expectations of their representative organisation grew massively. Members mandated the organisation to pursue a 50 per cent salary increase and to affiliate to congress. Members also decided to rescind the organisation's no-strike policy in an effort to strengthen the organisation's hand in negotiations. In addition, a belief among some members that the organisation's Executive was ineffective resulted in a campaign by a group of rank-and-file members to gain seats on the organisation's Executive Council in the late 1970s. Their success preceded more radical organisational changes in the mid 1980s when P.J. Madden, a new General Secretary, with a remarkably different perspective on strike action than those he succeeded, was appointed.

I. 'Something different is happening within the ranks of the INO'

INO members assembled in Bundoran, County Donegal, in 1978 for the organisation's Annual General Meeting. The theme of that year's gathering, 'change', could not have been more fitting. The mood among the assembled nurses and midwives was one of seething anger. One INO member recalled:

> We had one particular lady, she really stands out in my memory ... a widow who really worked hard all her life, had brought up her family and had to go back to work ... She got up and told her story. And it really was heart

breaking. [The widow spoke about] having to go back to work and starting with such a pittance of a salary. She really made a difference to that meeting … She really was applauded.[2]

The widow received almost unanimous support, but one attendee, a nun, addressed the meeting and asked: 'What [is] happening to nursing, there was a time [when] nursing was a vocation and why couldn't we continue like that,

ANNUAL GENERAL MEETING

The 59th Annual General Meeting and Seminar of the Irish Nurses' Organisation will be held on Friday, 22nd September, (Seminar), Saturday, 23rd September and Sunday, 24th September, 1978, in the Great Northern Hotel, Bundoran, and is open to all members of the INO.

PRELIMINARY PROGRAMME

Private Session—2 p.m. Friday 22nd to 11 a.m. Sat. Sept. 23.

Friday, 22nd September—Seminar—2-5.30 p.m./7.30-10 p.m.
Theme: "Change—The Future Development of the INO"
Speakers will include: Miss Catherine M. Hall, General Secretary, Royal College of Nursing of the United Kingdom; Miss Sheila M. Quinn, Chairman, Council, Royal College of Nursing of the United Kingdom.

23rd September—Business Session — 9.30 a.m. - 11 a.m.
Open Session—11.30 a.m. Sat. - 1 p.m. Sunday.
Motions and Resolutions— 11.30 - 5.20 p.m.
Presidential Address—Miss T. C. Taaffe, RGN, RM, RFN.
Nurse Admin. Cert. (Edin.)—5.20 p.m.
Sherry Reception—7.30 p.m.
Annual Subscription Dinner—8 p.m.

Sunday, 24th September—Open Session (continued)—9.30 - 1 p.m.
Motions and Resolutions—11.30 a.m. - 5.20 p.m.

The theme of the A.G.M. is "Change." For details re hotel bookings for official delegates, please contact Miss M. M. Brophy, Information Officer, at 20 Lower Leeson Street, Dublin 2.

The programme for the INO's infamous 1978 Annual Meeting in Bundoran. Courtesy INMO.

we were looking after the sick and it was a vocation?'[3] The nun received an unexpected response:

> [One member] got up and she said that it was easy for this lady to … say what she had to say about [nursing] being a vocation because she was a nun. She got up in the morning in her centrally heated convent and had her breakfast handed to her. She didn't have to go out to the supermarket and try and cope and pay for a flat or keep herself … it was time we acted like ordinary workers … She … got great applause.[4]

Reminiscing on the period, Ena Meehan, General Secretary, recalled unrest and unhappiness among the members.[5] Sensing the changed mood, INO President, Carmel Taaffe, took to the podium and remarked: 'Something different is happening within the ranks of the INO.'[6] In a remarkable volte-face for the organisation, Taaffe acknowledged: 'Nurses down through the years have adopted a non-militant approach in salary negotiations in order to ensure that patient care would not be put in jeopardy. They have paid dearly for this policy.'[7] The 1970s were an economically challenging decade that witnessed inflation soar to 20 per cent; oil prices alone rose tenfold.[8] The period also became synonymous with 'knock-on' strikes by workers keen to replicate the wage increases awarded to other sectors.[9] By the end of the decade, there was also growing unrest, including among white-collar trade unionists, at perceived injustices in the system of taxation. The system witnessed those who were taxed at source pay an inordinate and increasing amount of tax compared to farmers and large corporations.[10] Some 150,000 people marched in Dublin in 1979 in protest.

Also pivotal in the organisation's about-turn was the way in which nurses' and midwives' salaries were decided and the INO's exclusion from that process. Wage rounds ceased in 1970 and were replaced with a series of National Wage Agreements conducted by the Employer–Labour Conference. These were bipartite or tripartite agreements involving employers, trade unions and the government. The labour side was represented by the Executive of the ICTU; the INO, no longer being a member of congress, was not represented. Reminiscing on the period, Matron of Dublin's Coombe Hospital, Ita O'Dwyer, who spent over twenty years on the organisation's Executive Council – six of which she spent as President, recalled: 'Bad as it was, unions in ICTU had some say but the INO were totally on the periphery. It was demoralising to ballot members on a National Agreement, knowing the decision had already been taken.'[11]

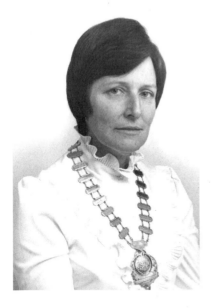

Ita O'Dwyer, INO President, 1981–5 and 1989–91. O'Dwyer is from Co. Tipperary. She spent time as a Midwifery Tutor including Principal Midwifery Tutor at St James' Hospital, Dublin, before becoming Matron at the Coombe Hospital, Dublin. Copyright Pat Sweeney Photography.

Members' frustration at the predicament resulted in the passage of a number of significant resolutions at Bundoran. The first of these was a resolution, endorsed by a number of branches, that the INO pursue a 50 per cent salary increase.[12] Secondly, and possibly emulating developments in Britain, where the RCN had just become a trade union,[13] Motion 61a, as proposed by the INO's Dublin branch, resolved that the INO affiliate to the ICTU. (There were ninety-five votes in favour and six against affiliation to congress.)[14] Ita O'Dwyer again: 'There was a sense of activity and change in the air. Nurses had developed a new awareness but we were still, as it were, looking at the change but not part of it.'[15] Thirdly, Motion 61b (i), as proposed by the organisation's Bantry branch in County Cork, resolved that the INO remove the no-strike clause from its by-laws.[16] With this new departure, the organisation had taken on the character of more mainstream trade unions, at least constitutionally.

I.I. A New Realisation: Militancy Yields Results

The INO's Executive Council was charged with a weighty responsibility following developments at Bundoran: achieving a 50 per cent increase in members' salaries, affiliating to congress and revising the organisation's policy on strike action. In order to achieve a salary increase of such magnitude, the organisation believed that a Committee of Inquiry was warranted. In an effort to exert pressure on the government to establish such a committee, 4,000 nurses and midwives marched from the INO's headquarters on 20 Lower Leeson Street, where the organisation had taken up residence in 1951, to Dáil Éireann on 21 November 1978. Following a 'good-humoured crush', nurses were admitted to the Dáil bar, restaurant and public gallery, where they put their case to TDs while the INO's leaders negotiated over 'tea and cake' with Minister for Health,

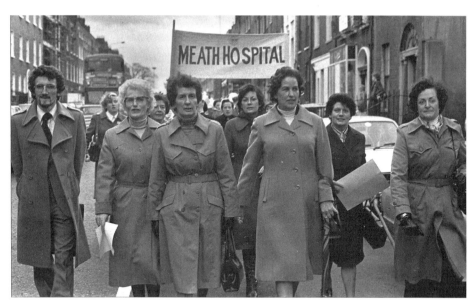

A delegation from the INO march in protest in Dublin in 1978. From left, front row: Kyran Lynch, INO Industrial Relations Officer; Ena Meehan, INO General Secretary; Carmel Taaffe, INO President; Maeve Keane; Patrice O'Sullivan is on the far right. Courtesy Derek Speirs.

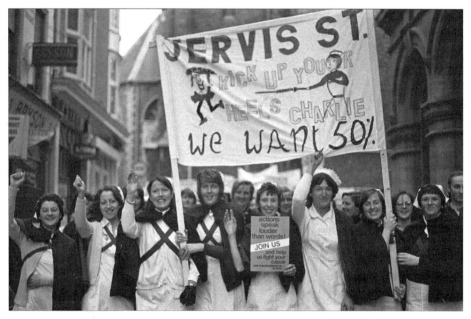

Nurses from the Charitable Infirmary, Jervis Street, Dublin, make known their demands for a 50 per cent pay increase during the protest march in 1978. Courtesy Derek Speirs.

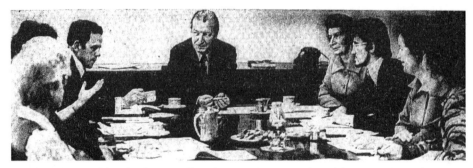

Minister for Health Charles Haughey (centre) meets with a delegation from the INO.
With thanks to Irish Newspaper Archives and the *Irish Press*.

Charles Haughey.[17] Pleasantries aside, the marchers' placards told their own
stories: one from the organisation's Roscommon branch referenced Haughey
and a popular television programme: 'Charlie's Angels Need More Money'.

The following day, when the Minister announced the terms of reference
of the proposed inquiry, the INO was vexed to learn that it 'did not refer
specifically to nurses' pay, in the manner anticipated'.[18] The INO convened a
Special Delegate Conference and, believing that the inquiry would not deal
properly with its pay grievances, decided to reject the proposal. Delegates also
resolved that if their salary concerns were not addressed to their satisfaction by
1 March 1979, mass resignation would occur. The threat of mass resignations
marked a real escalation in the INO's militancy and yielded immediate results,
with the establishment of a Special Conciliation Committee. The organisation
argued that its members' salaries were based on relativities that were now
outdated, and the Special Committee agreed to undertake work studies with
nurses from over thirty hospitals nationwide in order to establish the current
nature of nurses' roles. In the battle for improved conditions, some progress
had been made. But a parallel battle was also evolving, the results of which
were more immediate than those of the conciliation process. This was not a
battle with employers; rather, it was a battle within the INO.

II. The Unrepresentative Representative Organisation:
The INO and the 'New Policy Group'

Less than ten years after the INO's protest marches of 1970, members were once
again demonstrating in pursuit of better conditions, and some INO members
began to question the suitability for purpose of the organisation's Executive
Council as a result. The INO's executive in the period 1977–9 comprised

twenty-nine members: five nurses from junior managerial posts such as ward sisters; six nurses from senior managerial posts such as matrons, their deputies/ assistants or superintendent public health nurses; six nurses involved in nurse education, such as nurse tutors; four public health nurses and eight staff nurses/midwives.[19] The composition of the council did not reflect the overall nursing/midwifery staffing structure in Ireland, as staff nurses/midwives were proportionately under-represented.[20] Kathleen Craughwell recalled the INO at the time: 'It was kind of an elite thing ... the INO was for these senior people, it was for people who had arrived, if you like.'[21]

Reminiscing on this period in the organisation's history, some of today's nurses/midwives referred to the INO's Executive Council in disapproving and pejorative terms. Some used the phrase 'blue-rinse brigade',[22] and one described the executive as akin to a 'sewing circle' who tended to 'sit around and not do too much'.[23] Maureen McCann was one nurse who was distinctly dissatisfied with the INO. McCann commenced nurse training at Dublin's Mater Hospital in 1956 and was a member of the INO and a theatre sister at the same hospital in the 1970s: 'We weren't questioned as regards any [salary] offers [that] were made; everything was made at Executive Council level and then we were told what we were getting or otherwise.'[24] Some nurses also recalled the INO as not being especially amenable to the expression of discontent by its junior-rank members. Kathleen Craughwell recalled a hospital in which she worked that had no teaspoons: 'I do remember trying to feed a patient who had a stroke with a hard-boiled egg ... I don't know how I got it out of the shell, with a dessert spoon.'[25] She added that nurses who dared question such privation were branded agitators and suggested that they were more likely to be fired if they committed a subsequent misdemeanour. When asked if the INO would have been of any assistance in such a situation, she remarked 'It was people in the INO that were making those kinds of decisions.'[26]

The relatively high number of matrons on the Executive Council also had potential ramifications. The year of 1979 witnessed the publication of the *Attitude Survey of Irish Nurses*, which found that, of 1,364 nurses questioned, 64 per cent indicated that nurses feared, rather than respected, matrons.[27] This finding was echoed in members' testimonies. Lenore Mrkwicka was instrumental in establishing the organisation's Athy/Baltinglass/Carlow branch and recounted a 'fear factor' among rank-and-file members when formulating motions for the organisation's Annual Meeting: 'People would fear that back on the ranch you are going to be dealing with Matron who is on the Executive of the INO.'[28] This suggests that the composition of the organisation's Executive Council stifled the expression of discontent among members.

As a result of her frustration, McCann and a group of approximately twenty others decided that 'something should be done to change the INO to be more amenable to the members and not leave everything in the hands of the Executive Council'.[29] She recalled the grassroots movement that evolved:

> We met frequently in the Dublin area. There were two particular houses, one on the north side and one on the south side where people who wanted to make a change … We'd meet every so often and plan our strategy … We managed to get twenty people from right around the country [to run in the 1979 INO Executive Council elections].[30]

The would-be reformists labelled themselves the 'New Policy Group' and conducted their campaign similar to that of a general election, canvassing nationwide at INO regional meetings and in hospitals, and convening a press conference in Dublin in 1979 at which candidates alleged that the current Executive Council was 'inert' in its approach to negotiations on members' working conditions.[31] The group garnered widespread support and won twenty seats in 1979: the number of staff nurse and staff midwife representatives increased from eight to fourteen, mainly at the expense of those involved in nurse education, which fell from six to three. The organisation's Executive Council was now much more representative of the organisation's core constituency. Maureen McCann also recalled that the New Policy Group specifically recruited men to run for the election:

> We felt people don't listen to women, they listen to men … And we got a few men to run that time to make a change. I suppose things have changed now but at that time [the attitude was,] kind of, women … what have they to talk about? You know, there was an attitude [to] kind of forget about them.[32]

In the event, two men were elected to the organisation's Executive Council. This was in spite of the fact that, in 1972 there was only one male general nurse Branch Officer in the INO (based in Cork),[33] and in 1977 the INO had just thirty male members out of a total membership of 8,000.[34]

The New Policy Group had little time to bask in the glory of its success. In 1979, the conciliation process recommended a 16 per cent salary increase to nurses/midwives. The offer fell far short of the 50 per cent increase that members had mandated the Executive Council to pursue, and the council put it to a ballot without recommendation regarding acceptance or rejection.

Members exhibited a clear resolve and rejected the deal outright; the claim then proceeded to arbitration.

Fears regarding a nurses'/midwives' strike were heightened to such a degree at the time that the INO contacted An Bord Altranais to inquire as to its policy regarding the withdrawal of labour. The INO's line of questioning appears to have taken the board by surprise; the prospect of a strike had never been given any serious consideration and, apparently, was regarded as so outlandish that even the board needed to seek legal advice on the matter. It ultimately declined to issue a general statement on the subject and responded that each case would have to be considered individually.[35] Some members of the INO began to explore the acceptable parameters of industrial action, and one resolution by the organisation's Cork branch, at the INO's Annual Meeting in 1981, requested that 'the INO should urge An Bord Altranais to establish and publish a framework within which nurses must act in the event of an industrial dispute, in order to protect the vulnerable public'.[36] Such a framework had yet to be published by 1984, and this resulted in the INO publishing its own *Code of Ethics*. The code decreed that 'the withdrawal of essential services to patients as a means of resolving [conditions which violate justice] is unethical'.[37] In spite of changes to the organisation's by-laws that permitted industrial action on foot of developments at Bundoran in 1978, any such industrial action would clearly be of a limited nature.

The decision to proceed to arbitration proved worthwhile. The arbitration committee reviewed the evidence gathered in the work study analyses and recommended that general nurses' qualifications, duties and responsibilities were equal to those of assistant librarians and, more especially, psychiatric nurses. The comparison with librarians drew some ire from members of the New Policy Group. Remarks attributed to one member of the group went: 'An assistant librarian [has] no qualification and very little training … a staff nurse [has] three years' training and the responsibility of caring for the sick'.[38] The remarks drew a small avalanche of letters of complaint from disgruntled librarians to the national press, all of whom indicated the high level of education and training necessary for the post of assistant librarian.[39] Under arbitration, nurses and midwives were offered a substantial salary increase of 23 per cent with slightly lower increases for student nurses and slightly higher increases for managerial grades. The magnitude of the award supported the case that their pay had fallen far behind that of other occupations, and militancy or the threat of militancy had yielded results. The INO's Executive Council decided to recommend acceptance of the offer and put it to a ballot of members. The final outcome was relatively close, with 4,520 members voting to accept it and 3,928 voting to reject it.[40]

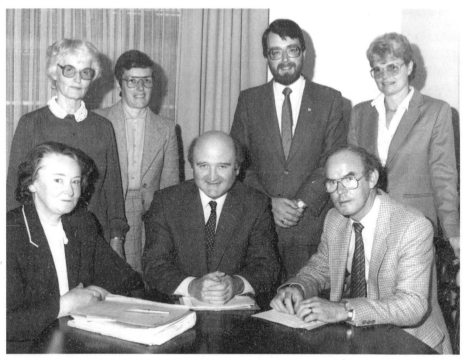

In 1984, an INO delegation met with the Minister for Health, Barry Desmond. From left, seated: First Vice-President Brigid Butler; Barry Desmond; Second Vice-President Patrick McGinty. Standing from left: outgoing General Secretary Ena Meehan; Executive Council Member Anna Monaghan; incoming General Secretary John Pepper and Deputy General Secretary Hilary Marchant. Butler, from Co. Waterford, trained in Cork's North Infirmary and served many years as Superintendent Public Health Nurse for Counties Carlow and Kilkenny, as well as fulfilling her obligations as a member of the Southern Health Board. She became President of the INO in 1985. Courtesy Fennell Photography.

III. The Path to Trade Unionism

The INO's return to the trade union fold was a somewhat clandestine affair, owing to the fear that other unions might attempt to frustrate its progress. P.J. Madden, who, in 1986, assumed the helm of the organisation as General Secretary, recalled: 'We had to go under the radar in the legal and technical procedure until we were sure that all of our own members bought into it.'[41] The INO began to explore the process of affiliating to congress soon after events at Bundoran, and it formally applied to affiliate on 8 November 1978. As ever, things seemed easier than they transpired. In 1949, in order to secure a mortgage for its office on Leeson Street, Dublin, a building it shared with a dental practice,

INO General Secretary P.J. Madden. Courtesy INMO.

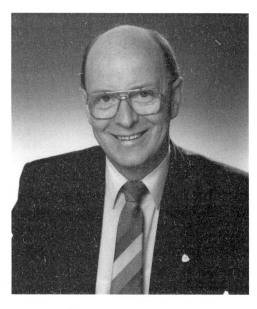

the INO was required to become a 'legal entity'.[42] It duly did so, and the INO's *Memorandum and Articles of Association* shows that the organisation was registered as a company, albeit with a caveat: 'That the Organisation shall not support with its funds any object or endeavour to impose on or procure to be observed by its members or others any regulations, restrictions or conditions which, if an object of the Organisation, would make it a trade union.'[43] This was a sticking point, and congress turned down the INO's application for affiliation:

> We do not consider it would be appropriate for us to accept a body which was not and could not become a Trade Union into affiliation with [the ICTU] … If, however, you do decide to form a body legally constituted as a Trade Union, and such a body applied for affiliation we should certainly consider such an application.[44]

This left only one option open to the INO: to form a new trade union, distinct from the existing organisation, and to fund it separately from the existing organisation. INO members provided the appropriate mandate to do so in 1980. Trade unions increasingly sought to represent general nurses at the time, which presented a challenge for the INO. It was forbidden for unions affiliated to congress to enlist members from other congress-affiliated unions, meaning that, as long as the INO remained outside of the ICTU, it could not prevent the poaching of its members. One present-day INO official, who, at the time worked for a different trade union, recounted a view among trade unionists that the INO was on its last legs – a skeleton that was having its bones picked by competitors.[45] Considering the unrest among some INO members, their sceptical and hostile view of the organisation's Executive Council, the fact that many remained unhappy with the 1980 arbitration award and the increasing competition from trade unions, the INO had little time to lose.

Efforts were underway to draft a trade union rule book by 1981. The new union was to be titled 'The Nurses' Union of Ireland', and an annual fee of £2 was levied on INO members from 1984 onwards. Some 6,600 members duly contributed the levy for the following three years, and the Nurses' Union of Ireland registered as a trade union in June 1986.[46] On 29 July 1988, the High Court, under Judge Mella Carroll (whom the INO would cross paths with again soon) ruled that the granting of a negotiating licence to the union 'would not be contrary to the public interest'.[47] P.J. Madden heaved a sigh of relief and recalled: 'I remember, and this is humorous, given that I am now a priest, but when we walked out of the High Court that day I said ... "I don't care what anybody else is doing, I am going over to Merchant's Quay to say a prayer of thanksgiving".'[48] But the organisation was not out of the woods just yet. The licence was issued with a proviso: '[that the union] works in close conjunction with the INO ... but is an entity separate and distinct from it'.[49] This created a legal and practical difficulty: if the INO was to remain independent of the Nurses' Union of Ireland, then the former would need to retain its excepted body status under the 1941 *Trade Union Act* in order to be recognised for negotiating purposes. In contrast, the latter could negotiate by way of its status as a licenced trade union. The proviso necessitated the organisation to think

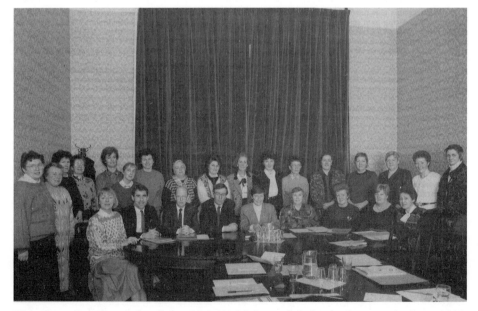

The Executive Council of the Nurses' Union of Ireland photographed in 1990. Courtesy INMO.

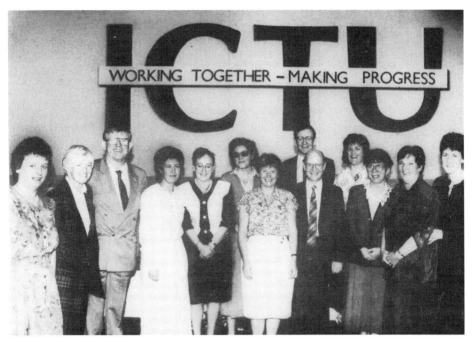

INO members and staff attending the ICTU Annual Congress in Killarney in 1991. Courtesy INMO.

outside the box. It did so, and in 1990, the Nurses' Union of Ireland craftily changed its name to the Irish Nurses' Organisation. The 'new' INO then proceeded seamlessly with all of the 'old' INO's activities with one important distinction: it was now a trade union.

Affiliation to congress, the INO's original aim, remained elusive. After years of economic recession, the government launched the Programme for National Recovery in 1987. This programme marked the beginning of over twenty years of tripartite social partnership between the government, congress and employers' representatives, but the INO was still not at the table. P.J. Madden met with a former president of congress in 1989 to ascertain the cause of the delay in granting the INO affiliation. Madden was informed that the 'biggest concern' was 'that the INO were opposed to strike' and could not take part in a general strike, should congress request one.[50] Madden assuaged these fears by furnishing the trade unionist with a copy of the INO's by-laws, which had been altered to permit industrial action following the pivotal meeting at Bundoran. Affiliation to congress was subsequently granted in 1990. The tortuous and protracted return to the trade union fray was not necessarily a bad thing, as it allowed members to accustom themselves to the 'new' INO. Liam Doran, who joined the organisation in 1983 as Student Officer and later became an industrial relations officer recalled:

> The biggest danger we face is getting detached from the average member, whatever, whoever the average member is. You can't be persuaded by the loudest in the room. They are not a barometer of what members want … You have got to look at the body of the room, you have got to look in their eyes almost and get a sense, what do they want most from their union at this time? … There is no point in pretending you are a leader if you look behind you and there is no one … there, right? We were always scared that while the delegates voted in [19]78 … are delegates fully reflective of your average member? … So it really was walk forward softly and walk forward gently, that we wouldn't frighten our own … Like we are still in the [19]80s and you are still talking about [19]80s Ireland and nursing; it is conservative … in the end, there was no internal dissension of any ilk but you were always wary of it so in that sense we proceeded very cautiously.[51]

As the INO was in the process of returning to its roots in trade unionism, members voiced their concerns as to whether the development would result in strike action. Their fears spoke to an age-old assumption that nurses' strikes and patient welfare were incompatible. This assumption was about to be tested.

IV. 'Is It Right? . . . 4 Patients In The Corridor': Health Cuts and their Ramifications

In time, the slogans on protesting nurses' and midwives' placards revealed a new source of discontent. At a protest march by nurses at St Luke's Hospital in Kilkenny, a placard read: 'Is It Right? . . . 4 Patients In The Corridor'.[52] The 1980s were characterised by a deep recession which resulted in severe cuts to the health service budget. Health spending, as a proportion of gross domestic product, fell from 7.72 per cent in 1980 to 7.04 per cent in 1985 and to 5.72 per cent in 1990;[53] the number of staff in the health service fell from 64,889 in 1981 to 57,275 in 1989,[54] and almost 3,500 acute care beds closed between 1983 and 1989.[55]

Cuts to the health budget in the 1980s affected nurses and midwives badly. Their own political ambivalence and relegation to a subordinate position within corporate power structures came home to roost. Student nurses were first in line for cuts and, in 1983, the North-Western Health Board proposed abolishing their meagre yearly salaries of £5,051 and paying them a training grant of £1,000 per annum instead.[56] By 1988, first-year student nurses had received a salary cut of £81, from £139 per week to just £58.[57] The move caused consternation. Indeed, cuts of this kind were partly responsible for a cohort of students staging a sleep-in on four wards at Beaumont Hospital, Dublin.[58] The INO challenged the pay cut, and the students ultimately had their original wages restored.[59] Over a decade after the *Report of the Commission on the Status of Women* recommended that women receive paid maternity leave, the Southern Health Board reportedly decided to 'disallow payment' of maternity leave to nurses.[60] Although the decision was reconsidered following protests by the INO, the Southern Health Board also reportedly declined to pay an ill, pregnant nurse during her sick leave because, in the board's opinion, pregnancy was 'not an illness'.[61]

Employers' ingenuity in cost saving knew no bounds, but it was the plight of patients that angered INO members the most. As early as 1926, the organisation's *Gazette* described an infirmary in England that employed

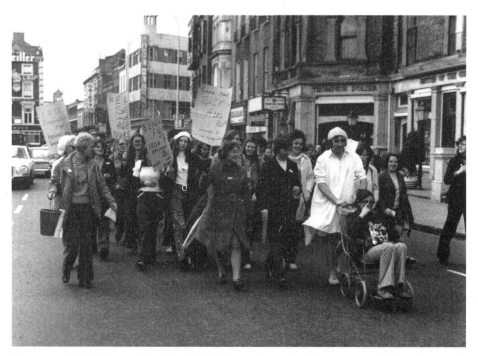

Marching in Dublin in aid of the INO's Benevolent Fund. Courtesy INMO/Copyright G.A. Duncan.

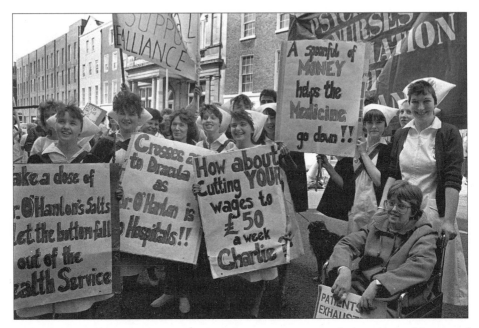

'How About?' A group of nurses and student nurses protest during the health cuts of the 1980s. The cut in payment to student nurses was particularly resented and is echoed in the placards. Courtesy Derek Speirs.

over thirty staff members for ninety-two patients. The piece noted that, in Ireland, some employers 'would faint if such numbers were suggested'.[62] Two patients were sharing one bed at Loughlinstown Fever Hospital, Dublin due to overcrowding by 1936,[63] and in 1943, there were reports of institutions with a bed-to-nurse ratio of 36:1.[64] By the early 1970s, reports of a 'row of beds' being placed in the middle of hospital wards were emerging.[65] The INO requested the establishment of a national bed bureau by 1976, and by 1977, it was furnishing the Department of Health with figures on overcrowding on a hospital-by-hospital basis.[66]

These years also witnessed the organisation's calling for the introduction of nurse-to-patient ratios and establishing a Committee on Overcrowding.[67] Kilkenny was a flashpoint; to ameliorate overcrowding of 'disastrous proportions' at St Luke's Hospital in 1978, the organisation proposed that only emergency cases be accepted, that an auxiliary hospital in Kilkenny be used to relieve the burden on St Luke's and that minor injuries be dealt with in casualty as opposed to the hospital's wards.[68] Nurses who were vexed at overcrowding at Kilkenny County Hospital also engaged in a work-to-rule and marched through Kilkenny City before delivering a protest letter to the South-Eastern Health Board. One nurse tried to capture the situation in a poem:

> We may seem to be hard when we hurry and fuss, But there's many of you, and too few of us. We would like far more time to sit by you and talk, To bath you and feed you and help you to walk, To hear of your lives and the things you have done; Your childhood, your husband, your daughter, your son. But time is against us, there's too much to do – Patients too many, and nurses too few.[69]

Some nurses feared that their institutions were so short-staffed that a patient might die yet remain undiscovered for a number of hours.[70] Unfortunately, the situation was not set to improve any time soon. In 1983, the Department of Health issued a diktat that two thirds of all vacancies arising in the civil service were to remain unfilled.[71] Facing unemployment, many nurses/midwives left Ireland altogether, and a number settled in the Middle East, earning the moniker 'Florence of Arabia'. The recruitment embargo and the flight of the nurses/midwives rendered the staffing problems more acute than ever.

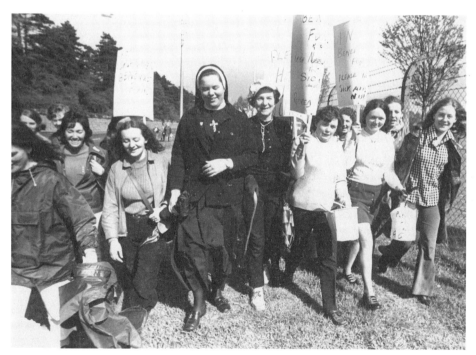

Marching in aid of the INO's Benevolent Fund. Courtesy INMO/copyright *Irish Press.*

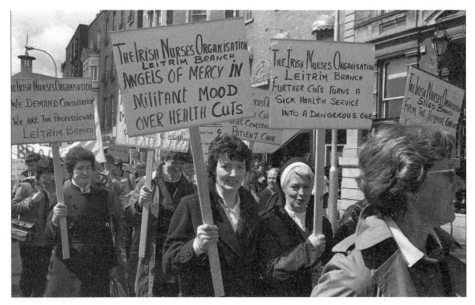

INO members protest over cuts to health services in the 1980s. Courtesy Derek Speirs.

As early as 1971, the INO submitted a resolution from its Annual General Meeting to the Minister for Health, Erskine Childers, recommending an examination of nurse staffing structures. The subsequent *Report of the Working Party on General Nursing*, not published until 1980, typified the snail's pace in these matters.[72] The INO's involvement in the report was clear, and many of its recommendations mirrored those that the organisation had been requesting for years: a more comprehensive nursing managerial structure, an increase in the number of public health nurses, the reorientation of public health nurses to a preventive health role and the employment of more ancillary staff. The publication of the report could not have come at a worse time, however, as the country was entering a period of dire financial straits. Minister for Health Michael Woods, addressing INO members in 1980, noted that his first intention was to commence a consultation process on the report's recommendations – his assurance that such a process did not merely represent kicking the ball further down the road was a case of protesting too much.[73]

The report's recommendation on staffing issues was particularly disappointing and concluded that it was 'not possible for the Working Party to be more precise [but] *nurse staffing levels should be more closely related to patient dependency needs and throughput and should be determined on a scientific basis*' [original emphasis].[74] Nurses and midwives were at a distinct disadvantage in meeting this recommendation. The Irish Nurses' Research Interest Group was formed in 1976, and the INO's efforts to inculcate members with an awareness of the scientific method was ongoing. The INO's *World of Irish Nursing* incorporated research reviews and a 'Research Corner' appeared in 1986. Yet, objectively derived data regarding the deleterious effects of short-staffing on patient outcomes remained many years away.

Staffing levels drove nurses' and midwives' dissatisfaction at the time, but a number of other annoyances also featured. Research into the adoption of the nursing process in Irish hospitals in the early 1980s showed that nurses were lamenting the demise of check lists and found care plans complex and difficult. Some also believed that mounting paperwork detracted from the provision of patient care: 'Care-plans that lasted for pages described an idyllic level of physical and psychological care … However, the prescribed two-hourly toileting for those confined to bed … often received a generous extension in reality. As the nurses … scribbled furiously the patients, unable to hold on, wet their beds.'[75] The organisation's exasperated Executive Council took an unprecedented step in 1982 and issued members with a proposal to refuse to accommodate patients on corridors from July 1982.[76] The decree rankled with rank-and-file members and was overturned at a meeting of branch representatives shortly afterwards.[77] This suggests that the organisation's new Executive Council was militant to an extent that was unpalatable to members. Said members evidently concluded that it was better to take care of patients in substandard conditions than to turn them away altogether.

Small wonder that stress in nursing soon became a subject of inquiry, and the Department of Health commissioned An Bord Altranais to conduct a study into the matter.[78] A total of 1,310 nurses were surveyed and, among the five most prominent stressors identified were 'inadequate staffing', 'being left short of staff at short notice' and 'being rushed all the time'.[79] The study recommended that 'the pressures (physical and psychological) under which nurses work must be recognised and steps must be taken to introduce procedures and methods to help nurses maintain standards of care'.[80] Revealingly, the study was never published, and representatives of the state largely continued to ignore or deny the INO's protests that cutbacks were having a deleterious effect on either patients or nurses/midwives. In an off-the-cuff remark in 1987, a representative of the Department of Health even commented on the 'many relaxed nurses' he encountered on his hospital visits.[81] What was the INO to do?

In the mid-1970s, student nurses from the Charitable Infirmary, Jervis Street, Dublin squared up against registered nurses from the same hospital in a charity football match. Funds raised contributed to the fledgling Faculty of

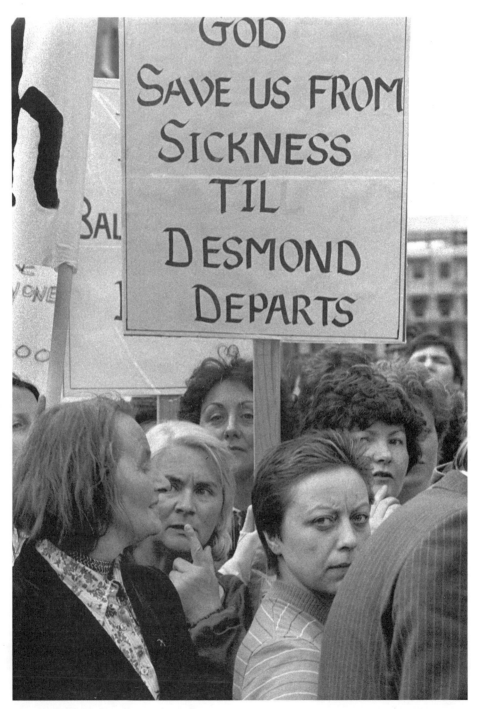

One protestor's placard at a march against health cuts in 1986 carried a personal message for the Minister for Health, Barry Desmond. Courtesy Derek Speirs.

Nursing at the RCSI. In a curious turn of events, the Chief Executive Officer of An Bord Altranais acted as linesman. In the years that followed, An Bord Altranais was to assume a different type of adjudication role. The board's 1988 *Code of Professional Conduct for each Nurse and Midwife* noted: 'Any circumstances which could place patients/clients in jeopardy or which militate against safe standards of practice, should be made known to appropriate persons or authorities.'[82] A breach of the code may have resulted in a nurse or midwife facing sanctions by the board's disciplinary or Fitness to Practise Committee. This effectively placed an obligation on INO members. Works-to-rule, marches and a multitude of coverage in the *World of Irish Nursing* had all failed to draw sufficient attention to the problem of short-staffing and effect a solution. The only option left was its most radical to date: a strike.

IV.I. St James' Day: The Dawn of Clinical Militancy

Frustration among INO members reached its peak at St James' Hospital, Dublin in 1989. That year, 98 per cent of nurses voted in favour of strike action at the 680-bed institution.[83] Reports suggested that some patients were spending up to twelve hours on trolleys and others could not leave the operating theatre for the want of an intensive care bed. One protesting nurse remarked: 'We are used to dealing with life and death; if the situation in the hospital continues it will be more death than life.'[84] The era of 'clinical militancy' had arrived. The INO had embraced the principles of scientific management in the 1960s, but in the recession of the 1980s, and amid severe short-staffing, the seemingly never-ending quest for efficiencies took its toll. In oral testimony, Kathleen Craughwell remarked:

> The patients at the beginning of my career [in the 1960s] were in hospital for months with, we will say, a urinary infection. I well remember old ladies there for a solid month ... Fast forward, the patients are hardly in bed now until they are discharged. The nurses hardly know their names ... The patient now becomes a series of things to be done ... Care is actually absent because they are not there long enough, most of them, for care ... the pressure on nurses to get things through the system is greater.[85]

Throughput and turnover became the new watchwords, with day-case activity rising from 2 per cent in 1980 to almost 40 per cent in the mid-to-late 1990s.[86] Indeed, the Manager of St James' is quoted as having described the institution as a 'factory where you turn the product over as quickly as possible and quality goes out of the system'.[87] In order to provide the requisite level of care, the INO requested the reopening of closed beds and the employment of fifty additional nurses. The hospital's managers made some accessions, but these were judged to be insufficient and the strike, which entailed the maintenance of emergency cover, proceeded on 18 July referred to as 'St James' Day' by the INO. The dispute was somewhat successful. The hospital agreed to establish a study on patient dependency levels, provide fourteen extra nursing positions, provide locum cover, convert a number of temporary nursing positions into permanent positions and reopen a ward in order to ease over-crowding.[88]

P.J. Madden was a key player in the organisation's increasing militancy. Madden was appointed General Secretary of the INO in the mid-1980s when his predecessor, John Pepper, left after two years in the post. He was a psychiatric nurse and former General Secretary of the Psychiatric Nurses' Association (PNA). As a young man he recounted being greatly influenced by a biography of James Larkin, subsequent to which he became active in trade unionism: 'I

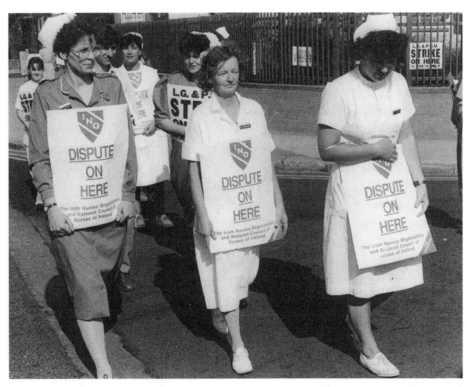

'St James' Day': INO members protesting on the picket line at St James' Hospital, Dublin. Courtesy INMO.

was young, I was brash, I thought I had the answer to everybody's problems including our own so I was essentially on what they would call the militant wing of the [Workers' Union of Ireland]' while working at St Brendan's Psychiatric Hospital, Dublin in the 1960s.[89] This informed a crucial difference between Madden and his predecessors, as he himself admitted: 'Key to understanding everything I stand for [is that nurses have] the right to withdraw [their] labour as any other worker has … I always insisted patient care, firstly, was a matter for management and, secondly, for those of us who are vicariously responsible on a daily basis.'[90] Madden also suggested an ulterior motive to the strike at St James' – that of reinforcing the INO's credibility as a trade union.

> On that morning we were outside St James' … a very well-known trade union official … drove his car along the picket line, stopped, opened his window and laughed across the road at us and then drove off. That was visible to everybody on the picket line that morning. That was the attitude that they had to us, that we were a joke.[91]

INO membership grew exponentially under Madden's leadership, from 9,000 in the mid-1980s to 23,000 in the late 1990s. The growth in members is all the more impressive considering that much of it occurred during a time of retrenchment in the health services. Growth was augmented by an expanding range of member services: indemnity insurance;[92] a salary protection scheme; a life assurance and car insurance scheme administered by Savings and Investments Limited (today known as Cornmarket Group Financial and still the primary provider of financial services to members); discounted health insurance rates; a low-interest rate loan scheme and, last but by no means least, discounted rail tickets which, evidence suggests, were tampered with by cash-strapped members in order that multiple trips could be taken on single tickets.

The organisation's new-found stridency also drove membership. Notwithstanding events at Bundoran in 1978, up to the late 1980s, nurses and midwives had broadly remained averse to strike action, with nurses assuming portering duties during a strike of porters at Dublin's Richmond Hospital in 1979[93] and INO members being among two cars of 'scab labour' that 'crashed the picket lines' during a strike at St Mary's Psychiatric Hospital, Castlebar, County Mayo, in 1983.[94] The latter incident was especially heated and ended up in court: those that passed the picket required a police escort off the campus and a nun was 'caught by the leg', 'abused', called a 'scab' and lost her shoe and handbag during the ruckus.[95] Bundoran was, therefore, something of a false dawn, as INO members remained conservative. It was only under Madden's leadership that a strike was first touted. Nonetheless, Madden remained aware that strike action still had the potential to unsettle members. When quizzed about his own qualms at the possible detrimental effects on patients of the strike at St James', he recalled vividly:

> I didn't show any of it publicly … However, when I did go home … I prayed intensely that night that no one would die in [St] James' on the day of the strike, that nobody would point a finger at a nurse and say, 'You allowed someone to die.' Because now I had my own inner conflict. But I knew we were doing the right thing … If management didn't see fit to meet the standards of care that we regarded as safe then we had a right to show that up … I would have never have been concerned in my conscience that I was responsible for the death of a patient. I just wouldn't want my members to live with the guilt or the fear that they had allowed it happen.[96]

The appointment of Madden to the position of INO General Secretary signified a changing of the organisation's old guard, reminiscent of the resignation of Kathleen Nora Price fifty years earlier. The decision to appoint a more vocal and forthright leader was an acknowledgement of the changing and increasingly challenging environment in which members found themselves. Madden was instrumental in beginning a much-warranted sea change among INO members with regard to employment rights. The *Connacht Tribune* once carried a story in which it was alleged that nurses at Galway Regional Hospital had been physically assaulted: 'Nuns have actually slapped student nurses across the face for minor misdemeanours.'[97] Elsewhere, the father of a student nurse at a Dublin hospital wrote to An Bord Altranais in 1978 and took issue with the 'indignity' caused by the 'inspection of girls' nickers [*sic*]' at the institution.[98] One student nurse was even likened to a prostitute and suspended for putting highlights in her hair, that is, until her mother, a journalist, showed up at the hospital's matron's office wearing her press badge and looking for answers.[99] These incidents underscored a need for increased education of INO members with regard to employment rights, and Madden instituted training courses in employment rights for INO representatives nationally. A rights-based approach to industrial relations soon took over, as recalled by Noreen Muldoon, INO Industrial Relations Officer in the Mid-Western Region:

> It was very, very hands on and the hours were extremely long [but] you had to put them in because you wouldn't get the work done otherwise … It was

extremely demanding ... It was like firefighting in a lot of senses because you got a call [and] you had to react to that immediately ... But it was extremely fulfilling ... You were utilising the law ... you were working within the law in a piece of legislation that you were using in taking [a] case. And I was very successful, I don't mind saying it myself ... I did achieve quite a lot for people at various stages throughout.[100]

Soon a more knowledgeable, belligerent and vocal INO began to appear. In the past, the organisation strove to resolve industrial relations issues as informally as possible: 'Everything was done and dusted over a cup of tea.'[101] This soon evaporated and one hospital matron, recalling her dealings with an INO Industrial Relations Officer, reminisced: 'I thought Jesus, what did I ever do to deserve you? Will no one here give me a break.'[102] Madden recalled with satisfaction: 'Now [members] began to see themselves as professionals with rights ... no longer women in service.'[103]

CHAPTER 10

Resemblance amid Rupture: The 1999 National Nurses' Strike, 1991–9

The writer and poet Micheál Mac Liammóir once remarked on his time as a patient at Dublin's Meath Hospital: 'Hospital is a purgatory-stage managed by angelic beings. One would hardly be surprised to see wings pushing their way through coats and aprons. In fact I believe I did on more than one occasion.'[1] Mac Liammóir's remarks were flattering and well-intentioned, but historic caricatures of nurses as angels are open to question. Unlike the overwhelming majority of nurses, the named angels in the Bible were male. Furthermore, not all angels were necessarily virtuous, with one third rebelling against God and falling from grace.[2] The analogy had been stretched to its absolute limit by the early 1990s. Reminiscing on what was a seminal decade for the INO, Lenore Mrkwicka, Deputy General Secretary of the organisation recalled: 'I don't know if it was on the back of a bus down in Clonmel or up on a pig lorry … I said … we are nurses, we are professional people. Being an angel, lovely, thanks for calling me an angel, but that doesn't pay the bloody bills.'[3]

I. Resolve Hardens: The Path to the Commission on Nursing

The INO affiliated to the ICTU in 1990. At that time, the congress, the government and employers were party to an evolving series of tripartite agreements referred to as social partnership. The particular agreement in operation in 1994 was known as the *Programme for Competitiveness and Work*.[4] The programme presented a challenge for the INO, as it stipulated that only 'a single cost increasing claim for an amount not exceeding 3 per cent of the basic pay cost of [a] group of employees' was permissible.[5] The INO had lodged a claim that included a salary increase of up to 19 per cent for staff nurses/midwives and 28 per cent for ward sisters. The organisation also lodged claims for a long-service salary increment, salary increases for those qualified

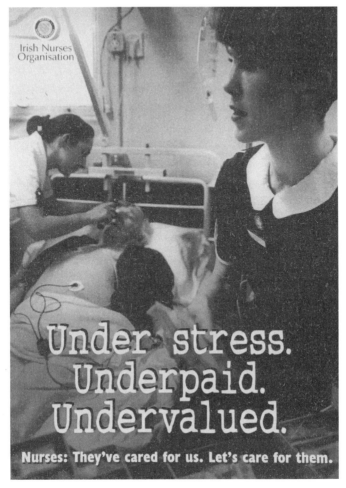

One of the iconic INO billboard posters used in the run-up to the 1999 national nurses' strike. Courtesy INMO.

in two divisions of the register,[6] allowances for members working in certain clinical areas, the introduction of a clinical specialist grade and changes to annual leave entitlements. The requested improvements to annual leave alone would account for 2 per cent of the overall payroll.[7] Liam Doran, who was slowly working his way up the organisation's ranks, remarked: '[the] difference between our perspective of this pay claim and Management's could hardly be greater.'[8]

INO members were not alone in their frustration, and a federation of trade unions, representing some 26,000 nurses and midwives, came together in pursuit of improved working conditions. The federation, known as the Nursing Alliance, comprised the INO as the largest affiliate, with the PNA, the Services, Industrial, Professional and Technical Union (SIPTU) and the Irish Municipal, Public and Civil Trade Union (IMPACT). In a continuation of the increased militancy of the INO, it balloted members seeking a mandate for a series of nationwide work stoppages, due to commence in March 1996. The Minister for Health, Michael Noonan, proved unflinching and reiterated that improvements in nurses' and midwives' conditions could only be achieved within the stipulations of the *Programme for Competitiveness and Work*. Nonetheless, the state advanced a new salary proposal in February that year. The proposal merely provided for cost of living increases for most and, in a ballot, over 99 per cent of INO members rejected it.[9]

The Labour Relations Commission then intervened, and a new proposal was devised. The proposal concerned salary and non-salary related matters including continuing education. The INO sent details of the proposal to its 20,000 members and the organisation's Executive Council, along with three other unions in the Nursing Alliance, recommended that it be accepted. Ninety per cent of members did not agree. A particular grievance was the plan to introduce a lower salary for newly qualified nurses and a lack of appreciable increase in staff nurses'/midwives' and nurse/midwife managers' salaries. Liam Doran recalled the turn of events:

> We became a victim of our own rhetoric ... I suppose it can be written about now, the thirty year rule could nearly apply ... [but] members told us quite clearly that they weren't having it, which of course made a final settlement all the more difficult to get because then you had the double whammy of the employer being offside with the members [and the union being] offside with the members. So who was their friend and where is that ring of confidence? ... So we were in the worst of all spaces ... Behind closed doors it obviously rattled us ... So yes it was a steep learning curve and a sobering event.[10]

A belief among members that the organisation's Executive Council vacillated in its pursuit of improved conditions, at this point, may have resulted in member attrition or defection to competitor unions. Doran was keen to assuage the concerns of the rank and file: 'The outcome of this ballot ... will only serve to strengthen the [organisation's] negotiating stance ... the message conveyed in this unprecedented rejection vote has been heard.'[11] Militancy continued to rise. At the organisation's Annual Meeting in 1996 (by then trading as the

Annual Delegate Conference), it was resolved to ballot members on a proposal to withdraw all but essential services, failing progress on the organisation's pay claim. This threat resonated with the government. Following the conference, an Adjudication Board was proposed to examine a number of grievances and to make non-binding recommendations. INO members were balloted on the proposal, and three quarters expressed their support for it.[12]

The board's recommendations, generally referred to as the *Blue Book Agreement*, were not quite as salacious as the title suggests, but its contents did represent something of a turn-on: significant salary increases for those in managerial, public health and teaching posts; restructuring and rationalisation of managerial posts; developments in education; an increased role for nurses/ midwives in policymaking and the move from temporary contracts to permanent contracts for some 1,700 nurses/midwives.[13] Liam Doran rightly referred to the recommendations as 'far-reaching' and a 'vast improvement' on the former offer.[14] After all, some nurses had been on temporary contracts for almost forty years:

> I qualified as a [general nurse] in 1960 and a midwife in 1962 … I have been on the temporary staff in [n. hospital] from 1973 to [1997] and in the intervening years applied four times for a permanent post and was unsuccessful … I feel I gave 100 per cent to my job whatever it was, going out in the ambulance to do emergency runs, delivering babies … looking after our elderly patients and I never had a complaint made against me so I can assure you my morale was very low after each time I was rejected.[15]

In spite of Doran's relatively upbeat assessment, the proposals were not far-reaching enough, and 60 per cent of INO members rejected them.[16] The level of vexation at the time among INO members was somewhat unique considering that the PNA and the SIPTU accepted the proposals. In total, 97 per cent of INO members balloted then voted to commence a national strike.[17] In the union's early days, the prospect of sympathetic striking detracted some from membership of the organisation. Now, in a remarkable turn of events, the PNA, the SIPTU and the IMPACT union issued strike notice in support of the INO. The Labour Court intervened and, on 7 February 1997, three days prior to the proposed action, issued a seminal recommendation, which noted that the 'size of the vote for strike is an indication of the anger and frustration felt by nurses, which cannot be ignored'.[18] The court conceded that nurses' '[salary] scales have fallen significantly behind other groups' and proposed a number of remedies.[19] Chief among these were a new salary scale for staff nurses/midwives including a long service increment and the conversion of 2,000 temporary posts to permanent ones. The most far-reaching of the court's recommendations concerned the establishment of a Commission on Nursing in order to investigate and make recommendations on a number of outstanding issues in the professions. P.J. Madden recalled:

> [It] went down to the wire … It was rather frightening actually to watch full page ads in the national [newspapers] telling people … there was now a strike by nurses going to happen … And at the eleventh hour [a representative of the Government] came to me and he said, 'I give you a Government Commission on Nursing … and I will give you someone that you believe in' … He knew I had a view on Mella Carroll which I had expressed at the time we received our [negotiating] license. He said, 'I will give you a High Court Judge to chair it, now I can't do more than that' … We debated it, there was a terrible tension at that meeting, but we eventually agreed we would call off the strike if we got the Commission on Nursing.[20]

The proposal that the INO rejected in early 1996 was worth £20 million. Later that same year, following intervention by the Labour Relations Commission, INO members rejected a revised proposal worth £37 million. In 1997, INO members rejected proposals arrived at by an Adjudication Board worth an estimated £53 million. Members had also voted overwhelmingly in favour of strike action. While their resolve and increasing militancy were clear, the organisation's Executive Council decided to defer the strike. Many members were unhappy with the decision and INO President, Anne Cody, recalled that the organisation's headquarters was inundated with complaints by members.[21] Yet, on that occasion, the Executive Council displayed a better judgement of members' mood, as the rank and file voted by a two-thirds majority to accept the court's recommendations.[22] But members' acceptance of the court's recommendations came with a proviso – that the Commission on Nursing's recommendations should be implemented in their entirety.

I.I. The Commission on Nursing

The advent of the Commission on Nursing was unlike the qualified successes that characterised the INO in the past. The commission, and the mammoth changes that ultimately flowed from it, owed mainly to the INO which, unlike other unions, rejected the recommendations of the Adjudication Board and set in train the threat of strike thereafter. It was fitting that P.J. Madden and Eilish Hardiman, an INO representative, were appointed as commission members. The INO's submission to the commission was a comprehensive one, almost forty pages of which concerned professional and educational issues such as nurses'/midwives'/care assistants' roles, skill mix, career pathways, An Bord Altranais, hospital planning and nurse/midwife management and education.[23] Twenty pages of the INO's submission also concerned pay and an appeal that 'the Commission must realise that the basic pay levels of nurses remains a very real issue' [original emphasis].[24]

The threat of militancy lit a fire under the commission's progress and, unlike the Working Party in the 1970s, it worked at remarkable speed. However, the commission's interim report, published in October 1997, caused some concern to the INO, which expressed its belief that issues regarding pay had not received sufficient attention. Liam Doran reminded the commission that the Nursing Alliance actively anticipated a revision of staff nurses'/midwives' salary scales and warned that 'the anger, frustration and disenchantment of nurses was put on hold by the creation of this Commission and will quickly return and re-surface if these long existing and widely known anomalies in pay and conditions are not addressed'.[25] The organisation also began readying itself in case members' pay was not given sufficient credence and, from 1997, a portion of members' subscriptions was diverted to a strike fund.

The following year, the organisation began to devise a national strike strategy. The organisation's Executive Council proposed that, in the event of a strike, routine home visits, elective hospital admissions and elective surgical procedures would cease, and outpatient appointments and day hospital activities would be suspended.[26] Members' involvement in the administration of intravenous medication would also cease. In a sign of the tensions that would soon become more apparent, some members expressed unease with a withdrawal from the administration of intravenous medication, which they believed was an essential service.[27] While overall militancy continued to rise, members clearly found themselves at different points on the continuum. As the commission produced its report, P.J. Madden resigned from the INO and Liam Doran assumed the position of General Secretary. Madden's wife had developed cancer, and this prompted him to take a step back from the busy schedule of trade union leadership. In his last editorial in the *World of Irish Nursing*, he quoted poet Alfred Tennyson: 'The old order changeth, yielding place to new'.[28] He could not have known that his choice of quote had a wider applicability. Soon the once strike-shy INO would be the central protagonist in one of the biggest strikes in Irish history.

II. The Prelude to Strike Action

The *Report of the Commission on Nursing* was presented to the Minister for Health and Children, Brian Cowen, in July 1998. Subsequent events suggested that the new Fianna Fáil-led administration, of which Cowen was a member, did not subscribe to the commission to the same extent as the previous administration. P.J. Madden recalled: 'The Department [of Health] essentially sold out the moment the ink was dry, I am certain of that. But then our experience in the Department all down through the years in negotiation has always been get us in, get us to a point where we believed something was going to be done and then they'd back off.'[29]

The report was the most insightful and progressive document ever to address nursing and midwifery issues in Ireland and made diverse and sweeping recommendations in the professional sphere. The role of An Bord Altranais would be revised; a pre-registration degree in nursing would be established; applications for pre-registration nurse education were to be made via a Central Applications Office; a National Council for the Professional Development of Nursing and Midwifery was to be established in order to oversee post-registration professional development; nurses and midwives would receive paid study leave; a clinical and managerial career pathway would be instituted and nurses/midwives were to be given greater responsibility and control.[30]

The report's recommendations in the industrial sphere were a little less tangible. Long service increments and annual leave were to be examined 'through the established structures',[31] and dual qualified and location allowances were to be referred to the Labour Court.[32] The commission found that 'current pay structures seriously mitigate against encouraging nurses to avail of promotional opportunities' and recommended that the issue of differentials between basic and managerial grades 'be examined as a matter of urgency, before the end of December 1998'.[33] While some of the commission's recommendations had a timescale, the rest were to be implemented 'as soon as practicable and in any event by the end of 2002'.[34] This remained some four years away, and the overall tenor of the report was, therefore, familiar to INO members who had grown used to their claims being long-fingered. Disappointment began to set in, but any industrial action was put on hold, pending the fate of three key grievances: an extension of the staff nurse/midwife salary scale through the addition of long service increments, improved allowances for those with dual qualifications or working in certain clinical areas and salary increases for managerial grades. Labour Court Recommendation 16083, issued in February

1999, recommended increases in the allowance paid to nurses in certain clinical areas and recommended an extension in the dual qualified allowance to incorporate midwives and sick children's nurses.[35]

Labour Court Recommendation 16084 was more equivocal and recommended further discussions between the Nursing Alliance and employers regarding long service increments and the salary of managerial grades.[36] The INO decided to partake in these discussions, and Doran again attempted to assuage members' concerns. In an editorial in the *World of Irish Nursing* in March 1999, he asked that members support the decision and reassured them that their 'anger and frustration' was understood.[37] It was labourist rather than socialist tendencies that led Doran toward a career in trade unionism. He recalls that his father contracted tuberculosis, underwent a pneumonectomy and spent two years at a Dublin Sanatorium in the mid 1950s. Upon discharge, and much weakened, his father assumed a number of kitchen and cleaning jobs, and the family moved to Surrey, England in search of employment in the early 1960s before returning to Ireland for good in 1974. Liam, an only child, recalled:

> My family, I am happy and proud to say, were the definition of … working class people … We lived in a two-bedroomed flat … we shared a toilet with people … and we came home to Ireland for six weeks each year on the boat [because we] couldn't afford the plane ... And I don't mean that in a God love us [way because I] never wanted for anything … [but] they were hard working people, paid every pound of tax … never on the dole … I suppose when I started work … I would immediately always veer on the side of what is the staff side's view[?] … It is just being brought up to appreciate the value of a pound … Am I convert to Lenin or Marxism, I don't really think so. It is more pragmatic with me.[38]

Media portrayals of Doran as strike-ready[39] are overstated. He is cautious and moderate and prefers conciliation to conflict: 'I am risk averse, although I might not look like it, but I am.'[40] At the age of forty-one, in the lead-up to the 1999 national nurses' strike, Doran was still learning the ropes: 'One of the things that will vividly live in my mind was waking up and getting the 6:30am headlines in the Mespil Hotel … I'm twelve months into a job as General Secretary. I am about to put … 32,000 people on strike … So yes you can sing it, I was extremely concerned, isolated, lonely.'[41]

The strike's occurrence was becoming a foregone conclusion, and Doran's attempts to mollify members were largely in vain – talks between unions and employers broke down after just one day. INO members' frustration grew, and some delegates had to be pleaded with not to walk out following an address by the Minister for Health and Children at the organisation's Annual Conference in 1999. The mood of members was synopsised by Anne Cody, INO President, when she declared: 'If, in order to secure [satisfactory remuneration] we have to engage in industrial action, then so be it.'[42] At the time, Cody was Theatre Sister at Dublin's Mater Hospital, where she also trained. She studied midwifery at the Rotunda Hospital, Dublin after qualification as a nurse. An avid poker player, she is from Roscrea, County Tipperary, and was the first INO president in many years to come from a non-senior managerial background. The changes in the organisation's leadership did not end there.

Dave Hughes joined the INO as Director of Industrial Relations in 1999. Hughes brought a wealth of experience in trade unionism, including militant trade unionism, with him and recounted that a branch of the ITGWU, for which he had once worked, was known as 'dial-a-strike'.[43] He recalls arriving at the INO during a 'revolutionary' period and rode shotgun to Doran and Lenore Mrkwicka during the dispute, the causes for which he asserts, were multifaceted: 'Like all nursing disputes pay is only part of it, it is never really just about pay. It is usually about a huge sense of demoralisation.'[44] Contributing to this was a consistent

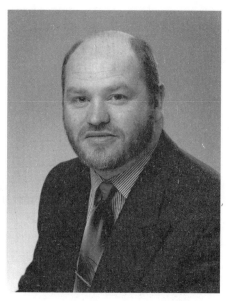

Dave Hughes. Courtesy INMO.

trend in employers procrastinating on or refusing to implement improvements in nurses'/midwives' conditions, even when those employers had previously agreed to them. Hughes, with characteristic candour, recalled:

> It is very hard to get [employers] to do what they agree in terms of nursing. Why, I still don't know, but … you have to fight with them to implement it … I was eighteen years a trade union official at that stage, and the idea that an employer would agree something and [not implement it] was an outrage to me … I was furious [at one such incident] and I can recall talking to Liam

Doran … and saying, 'these people have to be taught a lesson, your members are being treated like shite, nobody is going to do that to me … That is not going to happen, we are going to have to do something.' And Liam was already at that point anyway and we started working towards a national strike at that stage.[45]

Other issues were also exercising INO members' patience. Ireland witnessed a marked improvement in its economic fortunes in the 1990s and experienced economic growth of up to 9 per cent per year and a low rate of unemployment of 2 per cent.[46] Government budget surpluses became commonplace. But the 'Celtic Tiger' brought with it inflation and spiralling house prices. A host of public and political scandals were also emerging, chief among which concerned the former Taoiseach Charles Haughey. Haughey had been the subject of INO members' anger during the pay campaign of the late 1970s when he was Minister for Health. In the midst of that campaign, he made an infamous televised address to the nation in which he urged fiscal rectitude: 'We are living away beyond our means.' In spite of his utterances, in the late 1990s and in the middle of the INO's pay campaign, details regarding Haughey's own 'ostentatiously lavish way of life' began to emerge through a series of investigative tribunals.[47] It was claimed that he had spent £15,000 at an exclusive Parisian tailor , where the cost of a shirt, in 1999, was up to £350;[48] this exceeded the annual special allowance of £333 paid to nurses working in oncology and intensive care units. Moreover, it was reported that £15,000 of taxpayers' money had, over a period of time, been spent at an exclusive Dublin eatery by Haughey and that the then Taoiseach, Bertie Ahern, had signed the cheques to pay the bill.[49] This figure matched the £15,300 salary paid to newly qualified nurses in 1999. These revelations did little to placate nurses and midwives, who railed: 'When Brian [Cowen] and Bertie [Ahern] get shirty, we'll play dirty' and 'we only want what we deserve Bertie, we're not asking you to write a blank cheque'.[50]

The Labour Court issued fresh recommendations on 31 August 1999.[51] The recommendations represented a pay award valued at £100 million, including a £1,250 lump sum to every nurse and midwife in the state, conditional on the proposals' acceptance. It did not recommend any long service increment for staff nurses/midwives. Dave Hughes, likely remembering how badly the INO had misjudged its members' mood in the recent past, recalled:

On the morning when the Labour Court Recommendation came out … Liam said, 'what should we do?' I said, 'Liam we have no choice, this has to happen.

A Century of Service

This will not be accepted and if we go out with a recommendation for it we are going to split the membership … we have to keep them unified; they will be unified around a rejection, they won't be unified around an acceptance. It will just split them and we will never get them back.[52]

The INO's Executive Council recommended that members reject the proposals. The PNA and the SIPTU did likewise. All of the unions had correctly read the mood of their members. Nurses/midwives voted by a nine to one majority to reject the deal,[53] and 95 per cent of INO members who cast votes voted for strike action.[54] This was the most resounding endorsement of strike action of any of the unions in the Nursing Alliance.[55] Some 2,100 new members joined the INO at the time and the organisation's membership swelled to 25,000. A strike committee, comprising nurses and midwives, was established at each hospital in order to coordinate the deployment of services during the dispute, with a plan to maintain an unpaid nursing/midwifery service consistent with night-time staffing arrangements. The provision of essential and emergency services would be maintained as normal. Anne Cody recalled:

I was petrified. I was [INO] President at the time and I remember thinking, what are we leading them into and how do we lead them out of it? … There was this thing building up within the membership that we have to go on strike, we have to show our mettle … I remember when I became President [of the INO], the President of the International Council of Nurses, Kirsten Stallknecht,[56] … I remember talking to her and giving her the background to our industrial dispute … she said, 'From what you are telling me your members will not be satisfied until they go on strike, and once they've gone on strike they won't be rushing in to do it again.' And that's what happened.[57]

III. 'Black Tuesday'

On the eve of the strike, Brian Cowen wrote a piece in the *Irish Independent* declaring that the proposed action was an 'attack' on social partnership, that it threatened the Irish economy and reminded readers that any concessions made to nurses would incur 'a domino effect' in other occupational sectors.[58] Cowen's admission, however unpalatable, had substance: 'The conundrum that has haunted us,' attests Liam Doran, 'is called social partnership':

[because] whenever we tried to do something, which changed the relative position of nursing in the value chain, the walls of public sector bureaucracy

closes very rapidly to prevent anyone from moving up the value of the food chain ... The truth be known, [one day before the strike a representative from another union] said, 'Let it be known any increases nurses get out of this strike, we will come looking for, for other health professionals' ... So automatically then the government could say, well this isn't really about nurses, there will be consequentials.[59]

The strike commenced at over 1,000 locations nationwide at 8 a.m. on Tuesday, 19 October 1999, referred to as 'Black Tuesday' by the INO. A commentary piece in the *Irish Independent* in the days preceding the dispute noted: 'People will suffer grievously. Some may die.'[60] Few commentators thought to question why, if nursing and midwifery were of such critical life-or-death importance, nurses and midwives were not paid a salary that reflected such grave responsibility.[61] Concerns about the possible adverse consequences of the strike focused on two clinical specialities: oncology and paediatrics. The administration of intravenous medication was proscribed during the strike, and the care of patients requiring chemotherapy for cancer became a focal

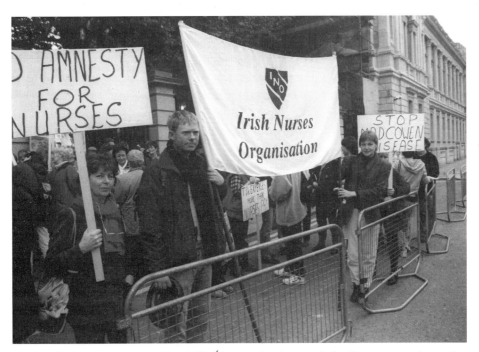

INO members protest outside Dáil Éireann in the week leading up to the strike. Courtesy INMO.

point. Two oncologists wrote to the national press: 'The strike, if it proceeds, will result in substantial physical and psychological suffering for many of our patients with cancer, and may hasten the deaths of others.'[62]

Our Lady's Hospital for Sick Children, Crumlin, Dublin, became the focus of intense media scrutiny. Dr Roisin Healy, a doctor at the hospital, spoke on *Morning Ireland*, Ireland's most popular radio news programme and, in light of nurses' withdrawal from intravenous duties, reportedly referred to doctors 'having to *stab* the children' [emphasis added] to insert intravenous cannulae[63] and questioned 'how nurses can ethically defend what is happening'.[64] Healy's intervention was attended by a small avalanche of media coverage concerning phlebotomy and cannulation in children. One piece referred to fears that children undergoing venepuncture would be deprived of the 'practised gentleness' of a nurse,[65] and one parent worried that a doctor, not a nurse, was going to take blood from her daughter: 'If they can't get a vein it will be very stressful.'[66] Liam Doran recalled Healy's radio interview and her choice of terminology:

> Let's be quite clear [here is where] the harder side of me comes out. I think that [comment] was totally unwarranted, totally untrue, totally unnecessary [and] totally misguided ... it got huge attention because it was Crumlin Hospital ... So then, and now, I didn't think there was any grounds for Dr Healy's comments. I will stand over anything and everything that every nurse did in Crumlin. I don't think you will find any nurse in Crumlin who doesn't put the child before anything ... So you can probably guess from me that I don't have a great deal of time for Dr Healy's strategies over those days.[67]

The strike was generating considerable public attention, dominating the main media outlets; media coverage was infused with hypothetical scenarios and highly emotive (if not alarmist) language that attributed both suffering and, possibly, death to nurses' and midwives' actions. Was this actually the case?

III.I. When is a Strike not a Strike?

At its first Annual Meeting in 1920, a spokesperson for the INU noted: 'There is no actual provision for a strike laid down in our rules and should drastic action be necessary ... in no case would the patient be allowed to suffer.'[68] By 1999, little had changed. Firstly, INO members defied the organisation's guidelines when they believed that it was in patients' interests. One recalled:

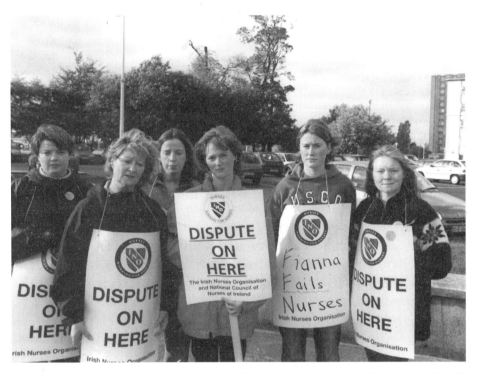

Striking nurses at St Vincent's Hospital, Dublin: Martina Meenaghan, Bernadette Farrell, Marian Fehily, Ciara Slattery, Olivia Kenneally and Susanne Williamson. Copyright Anne Henrichsen.

I found it to be a very difficult time … I worked in the area of oncology … and the agreement had been that nurses wouldn't give [intravenous medications] … [I] was assigned a patient who was very ill and who required [intravenous medications] … And this woman, I can still see her, she was only young, she was like twenty-five years old and she was miserable … I said, 'I am going to give her medicines' … [The patient] was so incredibly grateful … she said to me she understood the nurses were in a difficult situation … And I met her about a year later shopping … she came over to me and she said, 'I will never forget what you did.' Now, what was that worth? That was worth everything.[69]

Secondly, the roles that INO members jettisoned were those that could be performed by others; i.e., the strike was engineered to have as little impact as possible on patients. Liam Doran explains that the organisation 'had to err on the side of caution … The [intravenous medication] was one [role] where we always felt that the doctors could do them … [but] if that couldn't be done, say there wasn't enough [doctors] to do it, you would have to step into the breach … never losing sight that the patient wasn't to be blamed for the strike.'[70] Thirdly, much commentary in relation to the strike lacked substantiation. According to the *Sunday Tribune*, '*Consultants claimed*' [emphasis added] that nurses at Tullamore General Hospital, County Offaly, were refusing to prepare drugs for patients undergoing emergency surgery 'unless their hearts stopped'.[71] A piece in the *Sunday Independent* noted '*it's said that* nurses stood by as doctors fumbled to insert a tube into the chest cavity of a child who was struggling to breathe' [emphasis added].[72]

These anonymous reports are in stark conflict with others, which show, for instance, that midwives at Dublin's National Maternity Hospital maintained normal staffing levels, without pay, at the antenatal, neonatal and labour wards.[73] A girl who was involved in a road traffic accident and brought to Sligo General Hospital was ventilated and airlifted to a hospital in Dublin. She was accompanied on the flight by a specialist intensive care nurse who left the picket line to do so.[74] On the third day of the strike, some 10,000 nurses and midwives marched in protest in Dublin. As the march was about to begin,

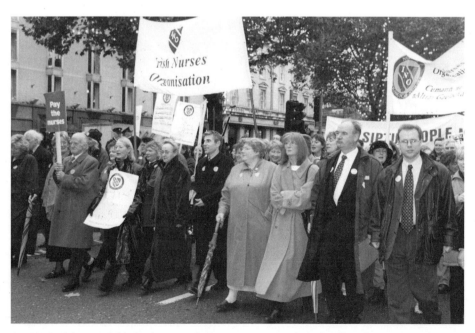

An INO delegation leads the way during a mass march and rally of 10,000 nurses and midwives in Dublin during the strike. Courtesy INMO.

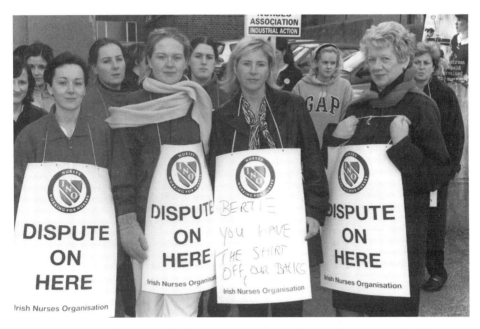

Striking INO members one of whom carries a personal and witty message for Taoiseach Bertie Ahern. Courtesy INMO.

some marchers reportedly tended to a pregnant woman they discovered haemorrhaging in a city restaurant.[75] One nurse interviewed following the strike maintained that some patients were unaware that a strike was even taking place.[76] INO President, Anne Cody, recalled:

> A [patient] was brought into [n. hospital] with chest pain and it turned out that he had a dissecting aneurysm. The nursing team that were on duty running the hospital were contacted immediately … [They] physically took that man and pushed him in his trolley up to the [Cardiac Catheterisation Laboratory] and he had his angiogram. Then [they] physically took him to theatre where he had his surgery and on to intensive care. Now I firmly believe that if it had been a normal working day, the [Laboratory] would have been busy [and] the theatre would have been busy.[77]

A patient receiving chemotherapy telephoned a popular Irish radio phone-in programme and maintained that, even if she died because of the strike, her family would still support the nurses.[78] One matron at a large teaching hospital recounted:

You are part of the management team and you are in a union. How do you function? I had that dilemma when I was Director of Nursing at [n. hospital] … But I did go out and stand outside with them on the picket line, took them out coffee … and was as much a part [with] them as I could be. With the result that when the strike was over there was no animosity because one of the things I truly believed in was, tomorrow, I was going to have to work with all of these people again.[79]

What is not apparent in the matron's testimony is a disproportionate concern for patient welfare considering the unfolding events:

I was in favour of the strike … provided no patient suffered … I don't think I slept a wink for that whole week … I would have to say I had concerns but I had great trust in the staff, I knew with hand on heart that there was no patient going to suffer … The [union representatives] were super … I would have to say it brought out the best in the nurses we had.[80]

P.J. Madden brought a markedly different perspective on strike action to the INO than his predecessors. Madden's wife, in a poignant turn of events, was critically ill and receiving chemotherapy during the strike. Madden explained plaintively:

During the year of the actual strike my wife died and during her last three weeks of life, during that strike, my wife was denied hospice nursing care in our home … I had to say this is exactly what it was all about, I couldn't claim any special privilege … but I will say this, that in an informal capacity, a wonderful woman, the President of the INO during the strike … Anne Cody … privately came to my home and dressed my wife's wounds when she wasn't on picket duty, which I will always be grateful for.[81]

Cody elaborated:

Yes I did. At the time, Lenore Mrkwicka was the Deputy General Secretary, and Lenore came to me and she said … 'What are we going to do?' And I said, 'You and I are going to deal with this' … The Public Health Nurses had left everything in the house, the dressings, everything that was required … and Lenore and I went out and did the dressings. Not many people know that, and I don't mind if people know it, they can say that the President [of the INO] broke the strike but I knew Mary Madden and I knew how ill she was and I said, 'No we can't leave this woman.' And I am sure if the truth be known there were nurses all over the country that knew similar situations and probably went in and did the dressings … You can't leave anybody suffering and I don't think patients were neglected because I firmly believe that other nurses did what I did but they are not saying it.[82]

The 1988 *Code of Professional Conduct for each Nurse and Midwife*, drafted by An Bord Altranais, stipulated that nursing 'demands a high standard of professional behaviour'.[83] It would be expected, strike or no strike, that any deviation from this high standard would result in nurses and midwives being reported to the board's Fitness to Practise Committee. After all, in 1983, 281 nurses were reported to the board for alleged misconduct – all of the nurses involved in an industrial dispute at one particular hospital were reported.[84] Yet the board did not experience the deluge of complaints regarding dereliction of duty that media commentary might have led the public to believe was taking place. In 1998, the Fitness to Practise Committee of An Bord Altranais considered applications into the fitness to practise of twenty-nine nurses.[85] In 1999, the year of the strike, the committee considered applications into the fitness to practise of eight nurses.[86]

IV. Exaltation Turns to Exploitation

'Nurses really got the bit between their teeth … They were the best I had ever seen at any union I had been in, they certainly learned very quickly, they formed really authoritative strike committees … They were very conscious of maintaining their high standing within the community', said Dave Hughes when recounting the strike.[87] He continued:

> There was still an awful lot of support for nurses, the public were still on their side, and they were very keen that they wouldn't lose that. So these were the things that preoccupied them … Our biggest fear was that patients would die and the Government would blame us. I still have a strong suspicion that Government actually would have liked something catastrophic to happen … and for us to be buried. Certainly at the time it felt that way.[88]

Members' efforts paid dividends, and the results of a survey undertaken by the *Sunday Independent* showed that 66 per cent of the public supported nurses in their decision to strike.[89]

The widespread public support for strikers suggests that they were in a strong bargaining position, but nothing could have been further from the truth, as the INO's decision to provide essential services, without pay, left members open to exploitation. Without so much as a smidgeon of hyperbole, a 'bedmaking crisis' of 'critical' proportions was reported at Mayo General Hospital and the County Hospital, Roscommon, where managers, it appears, fully anticipated that unpaid, striking nurses would continue to make beds as, in the managers' opinion, 'emergency care involved not only agreeing to admit seriously ill patients but agreeing to make all preparations necessary [including] getting a bed ready'.[90] The INO issued a swift rebuke and a reminder that making beds was not an essential service. Noreen Muldoon, INO Industrial Relations Officer, elaborated:

> Difficulties arose because management in some areas wouldn't accept that this was an actual strike and it was a withdrawal of labour and their expectations were totally different to what the unions, our members and us were going to provide ... it didn't matter to them that the service was being provided free ... That is what caused so much grief and it was difficult.[91]

There was also a gulf between some managers' 'concern' for the services and their actions during the strike. One INO Industrial Relations Officer, Clare Treacy, recalled: 'I can remember in [n. hospital] ... on [the] Friday afternoon seeing the General Manager getting into his car and driving away and I rang him and I said, "Where are you going?" He said, "I am going home", and I said, "You can't go home" ... they literally were just wiping their hands of it.'[92] Making beds constituted the thin end of the wedge. The INO's leverage, due to its decision to maintain essential services, was minimal enough, and it was only on the third day of the strike, following a protest march by 10,000 nurses and midwives in Dublin, that the government initiated discussions aimed at resolving the dispute.

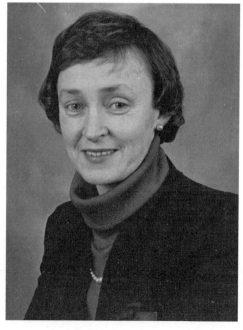

Lenore Mrkwicka. Courtesy INMO.

A collective unease characterised the INO's senior personnel at the time. Lenore Mrkwicka recalled: 'It was October and very, very cold ... people felt that notice would be taken and there would be ... a phone call to the General Secretary from the Department [of Health and Children but] three days went past and there were no phone calls ... It was freezing and there was no money, people were getting worried.'[93] Behind the militant rhetoric, some fifteen years after the fact, Liam Doran recalled his members' predicament:

> No matter how strong our rhetoric, no matter how robust our talk, at the end of the day the nurse or midwife is not going to walk away ... strike or no strike, pay or no pay ... [It is a] graphic illustration of the weakness of having a nurses' strike because patients come first and strikes come second ... So is that heroic or is that martyrdom? But it is what we are and we can't be not what we are ... [The strike] started on a Tuesday morning at 8 a.m. ... On the Thursday we had 10,000 people on O'Connell Street marching up and down and nobody was talking to us ... When I felt at my lowest ebb was on Saturday morning ... and I will be honest ... I hadn't seen [my] family for the week ... I was upset, the talks were not going well, there was no concessions coming ... they were still calling our bluff because we were providing services ... [So] there was no pressure on the other side to start finding solutions ... I said, 'I do not know how I am going to get out of this, I can't see a way forward at this point in time' and that was a real source of worry.[94]

Noreen Muldoon recalled the strike's solidarising effect:

> I can safely say that I saw home maybe twice throughout that nine days ... The care, the support, the attention that we, as [Industrial Relations Officers] got from [the INO's managerial team] was phenomenal ... I distinctly remember on one occasion going up to the Hospital of the Assumption in Thurles ... It was old, it came from the famine times ... you could smell the care when you went into it ... It was evening by the time I arrived ... This nurse came over and she went under the sink and she brought out a bottle of whiskey and she poured it into my tea and she said, 'You'll need that!' It was so funny. But that was the reciprocation of the care ... It was a really, really bad time in lots of ways but it was a very good time as well. That brought people together.[95]

Solidarity was beginning to wane, however, and back on the picket line, the mood was changing. 'The spirit on the picket lines was good on the first couple of days,' recalled Dave Hughes, 'then the weariness set in ... Some of our members [became] extremely hostile to the Union ... We had officials who were on the point of breakdown ... There was an awful lot of vitriol ... So whatever anger was there before the strike, the anger turned on us when it happened.'[96] Doran recalled this turn of events clearly and, in recognition of the slow progress being made in negotiations, the INO issued an ultimatum: '[If there is] no progress by Monday morning we are pulling people ... and you may get the consultants and doctors in from 8 a.m. on Monday morning because you will have no nurses. You haven't played ball.'[97] Doran's reference to strategy and the rules of engagement are fitting considering his previous life as a professional golfer at Canterbury Golf Club, England – a life he relinquished in 1976 in order to become a nurse.

But the prospect of a complete withdrawal of labour coming to pass was unlikely. Nurses and midwives were arranged at different points on a scale of militancy and, though a general upward trajectory was evident, it was slowly evolving, and the corps of INO members endorsed the strike only so long as essential services were maintained. Behind the rhetoric, a complete withdrawal of labour may also have been unpalatable to the organisation's leaders. When asked his personal view on an all-out strike, Liam Doran indicated:

> I have no difficulty in walking out provided I understood that there might be one or two of my colleagues left in ... it could be me left in that could respond ... in the event of something happening ... You are asking me my personal view, that is my personal view ... I think that is no less effective than an all-out but allows us to have a slightly higher moral position.[98]

IV.I. The Settlement

The threat of an escalation in the strike proved to be a turning point, and a number of grievances were referred to the Labour Court. Dave Hughes recounted the reception the INO received:

> The employers were sour as sour could be ... Every concession was resented. They could hardly look Liam in the eye. They probably hated me ... In the run up to the strike [someone described me and Liam] as being a lethal cocktail, because I had the industrial relations and the industrial dispute history behind me and Liam was all ... nursing ... and we felt like a lethal cocktail that day in the Court because they were absolutely vicious ... We were absolutely pariahs in everybody's eyes at that stage because we had ... kicked completely out of the water the prevailing national agreement.[99]

The court issued its proposal, Labour Court Recommendation 16330, on 27 October 1999.[100] The proposal was, of necessity, crafty, as the court was charged with establishing a concession that was specific to nurses/midwives and that would not lead to a deluge of similar claims by other occupational groups. It recommended that 2,500 new senior staff nurse/midwife posts be established and that this grade be paid 5 per cent more than staff nurses/midwives at the maximum of the existing pay scale. The court also recommended an allowance for those who undertook certain continuing professional development courses, a premium payment for unsocial evening hours and the creation of 1,100 junior managerial and 1,250 clinical specialist positions. All nurses and midwives were to receive a salary increase of 2 per cent with higher salary increases for some senior grades, and it was agreed to prioritise the implementation of the recommendations of the Commission on Nursing, ensuring a number of very significant developments in the years ahead. The INO suspended the strike, pending a ballot, and recognising the slim prospect of the government conceding any further, recommended acceptance of the proposed deal.

The haste with which the organisation acted was necessary, as financial strain was beginning to take its toll. Noreen Muldoon recalled: 'There was a [INO] fund set aside for people who were really in dire straits which I don't think has ever been made known ... I know a couple of people had their mortgage [repayment] paid.'[101] Anne Cody:

> I don't think the members would have thanked us if we took another three weeks [because] it took that length of time to get the information out and to explain it ... I don't think any sane union would ask their members to stay on strike for another three weeks while we get this information out to you and you can take an informed decision.[102]

The return to paid labour, pending a vote, was viewed as a climbdown and angered many: 'It is an insult to all nurses. There is a very strong feeling here that we should stay on the picket line until we have our say,' said one member.[103]

Liam Doran recalled the aftershow:

> Probably the most charged meeting I was ever at as General Secretary of the Union since I took the job was in St James' Hospital on the night of the 27 October 1999 ... that Thursday night in [St] James' was absolutely hypertension ... There must have been 400 people in a hall designed for 150 to 200 and they were not happy.[104]

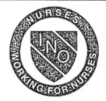

IRISH NURSES ORGANISATION

Information Meetings for INO members on the Labour Court Recommendation will be held at the following venues

REGIONAL MEETINGS

Galway - Friday, 29th October at 6.00 p.m. and 8.30 p.m.	Galway Bay Hotel, Salthill
Limerick - Friday, 29th October at 6.00 p.m. and 8.30 p.m.	Castletroy Park Hotel
Midlands - Friday 29th October at 8.00 p.m.	Tullamore Court Hotel
Northwest- Friday 29th October at 8.00pm	Southern Hotel, Sligo
Waterford – Saturday 30th at 6.00pm and 8.30pm	Bridge Hotel, Waterford

SECTION MEETINGS

Ward Sisters Section- Monday November 1st at 2.30pm	Liffey Suite, Ashling Hotel, Parkgate Street, Dublin 8
Super and Senior PHN Section- Tues 2nd November at 2.00pm	Liffey Suite, Ashling Hotel, Parkgate Street, Dublin 8

Notification will be issued locally on additional venues.

Notice of the highly charged post-strike regional meetings that the INO convened in order to disseminate the settlement package to its members. With thanks to Irish Newspaper Archives and the *Irish Independent*.

Doran's tone during the interview suggested that the 'hyper-tension' to which he referred could just as easily have referred to hypertension, the sometimes stress-related cardiovascular condition that had afflicted his predecessor Annie Smithson and witnessed her 'taking to the bed' for days on end. Much of members' unhappiness was attributable to the fact that, for the majority, i.e., staff nurses/midwives, the most immediate and tangible concession they gained, following a nine-day-long strike of 25,000 employees, was a 2 per cent salary increase; remember INO members were awarded a 23 per cent pay increase after 4,000 of them marched to Dáil Éireann and threatened mass resignation in 1978.

A belief that they had been exploited also rankled. In 1920, the union's first General Secretary, Marie Mortished, noted: 'I am not at all sure that the authorities do not take advantage of the nurses' devotion to duty.'[105] In 1999, having maintained all essential nursing and midwifery services for nine days without pay and having received a salary increase that many viewed as suboptimal, the narrative was very similar. Noreen Muldoon again:

> I knew that the nursing staff wouldn't let down their patients. I knew that they had so much care for them that they were never going to jeopardise anything got to do with patient care. I firmly believe that they were abused as a result of that ... that pure care was abused ... And nothing did happen, there wasn't one incident in the whole country that was as a result of nurses being on strike.[106]

INO members ultimately accepted the Labour Court's recommendations somewhat begrudgingly. One nurse from Mullingar Hospital, County Westmeath, remarked: 'I am against the [resolution] package but I will vote for it if it means that I dont' [*sic*] have to go back on the streets again and provide the kind of cover we gave during the strike.'[107] A series of national meetings and debriefings were convened with members and Anne Cody recalled: 'The sense that I got from those regional meetings was, "okay", we won't be doing this again ... It will be a long, long time before there is another national [strike].'[108] As a consequence of member feedback and annoyance, the organisation decided that members would never again work in an unpaid capacity. Crucially too, the organisation decreed that future strikes would entail an incremental withdrawal of labour.[109] Those who felt aggrieved at the strike may have found some solace in astrology. Horoscopes made an appearance in the INO's *World of Irish Nursing* in the 1990s and one pertaining to those with the star sign Libra was about to assume a wider applicability: 'A slightly depressed feeling persists [but] be determined to enjoy what's on offer and you'll be surprised at the results.'[110]

'Where There Were Patients, There Were Nurses': Three Nurses Reminisce

Anne McGowan: I was working in Sligo General Hospital at the time of the national strike in October 1999. I had become a hospital representative in 1993 and very quickly became involved an all activities of the union at local and national level. Strike action had been averted in 1997 but in the weeks leading up to 19 October 1999 there was a feeling of inevitability among members that the action would now go ahead – though this decision was not made lightly. In the weeks before the strike the in-house strike committee did an enormous amount of preparatory work under the guidance of the local Industrial Relations Officer Cora O'Rourke. I remember the huge attendances at meetings. There was a real sense of unity of purpose among the members and the feeling was that the strike was necessary in order to have our issues resolved. My main concern was that we were taking a huge leap into dark and unknown territory. Yes, we had done all the preparatory work but 'going live' with strike action was way beyond our experience. Still that was exactly what was about to happen.

It was with a very heavy heart and a knot in my stomach that I went in the door of the hospital on the morning the strike commenced. I remember being a little overwhelmed by the intensity of the media attention on us – every newspaper and radio station wanted a piece of the action. I was co-chairperson of the in-house strike committee with Ann Judge – another representative. At the time I was working as a Clinical Nurse Specialist in Cardiac Rehabilitation. This was largely an outpatient service and, thus, would not operate during the strike. This left me free to assume a leading role on the strike committee. The committee had a nurse/midwife representative from every area of the hospital. We held very regular meetings to discuss issues of concern and provide support and direction to members. Patient safety was the main priority. We also liaised with hospital management as the INO emphasised from the beginning that good working relationships were essential. Management provided us with very good facilities – a strike committee room, phones, fax machine, pagers, walkie-talkies and caravans with tea and coffee facilities at the hospital entrances for members on the picket lines. Our Director of Nursing at that time played a very supportive role. The direction from the INO was to provide and maintain essential services at all times. We had a Cardiac Arrest Team and a Rapid Response

Team available for emergencies. The scary part, for me, was that the strike committee was in charge of the hospital!

We worked so hard during the strike. I was present in the hospital every day. As the days went on members had increasing numbers of queries about the concept of essential services – no member wanted to do anything wrong. Working without pay became an increasing concern as we headed into the October Bank Holiday weekend; that weekend was the low point of the strike. Life on the picket line was not too bad. Retailers were very good to us with regular deliveries of soup, coffee and sandwiches. Ann Judge and I (we became known as the two Anns) went walkabout regularly to chat with and update members on the picket lines. Occasionally tempers were a little frayed but the anger was mostly directed at government. The rally in Dublin was a huge success and was attended by a busload of members from Sligo.

I will always remember Liam Doran's speech on the day; he quoted U2's Bono: 'we still haven't found what we're looking for!' My immediate reaction to the news of a settlement was relief. Members' responses were mixed – some grades had more gains than others. But all in all, everyone was glad that the strike was over. The strongest message from members at the post strike meetings was that they would never work for nothing again. On occasions since, when the hospital has been having bed pressures, I have been asked by several consultants to reinstate the strike committee – the reason being that 'everything ran so well when ye were in charge' – a rare compliment indeed![111]

Madeline Spiers: I was a theatre nurse in St Columcille's Hospital, Loughlinstown, Dublin during the strike, and I never worked so hard in my life. The Commission on Nursing served as a blueprint but its delivery was at a snail's pace; we remained undervalued and underpaid. The INO brought vision and an action plan, and we believed that justice and right was on our side. We organised a strike committee and manned the hospital gates. I recall the march in Dublin and the camaraderie of my colleagues and, yes, we worked for free. Indeed, I believe that the state would have been happy to allow strike committees run the health service until we could no longer afford to work.

I remember standing at the hospital gates with a placard and a couple stopped their car and gave us coffee. You see, the public recognised the legitimacy of what we were demanding and saw us delivering emergency care regardless of the dispute. Employers sought reassurances that our pay demands would be ring-fenced to nurses and midwives but other unions would not agree; so much for solidarity. We rattled the system. I was both angry and relieved when it ended; you win some and you lose some. At the end of the day we cared about patients, the management of the service cared about the cost. This remains a core problem we have yet to reconcile.[112]

Teresa Hayes: Tallaght was a new hospital, just shy of sixteen months open, and this was its first major industrial dispute, albeit a national strike. As a result, management were keen to keep good relations with nurses intact. To be fair we had a very supportive Director of Nursing and Chief Executive Officer. I was a Nurse Manager on a busy medical ward and also served as the Chairperson of the Strike Committee; everyone rallied to the call. Rosters were drawn up, scrutinised and redrafted. Our mantra was simple, 'where there were patients, there were nurses'. No one was going to depict us as putting patients at risk; after all, we were providing our services free of charge. We dealt with any patient safety issues in a reasonable, pragmatic manner and I am proud of how INO members portrayed themselves, professionally and with dignity, while at work and on the picket line.

The public support was unwavering; one day an elderly man arrived with a cheque for £25 made payable to the striking nurses. What a lovely touching thing; it was symbolic of the support we received on the picket line and it will always stay with me. I remember the camaraderie, the friendships and the unity of purpose among the nurses on the picket. However, those on the wards were fraught with hard work, and the minimum cover provided only

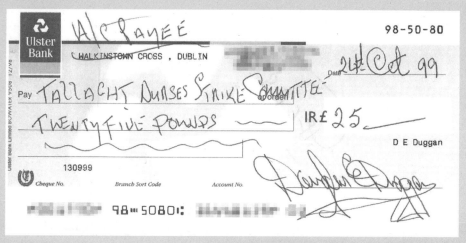

A cheque to the value of £25 kindly donated to the striking nurses at Tallaght Hospital, Dublin, by Douglas Duggan. Courtesy INMO/Áine Duggan.

made the burden of pressure greater on ourselves. We quietly gave additional support from the picket line without management's knowledge; after all, we had to look after our own. But there was no doubt about it – it was a very lonely and stressful time on the wards. We rotated between picket duty and the wards on a four-hourly basis. The hardest part was not knowing when it was going to end, and the word back from headquarters was not encouraging either. The weather didn't help; it was dreary and cold and the dark evenings were upon us. Management didn't hang around either, heading off for the long weekend and making it clear that we were in it alone and for the long haul. It was exhausting and the loneliest nine days of our working lives.

Was it worth it? At the beginning it was hard to see the benefits, but with the passage of time I see it as seismic – without realising it, nurses and midwives determined that never again would the employer take our services for granted and never again would we be handmaidens. The 1999 strike will live long in the memories of all those nurses and midwives involved.[113]

CHAPTER 11

From Aftershow to Afterglow, 2000–8

Lasting for nine days and involving 30,000 workers, the 1999 national nurses' strike was a dispute of enormous proportions. Why, then, has the event not entered the annals? Perhaps it is because the strike did not fit the typical definition of a strike; after all, no hospital closed. Alternatively, perhaps the event fell foul of the invisibility of women in Irish history. Maybe it came a cropper because it did not fit with the Irish penchant for political and nationalist history. Or could it be that nursing/midwifery historians remain as transfixed as ever with education and registration and believe trade unionism a little too pedestrian? Or maybe the dust has simply not yet settled on the event. The dispute's outcomes, and the INO's role in driving these, have also been overlooked. Lest anyone forget, it was INO members, in the main, who rejected the recommendations in the *Blue Book Agreement*, and an astonishing 97 per cent of them threatened to take strike action. This, in turn, led to the establishment of the Commission on Nursing and it was the subsequent strike, to which the INO was the largest party, which ensured that the commission's recommendations were implemented. This marked the beginning of something of a 'golden age' in nursing and midwifery in Ireland in which the INO was the central protagonist.

I. What's in it for You?

One day after the suspension of the 1999 national nurses' strike, the INO attempted to convey the outcome of the dispute to its members. Liam Doran, suffering from the opposite of writer's block, put pen to paper, and Dave Hughes recalled the document he drafted:

> I came into Liam and he had written about ten pages to explain all that had happened and I said, 'No you can't do that.' And this is what we produced in the end which is one page: *What's in it for you?* I said, 'No, this has to be very simple, you have to say to people what they got out of the strike.' And that is

THE IRISH NURSES ORGANISATION

THE TOTAL PACKAGE
WHAT'S IN IT FOR YOU - AT A GLANCE

STAFF NURSE	PROMOTIONAL GRADES
➢ £1,250 lump sum; ➢ *2,500 new Senior Staff Nurse posts (determined by length of service - **no** supervisory role) at 5% above Staff Nurse rate; ➢ *1,100 new CNM1 posts; ➢ *1,250 new CNS posts; ➢ *2% salary increase from 1st July 1999; ➢ Annual Leave - 3 days extra based on service; ➢ *Time plus one-sixth from 6.00 p.m. - 8.00 p.m.; ➢ Allowances from £328 to £1,000 or £1,500; ➢ *Location allowance (£1,000) now payable in designated areas of Mental Handicap and Psychiatry; ➢ *All category 2 courses, or equivalent, as approved by An Bord Altranais will, in future, attract the specialist allowance when the nurse is engaged in such duties; ➢ The extension of the dual qualified scale to midwifery and sick children.	➢ New salary scales (+10% in 2 phases); ➢ *2% on all points from 1st July 1999; ➢ Lump sum of £1,250; ➢ *Lump sum of £1,000 for role in implementing action plan for Commission; ➢ *Post-Partnership review of differentials; ➢ 4 days extra leave related to service ➢ *Confirmation of reporting relationship related to Director of Nursing; ➢ *Allowances - Time plus one-sixth where applicable; ➢ Increased specialist and location allowances where already held i.e. Junior Ward Sisters and Ward Sisters working in known designated areas including A&E; ➢ New CNM3 post salary increased to £29,600.
PUBLIC HEALTH NURSING GRADES	NURSE TEACHERS
➢ PHN - New salary scale (6% at max); ➢ Personalised allowance of £900 per annum; ➢ Senior PHN - New salary scale (10% at max). *PHN & Senior PHN:* ➢ *Specialist qualification allowance of £1,500 per annum; ➢ Additional leave (up to 4 days); ➢ £1,250 lump sum; ➢ *Post-Partnership review of differentials; ➢ *2% on all points of scale from 1st July 1999.	➢ *Salary increase (10% at max); ➢ *2% on all points from 1st July 1999; ➢ Lump sum of £1,250; ➢ *Immediate discussions on future conditions of employment.

*Denotes improvements achieved since strike action began.

What's in it for you? Courtesy INMO.

what we put out and ultimately that was what people did get and was what they voted on.[1]

The document laid bare the large number of industrial concessions that the strike and its preceding campaign had yielded: salary increases, lump sums for promotional grades, the advent of the senior staff nurse/midwife grade and vastly improved allowances. But to focus on industrial successes alone is to sell the organisation short. A vast amount of progress in the professional and educational realms had also been won. The INO had historically taken issue with the relegation of the nursing/midwifery perspective in the corporate structure and with the lack of promotional opportunities in the professions. In its submission to the Commission on Nursing, it argued that the ward sister role was essentially a clinical nursing/midwifery management role as it incorporated both a patient and general managerial remit. It also argued that nurse/midwife managers be given more autonomy, especially in relation to budgetary matters, and that a tiered managerial career pathway be introduced.[2] The commission took heed and rebranded ward sisters as clinical nurse/midwife managers, established a staggered career pathway and recommended that the new grade be given a greater say in budgetary arrangements.[3]

The INO also argued that its members' roles could be expanded if an appropriate structure for doing so existed.[4] These sentiments resonated with rank-and-file members who, in submissions to the commission, expressed concerns that the absence of formal scope of practice guidelines, like those that existed in Britain, resulted in uncertainty regarding whether or not they were permitted to adopt new and extended roles.[5] The commission, in response, urged An Bord Altranais to address the situation, and the *Review of Scope of Practice for Nursing and Midwifery* document was published by the board in 2000.[6] The document's decision-making framework brought clarity to the limits of nurses'/midwives' practice in a prescriptive rather than restrictive fashion, and, over time, significantly broadened the actual and potential practice parameters of both professions.

Aligned to the expansion in nurses' and midwives' roles was debate regarding specialist practice. The INO drew the commission's attention to the continued rise of specialisations within the professions and to the proliferation of nurse- and midwife-led services. The INO suggested that a national framework was necessary to support further developments. The commission responded and recommended, as a priority, the introduction of a three-tier clinical career pathway comprising staff nurse/midwife, clinical nurse/midwife specialist and advanced nurse/midwife practitioner. The national framework for the further development of specialist roles was to come from the National Council for the Professional Development of Nursing and Midwifery – a new body charged with the post-registration development of nursing and midwifery; the INO had always been at the forefront of post-registration education, but now its efforts had been augmented with the establishment of a body to oversee further progress. Some 600 new nurse/midwife specialist posts had been approved by 2001,[7] and the INO urged the speedy creation of further such positions.

Developments in the advanced practice sphere were driven by the labour and clinical backdrop: a European Working Time Directive, which necessitated a reduction in the length of the working week of non-consultant hospital doctors, merged with ongoing overcrowding in the country's Emergency Departments. Tallaght Hospital, Dublin ran out of trolleys to accommodate emergency patients on one occasion and an INO campaign, 'Enough is Enough', distributed postcards to the public and invited them to relay to the Minister for Health and Children, Mary Harney, their experiences of Emergency Departments: 'Would you like to watch your husband dying on a trolley from terminal cancer … waiting to get pain relief due to shortage of staff?' went one.[8]

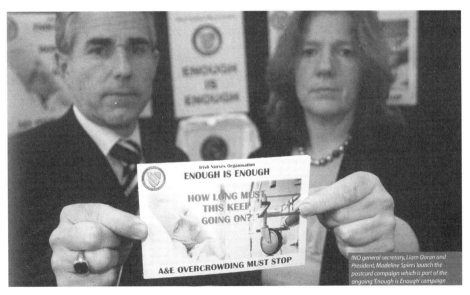

INO General Secretary Liam Doran and INO President Madeline Spiers launching the 'Enough is Enough' postcard campaign in 2006. Spiers trained at the Royal City of Dublin Hospital, Baggot Street, in the mid-1970s and worked at home and abroad as a theatre nurse. She has published extensively on the areas of health policy and health service management. Courtesy INMO.

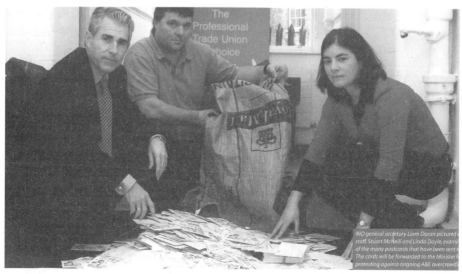

Liam Doran and INO staff members Stuart McNeill and Linda Doyle sift through a deluge of 'Enough is Enough' postcards in 2006. Courtesy INMO.

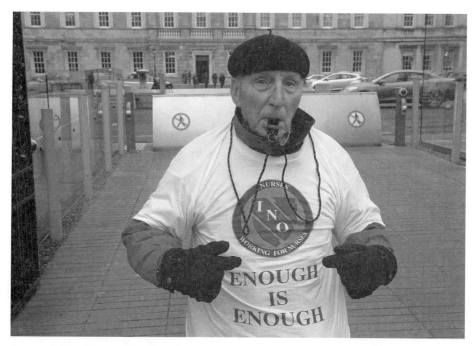

A member of the public rows in behind the INO's 'Enough is Enough' Campaign. Courtesy Lisa Moyles/INMO.

Harney soon admitted that the state of affairs constituted a 'national emergency'.[9] While addressing the INO's Accident and Emergency Section Annual Meeting, she indicated that advanced nurse practitioners were one of a suite of initiatives needed to remedy the problem.[10] Ireland's first nurse practitioner was appointed at the Emergency Department at St James' Hospital, Dublin, in 2002. By 2005, a total of seventeen advanced nurse/midwifery practitioner posts in areas including emergency nursing, sexual health and diabetes had been approved, and forty more were in the offing.[11] The pioneering nurse practitioner at St James' recounted her authority to independently assess, diagnose and discharge patients in her care.[12] Between 2005 and 2012 the advanced nurse practitioner in gastroenterology at the same hospital carried out almost 4,000 endoscopy procedures.[13] By 2009, the midwife-led unit at our Lady of Lourdes Hospital, Drogheda had delivered its 1,000th baby.[14] Further expansion in nurses'/midwives' roles was also underway.

An extensive review of nurse and midwife prescribing, undertaken by An Bord Altranais and the National Council for the Professional Development of Nursing and Midwifery was completed in 2005. The INO was represented on the Review Board and identified a number of potential benefits of extending prescriptive authority to its members: safety, patient satisfaction, convenience, compliance and cost-effectiveness.[15] The review found favour with Mary Harney and, in 2005, she announced her intention to introduce, at least initially, prescribing for specialist and advanced nurse and midwife practitioners.[16] The INO took some issue with the plan and, in a submission to the Department of Health and Children, argued that, provided prescribers were appropriately educated and competent, prescriptive authority should be extended to all nurses and midwives and that they be able to prescribe from an open as opposed to a limited formulary. The thrust behind the organisation's relatively radical submission was its view, informed from its growing knowledge of developments in other jurisdictions, that confining prescriptive authority to a small subgroup, or to a limited range of medicines, would limit its benefits and might necessitate revision at a future date.[17]

One of the drivers of nurse/midwife prescribing in Ireland at the time was Elizabeth Adams, who was appointed as Professional Policy Advisor to the INO in 2006. A theatre nurse, Adams cut her teeth in policy matters in Western Australia where, as Principal Nursing Officer at the Department of Health, she was influential in having prescribing authority extended to nurse practitioners working in rural areas. She recalled: 'My role involved negotiating the smooth passage of the legislation through both houses of parliament and successfully developing and delivering a State-wide implementation and evaluation framework for the expanded scope of practice.'[18] Adams received the Government of Western Australia Award for her endeavours and continued: 'Due to my experience with the development of the legislation and implementation of prescriptive authority in Australia ... I grasped the opportunity to make a difference in Ireland.'[19] The INO's argument was ultimately successful and prescribing, for all nurses and midwives that undertook the appropriate post-registration education, and from an open formulary,[20] was introduced in 2007. The National Maternity Hospital was the first institution to employ a nurse or midwife prescriber, and in her first weekend in the role, she wrote some fifty prescriptions.[21]

Nurse and midwife prescribing is a microcosm of how the INO functions in driving change in the professional arena, in consensus seeking and in liaising with other stakeholders. The Department of Health and Children established a steering group on the matter; a number of laws required amending; a syllabus leading to the award of nurse/midwife prescriber was formulated and an updated set of *Nurses' Rules* were drafted. Annette Kennedy, soon to be introduced more formally, was employed as the organisation's Education and Research Officer in 1993 and too had a major hand in nurse and midwife prescribing. She remarked:

> Liam [Doran] and myself probably worked well [because] it was like good cop, bad cop. He was the guy who went out and pushed the Government into doing things ... and then they would talk to me because ... I was professional rather than industrial. ... I believe in my heart and soul that everybody has the same goal ... we are all looking for the same thing but we might have different ways of coming at it ... that happened in prescribing. We had the regulators, we had the universities, we had the Department [of Health and Children], we had the union and the health service ... we all wanted to get it through. [Mary Harney's enthusiasm for prescribing acted as a] window of opportunity ... we wouldn't have got it through at any other time ... I would say the INO is the chief instigator of getting that through ... I am very proud of prescribing ... it is needed, very needed.[22]

None of the vast changes that were taking place in the professional arena would have been possible were it not for significant groundwork by the INO in relation to nurse and midwife education in the previous years. The organisation remained underwhelmed with the performance of An Bord Altranais: relations with the board had gone from simmering in the 1960s, to bubbling in the 1970s and were, by the 1990s, approaching boiling point. In 1993, Kathleen Craughwell,

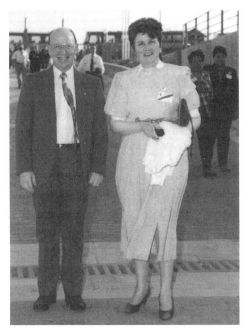

Kathleen (Kay) Craughwell photographed with P.J. Madden at the ICN Congress in Madrid, Spain, in 1993. Craughwell is from Co. Galway where she trained as a nurse. She then trained as a midwife in Scotland, public health nurse in Cork and children's nurse in Dublin. She worked as a paediatric Ward Sister in Galway, as Matron in Mallow, Co. Cork, as Director of Nursing/Midwifery in the Regional Maternity Hospital in Limerick and, more recently, as Director of Nursing in Sligo General Hospital. Courtesy INMO.

INO President, described the board as a 'dismal failure' in relation to post-registration education, and the INO took matters into its own hands.[23] That same year, the INO established the Education Resource Centre, later branded the Professional Development Centre and employed Annette Kennedy as its Education and Research Officer. Described as a maverick by her colleagues, Kennedy was a general nurse and midwife who, in

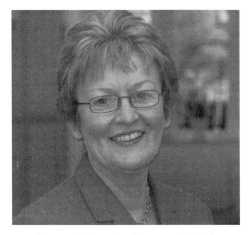

Annette Kennedy. Courtesy INMO.

the early 1980s, was ward sister at the Intensive Care Unit (ICU) of Dublin's Richmond Hospital:

> There was no such thing as ICU courses then, no such thing as any type of course really, which is what probably led me into the area of education here in the INO. No, the unit Sister taught you as much as she could and your colleagues taught you as much as they could … I took over the job of opening [a new neurological ICU] and running it … I got nurses who had never been in ICU … So you can imagine what that was like, trying to teach them and trying to organise a unit [so we] decided that we would have a combined neuro/ICU course and we set it up ourselves … I was sent on a day release to the [RCSI] because they had started up a management course … So a lot of the courses that were set up started … off by [Ward Sisters and] nurses realising that if they wanted to have confident people in their unit and they wanted to have them skilled they had to start the courses themselves.[24]

Kennedy soon became restless and was seconded to undertake the Nurse Tutor course at University College Dublin. She returned to the Richmond, by her own admission, as a somewhat unconventional teacher and, in light of the strict discipline imposed on student nurses, recalled: 'I spent a lot of time trying to tell [students] how to survive within the hospital scheme of things and how not to get themselves into trouble and to always smile and say they were sorry and all that kind of thing.'[25] It was at about this time that Kennedy was alerted by a friend to the fact that the INO was seeking somebody to head up its expanding professional and educational remit. Kennedy was interviewed and got the nod. In the absence of any formal job description, she was given carte blanche at the organisation: 'I had no idea what I was supposed to do, no idea.'[26] The lack of formal educational preparation for her managerial position at the Richmond remained to the fore of her thoughts, however, and she set about establishing a managerial course as her first priority:

> At that time Plassey Management was linked to the University of Limerick … They were running practical courses for general organisations … they would teach first line and second line managers how to manage … I liked their stuff … so we set about actually writing the modules for the management course … It took us the guts of a year, maybe longer. And we had all of that organised [when] I got a call … saying [Plassey Management] had gone into liquidation. I think that was the worst day of my life because I had asked the

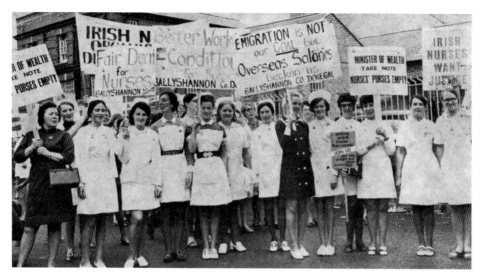

Nurses from Donegal and Leitrim join their colleagues in Sligo to march in protest at their conditions, 1970. Digital content created, published and reproduced courtesy of Digital Library, UCD.

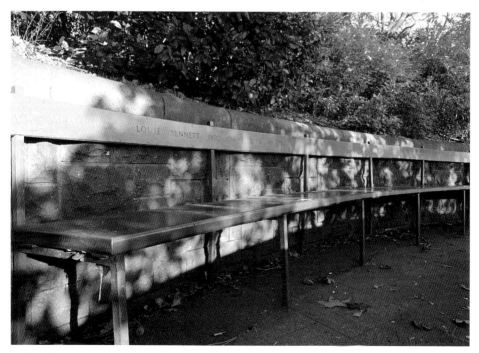

A bench dedicated to the memory of Louie Bennett at St Stephen's Green, Dublin. Courtesy Lisa Moyles/INMO.

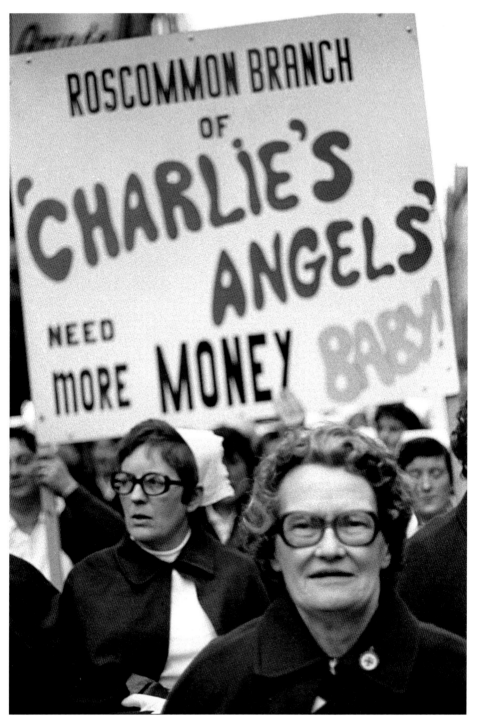

'Charlie's Angels': nurses protest in Dublin in 1978. Courtesy Derek Speirs.

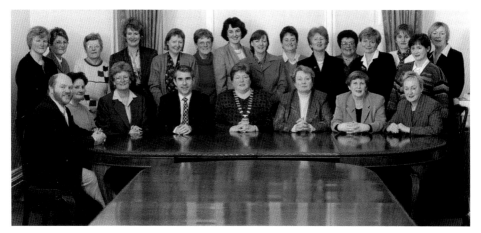

The embattled INO Executive Council of 1998–2000. Back standing left to right: Catherine Tormey, Kathleen Craughwell, Anna Monaghan, Patricia Flynn, Rita Corcoran, Mona Clancy, Ita Tighe, Mai Murphy, Joan McDermott, Kay Kennedy, Winifred Collier, Brigid Burke, Patricia Dolan, Maura Hickey, Dorothy Mullarkey (Administration Manager). Seated left to right: Dave Hughes (Director of Industrial Relations), Tess O'Donovan, Annette Kennedy (Director of Professional Development), Liam Doran (General Secretary), Anne Cody (President), Imelda Browne (First Vice-President), Clare Spillane (Second Vice-President), Lenore Mrkwicka (Deputy General Secretary). Other members of the Council not included: Tina Howard, Regina Buckley, Loretta Crawley and Mary Wynne. Courtesy INMO.

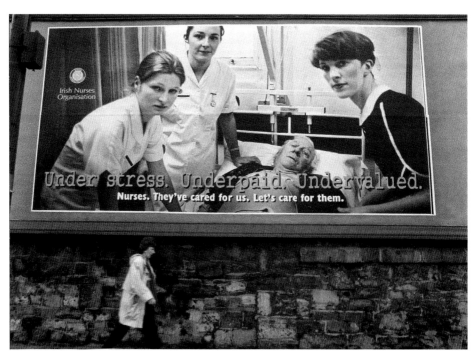

One of the iconic images used as part of the INO's campaign in the lead-up to the 1999 national nurses' strike. This image was on a billboard in Dublin. Courtesy Derek Speirs.

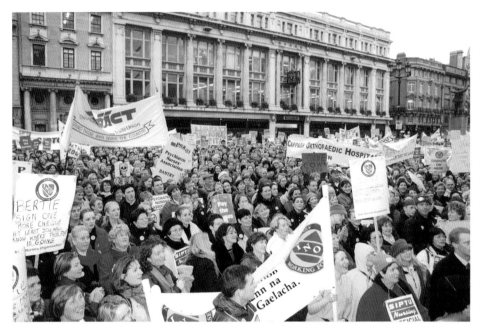

A portion of the crowd that gathered on Dublin's O'Connell Street in support of nurses during the 1999 national nurses' strike. The iconic statue of James Larkin, arms outstretched, is visible on the extreme right of the image. Courtesy INMO.

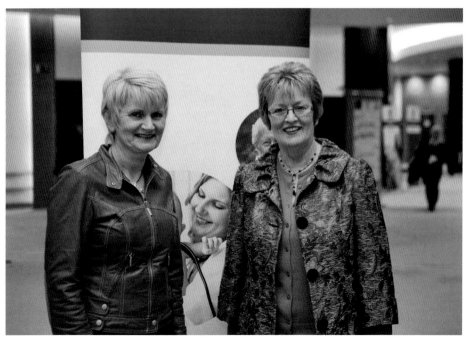

Marian Harkin, MEP (left), with the INO's Annette Kennedy in 2010. Courtesy INMO.

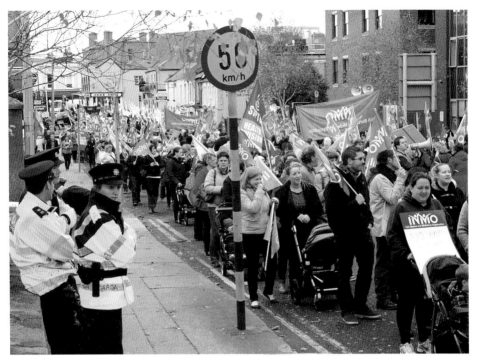

Hundreds of INMO members protesting outside the headquarters of the Nursing and Midwifery Board of Ireland in opposition to a rise in retention fees, 18 November 2014. Courtesy Lisa Moyles/INMO.

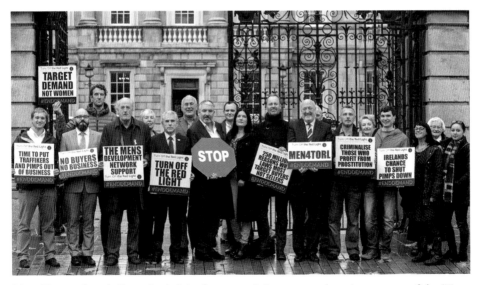

Liam Doran, fourth from the left in front row, joins many others in support of the 'Turn Off The Red Light' campaign in 2015. Courtesy INMO.

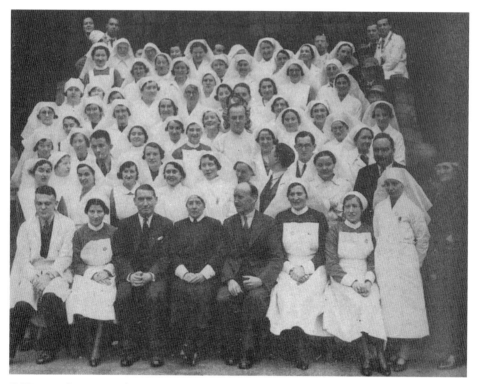

INO members attending the Organisation's first refresher course for nurses at the Richmond Hospital, Dublin, in 1938. The Matron, Miss Hazlett, is seated in the centre of the front row and the INO's Kathleen Nix is standing on the far right of the image. Courtesy INMO.

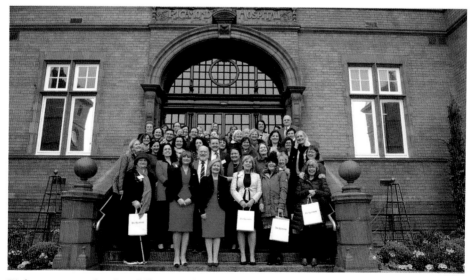

Eighty years to the day following the Organisation's first refresher course for nurses at the same hospital, the Richmond reopened on St Valentine's Day 2018 to host a seminar for members. Courtesy Lisa Moyles/INMO.

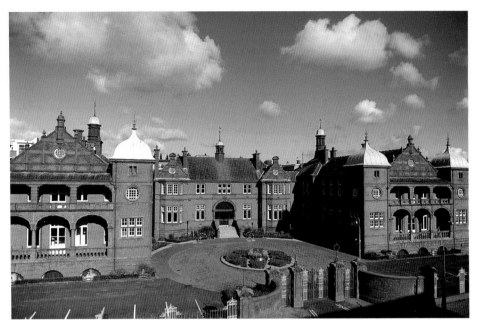

'From small acorns …': the landmark Richmond Hospital on Dublin's North Brunswick Street. The iconic building became home to the INMO's Education and Event Centre in 2018. Courtesy Lisa Moyles/INMO.

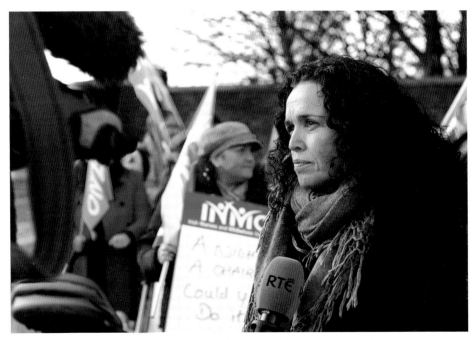

Phil Ní Sheaghdha on assuming the leadership of the INMO in 2018. Courtesy Lisa Moyles/INMO.

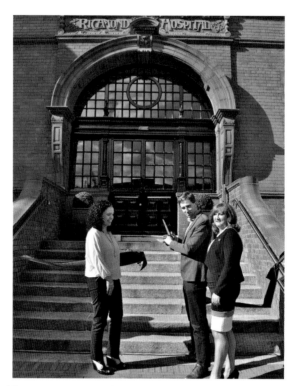

Minister for Health Simon Harris officially opening the INMO's Richmond Education and Event Centre in April 2018. Pictured with the Minister are INMO General Secretary Phil Ní Sheaghdha (left) and INMO President Martina Harkin-Kelly (right). Courtesy Freda Hughes/INMO.

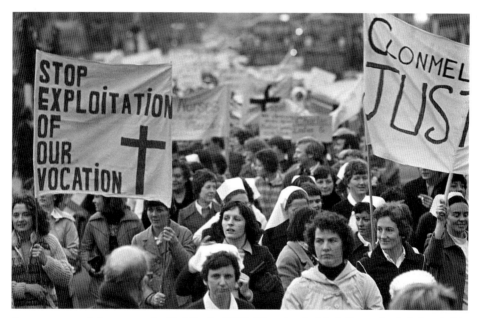

A protest march by nurses in Dublin in 1978. The sign held aloft on the left-hand side of the image speaks volumes. Courtesy Derek Speirs.

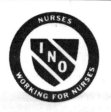

'Available throughout Ireland with no time off work required'

FIRST LINE MANAGEMENT DEVELOPMENT FOR NURSES

Certificate Programme through Open Learning

UNIVERSITY
of
LIMERICK
OLLSCOIL
LUIMNIGH

- developed by the Irish Nurses Organisation (INO) and Plassey Management and Technology Centre specifically to meet the needs of first-line nurse managers in the Health Sector in Ireland

- provides individual nurses with the knowledge, skills and abilities to excel in a management role, thereby enhancing their career prospects

- provides individual nurses and health sector organisations with a flexible approach to first-line management development

Awarding Body University of Limerick*

Entry Requirements? Open Entry for front-line nurse managers with a minimum of three years post-registration experience

How Do You Study? Through Open Learning; in your own time, at your own pace, with no time off work required

How Long is the Programme? Approximately 10 months, comprising 2 stages

Study Hours Per Week? Approx. 5 hours

When Do You Register? By 20th October 1995

Fee? Stage One £780; Stage Two £730
(for INO Members Stage One: £680; Stage Two: £630

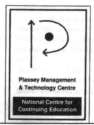

Plassey Management & Technology Centre

National Centre for Continuing Education

Who to contact

Plassey Management & Technology Centre
University Campus
Limerick
Tel: (061) 202003/202130
Fax: (061) 202532/330872

(Subject to final confirmation)*

An advertisement for the course that nearly never was. Courtesy INMO.

INO to invest money in this and when I told P.J. Madden he said, 'I had to go through the Board to get a kettle, and we have invested money on your say-so in this.'[27]

Notwithstanding his initial frustration, Kennedy recalled that Madden was exemplary in handling the situation, and a series of intense negotiations ensued before the course was ultimately adopted by the University of Limerick in 1994: 'It was one of the greatest successes at the start considering it nearly went down the Swanee.'[28] The course was conducted by distance learning in order to meet the demands of members, most of whom were women and, arguably, subjected to the demands of the 'second shift' – not to mention the first one: 83 per cent of nurses found it difficult to access education and half reported not being permitted time off work in order to undertake exams.[29] Examinations for the

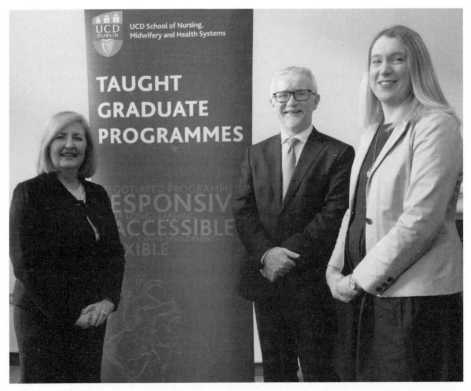

Elizabeth Adams, INMO Director of Professional Development, with Dr Martin McNamara, Dean of Nursing and Head of School, and Breda Connaughton, Lecturer and Clinical Tutor, UCD School of Nursing, Midwifery and Health Systems. Courtesy Lisa Moyles/INMO.

Certificate in Management were conducted at the INO's headquarters and, by 1997, those who completed the course were eligible to undertake a Diploma in Health Services Management – also a joint venture between the INO and the University of Limerick. The INO's Professional Development Centre was soon delivering courses to members on topics as diverse as assertiveness training, personal development and legal issues. University College Dublin had resisted the INO's advances in the 1940s, but soon a formal relationship was forged between both bodies which witnessed INO members who had completed a number of courses at the organisation's Professional Development Centre being eligible to pursue a University-based Certificate in Enhancing Clinical Practice.

Ongoing increases in the INO's membership, staff and remit meant that it had long since outgrown its office at Leeson Street and, by 1987, there was a concerted effort to find a bigger abode. All previous attempts to up sticks had come to nothing until P.J. Madden was approached, out of the blue, by a buyer keen to acquire the organisation's premises. As luck would have it, the building formerly occupied by An Bord Altranais, 11 Fitzwilliam Place, had just been vacated, and the INO acquired it. The new premises was a short hop from the old, but the potential that it conferred on the organisation was a giant leap. Chief among its strengths was a mews building at the rear and, amid much fanfare and a reception attended by over 100 members and sponsors, the organisation's Professional Development Centre moved to the renovated mews, equipped with office space and a classroom, in 1997. The mews was once home to feminist author Mary Lavin – no doubt Louie Bennett and Marie Mortished would have approved. The organisation had amassed a range of books and journals through exchanges with other nurse/ midwife representative associations over its lifetime. These volumes had never been arranged sequentially and, working quickly, a newly appointed librarian bound and catalogued the collection and established a comprehensive library facility for members by late 1997.

The library was officially opened by the Minister for Health and Children, Brian Cowen, in April 1998, the year that the organisation 'went live' on the World Wide Web; all of this from an organisation that, at one point in the 1940s, could not procure as much as a filing cabinet.[30] The early professionalisers who had once disparaged the organisation would have baulked; substantial changes in nurse and midwife education were now being driven by the INO, suggesting that trade unionism and professionalism were not at odds after all. But for all the changes happening in post-registration nurse and midwife education, more still were afoot in pre-registration education.

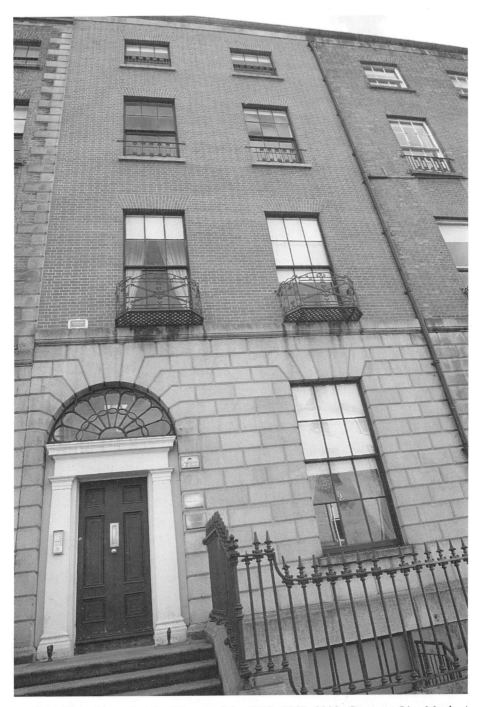

11 Fitzwilliam Place, Dublin. Home of the INO, 1987–2003. Courtesy Lisa Moyles/
INMO.

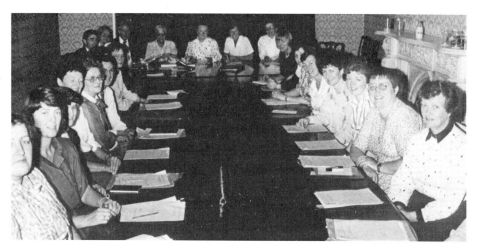

The INO's Executive Council pictured in the Board Room of the INO's new headquarters at 11 Fitzwilliam Place, Dublin, in 1987. Courtesy INMO.

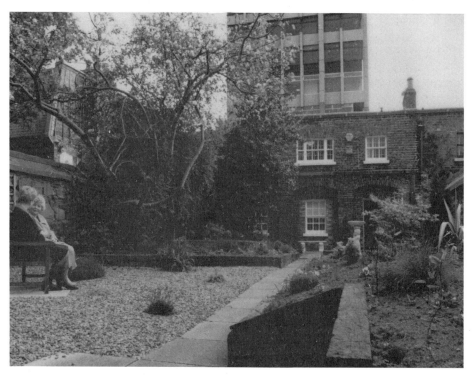

The Mews: home of the INO's new Professional Development Centre. Courtesy INMO.

I.I. From Apprentice to Academic and Everything in Between

The 1970s had brought changes to the apprentice system of nurse training, with diktats from Europe driving changes in clinical placements. The INO fought to enforce and optimise these changes, but by then it also harboured a more aspirational plan for student nurse education, as indicated by Carmel Taaffe, the organisation's President. Referring to the dual aim of increasing both the status of nursing and the quality of patient care, Taaffe noted: 'These goals can most effectively be achieved if basic nurse education is brought within the gambit of university education, where educational expectations and practices differ considerably from those pertaining in many traditional hospital schools.'[31] The likely impetus behind the change in the INO's position was developments in nurse education in Britain, where a number of institutes of higher education then offered degree courses in nursing as well as registration. INO members put forward a motion at the (now infamous) Annual Meeting in 1978:

> That the system of nurse education be changed from an apprenticeship to a collegiate programme. We will then see a more self-confident nurse who will have benefitted from the opportunity of personal development as well

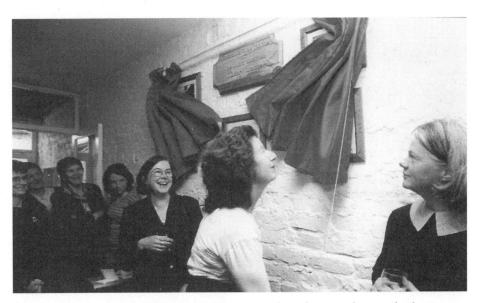

Mary Lavin's daughter, Valentine McMahon, unveils a plaque to her mother's memory at the INO's new Professional Development Centre in 1997. Also pictured are McMahon's sisters Caroline Walsh and Elizabeth Peavoy. Courtesy INMO.

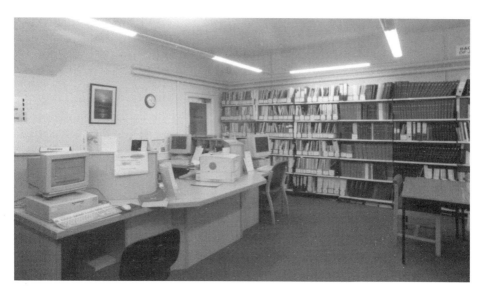

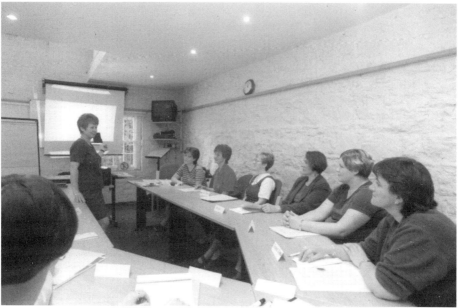

An education session with INO members at the organisation's new Professional development Centre (bottom). Also pictured is the INO's new library (top). Courtesy INMO.

as a deeper educational experience. An inquiring individual who will expect improved working conditions as well as monetary rewards for a high standard of professional service.[32]

The resolution was referred to the Working Party on General Nursing which was, by then, regarded as a panacea for every ill affecting the profession. But the Working Party's recommendations regarding pre-registration nurse education were by no means radical; they included the amalgamation of training schools, a teacher to student ratio of 1:15 and the use of key learning objectives, all of which were to be deployed within the existing apprenticeship model, as opposed to at degree level.[33] The majority of nurses were not too perturbed by the Working Party's failure to throw its weight behind a pre-registration degree programme, however, as an *Attitude Survey of Irish Nurses*, undertaken at the time, showed that 89 per cent of nurses believed that nursing was best learned in a hospital.[34] The report's recommendations stifled the INO's prospects of securing the transfer of nurse education to third-level for another decade, and the organisation again returned to its goal of improving the apprenticeship model. European Community Directive 89/595 stipulated that one third of nurses' training be theoretical, meaning, by the organisation's Tutors' Section's reckoning, an increase from twenty-eight to forty-eight weeks of classroom instruction. The tutors argued that the existing number of tutors was insufficient to implement the new rule and planned to boycott teaching from 1991 in protest.[35] The organisation was successful and the Department of Health sanctioned the employment of fifty extra tutors to deal with the increased workload.[36] By then, however, the sands were beginning to shift beneath the apprenticeship system once and for all.

Research carried out in the early 1990s showed that a growing number believed that would-be nurses should be full-time students, not apprentices, and that a university degree should be the standard mode of entry to nursing in Ireland.[37] The findings mirrored a mounting body of opinion that nursing, in spite of its practical leaning, had theoretical underpinnings and that such underpinnings needed to be buttressed if nurses were to meet the challenges of providing comprehensive care in the future.[38] Students themselves were also beginning to question the apprentice model, and a group of them penned a letter to the Minister for Health, Brendan Howlin, in 1993:

> We are a group of student nurses having just completed our General Nurse Training in November 1993, and have now just signed on in the Dole Office … It would appear that the only reason we were taken into training was for the amount of service we could provide during our three years. At all times, our education seemed to be secondary to the hospital's service needs … Unlike students in other sectors we received no educational recognition on completion of the course.[39]

An Bord Altranais read the signs, commenced a review of the system of pre-registration nurse education in 1990 and produced its findings, *The Future of Nurse Education and Training in Ireland*, in 1994.[40] The report recommended student status for trainee nurses, a severance of students' status as employees of the service, the establishment of colleges of nursing with links to third-level institutions and a more structured approach to post-registration education. The report was silent in relation to the exact nature of the academic award made on completion of any new course of education, but developments in Galway were about to provide clarity. No sooner had An Bord Altranais published its report than Howlin announced an experimental system of nurse education, a joint venture between University College Galway, the Western Health Board and the Department of Health, leading to the award of a Diploma in Nursing and registration as a nurse. Graduates had the option of undertaking an additional year's study in order to gain a degree.

The 'Galway Model' brought with it manpower ramifications. The state's reliance on the labour of nurse apprentices was enormous. Now, apprentices were a dying breed, and the INO had concerns about the consequences. The organisation reached agreement with employers regarding their replacement with a defined number of nurses and ancillary staff in 1995.[41] The Galway Model also caused the INO some concern regarding the emergence of two tiers of nurse in Ireland: those educated to registration level and those educated to registration and diploma/degree level. The organisation was inundated with requests by members that they be able to revise their qualifications and, in 1996, following extensive negotiations between the INO and the Department of Health, Dublin City University launched a course through which registered nurses could pursue a degree in nursing. Furthermore, after lobbying by the organisation, it was soon announced that employers would pay the third-level fees of all nurses wishing to undertake a degree.[42] The Galway Model was intended to be experimental and subject to formal evaluation and review in 1996. Concerns were aired regarding the model even before this review was complete: some believed that it perpetuated the theory-practice gap, that the syllabus was front-loaded and that it lacked time for self-directed learning.[43] The student experience was also suboptimal. One student shared a page of her diary:

07.40: Arrive to ward
07.45: Report – I do not understand a lot of the abbreviations
08.00: Allocated to staff nurse, who disappears …
08.45: I spot staff nurse doing drug round. Up to my neck in bed-bath and bowels

09.30: ... Start the vital signs

10.00: Go to break with rest of students on ward and no-one is happy

10.20: Return from break. Approach staff nurse ... She asks me to do Bed 7's dressing ... Point out that I have never seen the dressing before. Am told to check the wound chart and shout if there are any abnormalities. Proceed to do the dressing unsupervised ...

12.00: ... Feeling absolutely useless at this moment

14.15: ... Clinical placement co-ordinator arrives to find out if I have had my first [proficiency assessment]

14.50: Why is everyone looking for commodes now?

15.15: Ward sister sees me leaving and says she will do my [proficiency assessment] this week

3 weeks later: Receive my first [proficiency assessment].[44]

In spite of its shortcomings, amid the militancy and strike threats that characterised nursing and midwifery in the mid/late 1990s, the Galway Model was rapidly extended and, by 1996, twelve schools of nursing had adopted it. The INO's General Secretary, P.J. Madden, recounted:

The Minister of Health of the day chose to hold a press conference as the balloting was about to commence on the second set of [1996] proposals at which he announced unilaterally the extension of the Galway initiative. Now there was no academic input into that judgement. It was purely a political judgement and the consequences of that are what we are landed with today.[45]

Madden's testimony suggests that the Galway Model was extended partly in order to appease the INO and, barring its faults, this may have been strangely opportune when looked at with the benefit of hindsight. The Commission on Nursing recommended that, from 2002 onwards, nurse education be conducted nationally at degree level.[46] The earlier nationalisation of the Galway Model meant that this was not the major undertaking that it otherwise would have been. After all, links had been established with third-level institutions and the transition from diploma to degree was far less arduous than that from registration alone to degree.

To diminish or deny the pivotal role that the INO played in these changes is an oversight. The mere fact that the Commission on Nursing recommended degree-level education meant little in the absence of the show of industrial muscle that the 1999 national nurses' strike represented. Those that think otherwise would do well to reflect on the fate of some of the recommendations of the commission's forerunner, the 1980 *Report of the Working Party on General Nursing.* That document recommended the establishment of a common core nurse-training programme followed by specialisation in the student's chosen branch of nursing. Such a move was not implemented and provided ample evidence, if any were needed, that reports came and reports went and were just as likely to be ignored as realised. In the same vein, it is too easy to conclude that the abolition of the apprenticeship model was a foregone conclusion hastened by the fact that European Union Directives meant that salaried nurse apprentices were spending more time in class – making them a more expensive source of labour than they had been. Degree-level education, in itself, necessitated the state to find £176 million to build schools of nursing at the country's third-level institutions, so economics was not the only variable at play.[47] Liam Doran has the weight of history on his side when, unusually animated, he asserts:

> [I] don't care – they could hold their breath dying for the want of air but they would still be at best in a quasi-diploma/apprenticeship model of training. They would never have put in the money to develop the capital infrastructure at campus level … never in a month of years … I don't care what anyone says, [it] wouldn't have happened without the political wind to make them happen on the back of a dispute and the argy-bargy that goes with it.[48]

Annette Kennedy recalled the challenges that the move to degree level education brought for the INO:

> There were two problems in relation to moving into third-level: One, there wasn't enough tutors. [Two], the vast majority of tutors only had a degree [and] wouldn't be accepted into third-level, into universities, at that time without a master's. We were [also] negotiating at the time the fact that they would be taken on as lecturers rather than [as] a lower grade nurse tutor … That was a very, very hard fought battle particularly with the universities … I remember Liam [Doran] saying to one of the [university] Deans: 'If Jesus Christ was here and wanted to get over the bar what would he have to do?' … The Department [of Health and Children] were on our side [and] decided they would fund a number of nurse tutors who wanted to do the master's [but] we couldn't get the universities here to come on board … So then we went to Coleraine and went to the University of Ulster [and] they came down and they worked out of the [INO's] mews building every weekend to put so many people through the master's programme. That was a major feat for the INO.[49]

It was also a clear demonstration of the organisation's ability to find solutions to problems. The traditional indicators of professional status that nurses and midwives had failed to live up to in the 1960s were increasingly being realised, thanks in large part to the INO. Third-level education had been achieved, which, in turn, brought a focus on nursing and midwifery research, and the organisation launched its own journal, *Nursing Research*, in 2001. A research website, Nurse2Nurse, followed in 2002. It was important that the organisation's reach did not begin exceeding its grasp, however, and a newer, larger headquarters was now warranted. The former Whitworth Hospital on Dublin's North Brunswick Street fit the bill and was purchased as the INO entered the new century. The building's 17,000 square feet replaced the 6,500 square feet premises at Fitzwilliam Place. The Whitworth allowed for a

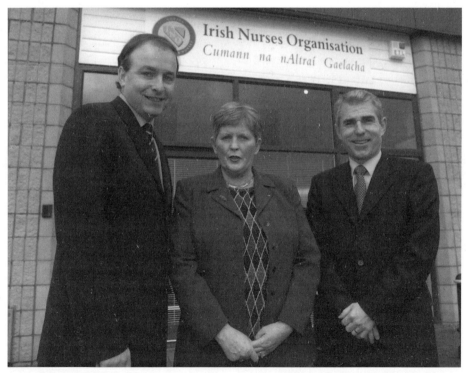

INO President Clare Spillane (centre) pictured with Minister for Health Micheál Martin (left) and INO General Secretary Liam Doran (right) at the organisation's Cork office. From Portlaoise, Spillane trained as a nurse at Harefield Hospital in Middlesex. She later specialised in tuberculosis nursing and became a midwife. She returned to Ireland and worked as a midwife and then as a nurse most recently at Carlow District Hospital. Courtesy INMO.

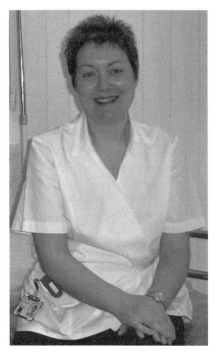

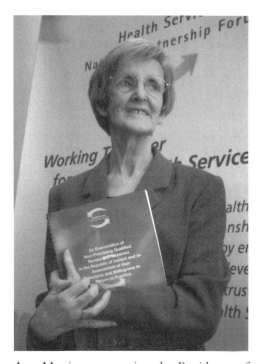

Eilish Corcoran acted as INO President following Clare Spillane's death in 2003. Corcoran trained at the South Infirmary, Cork, in the late 1980s and later specialised in emergency nursing at St James' Hospital, Dublin, before returning to the South Infirmary. Courtesy the author.

Ann Martin on assuming the Presidency of the INO in 2003. Martin trained as a nurse and midwife in her native Galway and, before her election to the position of President, was Clinical Midwife Manager at the Maternity Department of University College Hospital, Galway. Courtesy INMO.

significant expansion in library facilities as well as ample office and meeting space. For the twenty founding members who squeezed into the union's one-room shared office on South Anne Street over eighty years previously, the new digs could scarcely have been imagined and, in a bittersweet turn of events, was opened by the organisation's President, nurse and midwife Clare Spillane, just days before her untimely death in 2003.[50]

I.II. The Professional, the Political

The INO's professional remit is vast and varied, a veritable broad church. The organisation once took issue with fast-food giant McDonald's when a television

advertisement depicted a nurse, in full uniform, eating a burger at one of
its restaurants.[51] It might have been anticipated that the organisation would
have been happy that the nurse got a meal break at all, but it appears that the
sight of a nurse wearing her uniform outside the hospital setting was just a
little too improper. So what exactly constitutes the INO's professional remit?
Annette Kennedy recounted 'being part of the policymaking arena' as one of
the INO's professional preoccupations.[52] The organisation had long been active
in this regard, but the advent of the Professional Development Centre brought
renewed focus and vigour to its professional and educational endeavours. A
Chief Nursing Officer was appointed at the Department of Health and Children
in the run-up to the 1999 national nurses' strike. The gesture was too little for
the INO, however, as the post was pegged at the fourth rung from the top in
the department's hierarchy. The organisation persisted and was successful in
having the status of the Chief Nurse revised. Liam Doran recalls: 'The only
reason we have a Chief Nursing Officer at the Assistant Secretary level in the
Department now is the [INO] ... I was told it would never happen ... And it
has now happened ... I now have them [on the] second rung on the ladder at
the same level as the Chief Medical Officer.'[53]

Influencing policy matters was also contingent on the INO reappraising
its stance on political engagement. The organisation had failed on more than
one occasion to win representation in the Senate through the years. History
offers an insight as to why. The electoral panel to the Senate effectively
precluded many organisations that represented women from the nomination
process.[54] This was to the detriment of nurses and midwives; after all, the
former General Secretary of the Irish National Teachers' Organisation, T.J.
O'Connell, used his position as an elected member of Dáil Éireann to highlight
the need for improvements in teachers' working conditions, from pensions[55]
to accommodation.[56] A number of Liam Doran's editorials in the early years
of the new century addressed the need for members to become more political.
Doran had, at the very least, a light breeze at his back, as independent and
single-issue candidates were making steady ground in electoral politics in
Ireland. In addition, 2012 would witness the introduction of gender quotas,[57]
and the advent of third-level education conferred many nurses and midwives
with Senate voting rights for the first time.

But while the breeze was at his back, the gale was at his face: nurses and
midwives remained unusually ambivalent on matters of politics. In a recent
election to the board of An Bord Altranais, conducted online, just 3.6 per cent
of nurses and midwives cast their ballot.[58] Their seeming disinterest is a little
unusual when contrasted with doctors, almost 17 per cent of whom voted in

elections to the Medical Council in 2013,[59] and when compared to teachers, just over 23 per cent of whom voted in elections to the Teaching Council in 2016.[60] Ambivalence is not the only problem. An advertisement for the Fianna Fáil party appeared in the *World of Irish Nursing* ahead of the general election of 2002.[61] Considering that Fianna Fáil had been in government during the national nurses' strike three years earlier, the advertisement drew a disapproving response from members, who penned letters of complaint to the INO, suggesting that political party allegiance remained unpalatable.[62] Doran becomes exercised on the topic of politics:

> We have to get off the pot on this one … we want to get elected at everything but we don't want to be political about anything … Politicisation begins from the bottom up … Just because we are supporting [a nurse or midwife] who is Fine Gael or Fianna Fáil or Labour … doesn't mean [the INO] support[s] Fine Gael or Fianna Fáil or Labour. It means we want a … nurse [elected] so they can bring [up] nursing things … It is about getting nurses political but it is also about getting this organisation to be less pernickety because the chances of an independent nurse getting elected to anything are [small] … We can't beat the political system, we have to join it.[63]

Globalisation and Ireland's membership of the European Union also necessitated the INO to assert its influence at international level. Annette Kennedy was elected as President of the European Federation of Nurses' Associations, an umbrella body representing over six million nurses, in 2005. The value of the INO's association with international organisations was, and is, most likely not recognised by rank-and-file members who, understandably, remain more concerned with developments at local level. Yet, international developments were increasingly playing a role in local ones and, amid a shortage of nurses/midwives that necessitated large-scale migration to Ireland, the federation lobbied on issues such as the need for consistent educational standards for nurses throughout the European Union. Similarly, the looming accession of a number of new countries to the European Union generated debate regarding the reciprocal recognition of midwives' qualifications.[64]

If these issues appeared lofty to the average INO member, issues of a more practical nature were also pursued on the international stage. Health service staff across Europe sustained one million needle-stick injuries per year at the time; one nurse suffered a needle-stick injury whilst putting a used needle into a sharps bin and later tested positive for human immunodeficiency virus.[65] The European Federation of Nurses had lobbied the European Commission on the issue from as early as 2004,[66] and Kennedy took up the cudgels, lobbied members of the European parliament (MEP) and spearheaded the federation's efforts to have sharps injuries addressed further. Her efforts soon attracted the attention of Irish MEP Marian Harkin, who adopted the case.[67] European Directive 2010/32 subsequently outlawed the re-sheathing of needles and necessitated the use of sharps with inbuilt protective mechanisms.[68] Nor was the organisation's growing internationalism just of benefit in professional matters. The organisation won a seminal case in 2015 when it took a case to the European Commission on behalf of two nurses who, in spite of their tenure and experience in another European member state, had been placed on a less favourable new entrant salary scale.[69]

The vast array of changes that had taken place in nursing and midwifery engendered hope that the relative 'worth' in terms of salary of nurses and midwives would increase accordingly. Nurses and midwives had assumed new managerial and clinical roles with vastly expanded responsibilities, and all new entrants to the professions were to be educated to degree level. As Ireland basked in a period of economic optimism, a new mechanism, known as benchmarking, was touted as a means through which the worth of nurses, midwives and all public servants could be evaluated. A comprehensive review of the nursing and midwifery role was to take place, historic relativities were to be dispensed with and INO members were to receive their long-sought dues. This, at least, is what they thought.

II. Well Travelled, Better Prepared

Benchmarking sought to gauge the worth of public servants' labour against their colleagues in the private sector and to adjust public sector pay to the market rate. This seemingly placed nurses/midwives in a strong bargaining position, as Ireland was in the grip of a nursing/midwifery shortage. Working visas for foreign nurses and midwives needed fast tracking; nursing vacancies rose to 1,200 in Dublin alone,[70] and by 2002, there were 3,000 nurses from outside the European Union working in Ireland.[71] However, these much-needed arrivals did not receive the *céad míle fáilte* that might have been expected. Some were housed in accommodation with broken windows and rising damp, and others found themselves sleeping six to a bedroom or, indeed, sharing a bed. One INO representative took it upon himself to investigate their lodgings only to have the floor give way when he entered.[72]

The INO, as part of the Nursing Alliance, put forward a 75-page submission to the Benchmarking Body, ably arguing in favour of significant improvements in members' terms and conditions.[73] First and foremost, the alliance made a case (to the male-dominated body) that nursing/midwifery labour, being (stereotypically) women's labour, was undervalued. It also argued that nursing and midwifery were regulated professions requiring significant clinical, managerial and teaching skills in addition to the need for continuing education. The alliance also pressed home a claim for improved allowances, an allowance for those working in Dublin and a 35-hour week. The alliance's main goal was parity with therapy grades such as physiotherapists but for all of its talents, arguing for an increase in salary at the same time as a decrease in working hours was a tactical error. It provided ample opportunity for detractors to advance a 'more for less argument', which they did with gusto.

Nonetheless, INO members remained hopeful as to the outcome of benchmarking, but their optimism soon proved fruitless. Benchmarking failed to deliver a shorter working week, improved allowances or a Dublin weighting allowance. To add insult to injury, the salary increase recommended to nurses and midwives was small enough to erode the slight move toward parity with therapy grades that the increases of the 1999 national nurses' strike had won. Benchmarking offered therapy grades a 12 per cent salary increase at basic level and a 14 per cent increase at senior level, while staff nurses/midwives received an increase of 8 per cent and middle ranking clinical nurse/midwife managers received an increase of 12.2 per cent.[74] In fact, benchmarking created new anomalies and, in the intellectual disabilities sector, (sometimes) unqualified staff were now touted to earn more than registered nurses, despite nurses carrying more managerial and clinical responsibility.[75] The INO struggled to see the logic in the body's recommendations and requested evidence of its deliberations. This, revealingly, was not forthcoming. On finding out that the body had disbanded, one of the organisation's columnists, Moira Cassidy, deduced: 'It doesn't exist anymore – a bit like a three-card, travelling huckster whose cover has finally been blown, it packed up shop and ran for the hills once the report was issued.'[76] Over a decade on from benchmarking, Liam Doran is philosophical:

> Benchmarking ended up being a massive exercise to restore the status quo into public service pay relativities post the nurses' dispute of '99 – nothing more and nothing less. And that is why we only got 8 per cent at the staff nurse grade and the [therapy grades] got 11 per cent ... It can be dressed up all it likes, but that is what it was ... Machiavellian in the extreme.[77]

A new national pay deal was touted in 2004 that promised a further benchmarking exercise by the end of the decade. Issues such as the anomaly in the intellectual disabilities sector and the 35-hour week had not gone away, but made wary from past experience, the INO's Executive Council doubted whether a second such exercise would be any more beneficial than the first. They warned members against it, who reciprocated by a three to one majority against,[78] and the organisation lodged its claims directly with employers which, in turn, found their way to the Labour Court in 2006. Notwithstanding past differences between the INO and unions that represented psychiatric nurses, the organisation found an increasingly close ally in the PNA at the time, and both unions held a rally of 1,200 activists at Dublin City University's Helix Theatre while the court was deliberating. Labour Court Recommendation 18763 was yet another setback and recommended that nurses and midwives engage in the touted second benchmarking process.[79] The INO thought differently, and in a case of well travelled, better prepared, hit upon a protest strategy that would not affect members' pay. A 35-hour week had become a

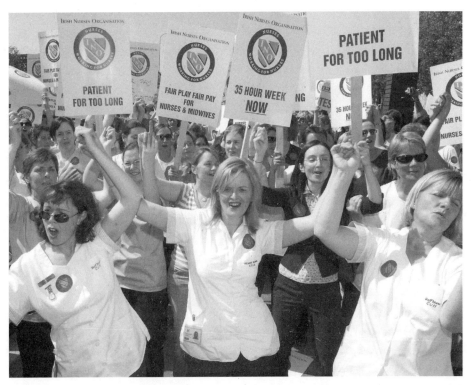

INO members sing a protest song at Cork University Hospital during their campaign for a 35-hour week in 2007. With thanks to Irish Newspaper Archives and the *Irish Independent*.

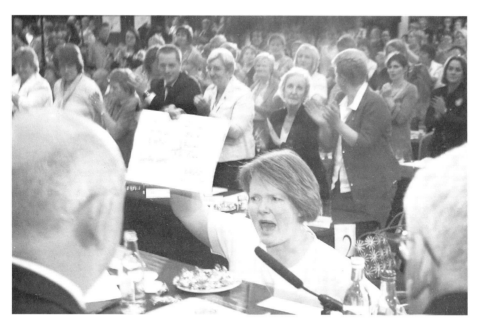

'Do the sums': tensions boil over when an INO member charges the top table during the organisation's 2007 Annual Delegate Conference to make her point known. Photo by Mark Stedman. With thanks to Photocall Ireland, Irish Newspaper Archives and the *Irish Independent*.

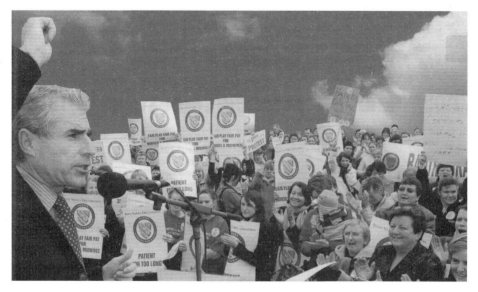

Liam Doran addresses INO members during the 2007 campaign for a 35-hour week. Courtesy INMO.

priority and 96 per cent of members endorsed a series of lunchtime protests and a work-to-rule in its pursuit.[80]

The work-to-rule lasted for six weeks and proved a partial success. A 37.5-hour week was proposed by employers, and this was accepted, albeit narrowly, by INO members.[81] Crucially, and in a rare turn of events, the reduction in working hours was not replicated in other occupational sectors, meaning that it was a specific gain for nurses/midwives. Moreover, it was the first reduction in the working week of any group or category of worker in over forty years, proving that striking was not the only weapon in the organisation's armoury. The INO had clearly learned a lesson from the 1999 national strike – a lesson that had been added to its corporate memory. Nonetheless, the round-the-clock nature of nursing and midwifery work, the lack of support staff and nurses' and midwives' inherent service obligation meant that even a work-to-rule was challenging, as Liam Doran discovered under the most poignant of circumstances:

My mother was dying in the middle of the work-to-rule ... Mammy was in long term care and we had issued a ban on non-nursing duties [including] admin[istration] duties, non-essential duties, i.e. household, portering staff duties [and] making tea and toast ... Stop all that lark. So I was called at 11:00 p.m. at night, down to St Columba's Hospital in Thomastown ... brilliant staff [and] mammy's home for the last four years. I got down there about 3:30 a.m., mammy passed away at 5:30 a.m. ... No healthcare assistant on, two staff nurses on, and what is the first thing they said to me? 'Do you want a cup of tea Liam?' ... I am an only child, I was two hours on my own with my mother as she was entering her final hours ... The [nurses] gave me tea and toast twice, giggling and saying, 'Non-nursing duties Liam' and all the rest to break the ice! ... In the middle of it all I realised what a load of garbage [it was]. What is a non-nursing duty? I am a son watching his mother die ... I am hanging out for a cup of tea, having driven 120 miles at 100 miles an hour to get down in case anything happens ... I get tea and toast ... Now the physiotherapist wouldn't get me tea and toast, the dietician wouldn't get me tea and toast, the occupational therapist wouldn't get me tea and toast ... but there is no point in saying the nurse is not going to get you tea ... It is in [a nurse's/midwife's] soul to do it automatically without thinking [regardless of what] the union directive says ... that is pure priceless. The trouble is a pay bargain determination system that doesn't value that.[82]

Doran continued that nurses/midwives are:

> All too often evaluated by the lowest common things that they do in the food chain which is, do you make the tea and the toast? Do you clean the bed? Do you wipe down the bedsides? Do you wipe down the bed table? ... Whereas the physiotherapist diagnoses muscle strain and implements a care plan to repair the muscle strain. The dietician observes the calorific intake of the patient ... whereas the nurse feeds them. Which is more important? There is not much point watching my calorific intake if I'm starving ... 'cos no one's feeding you.[83]

There is a hierarchy of caring hinted at in Doran's testimony. It is a hierarchy that pits mental and manual labour at opposite ends of the spectrum. This hierarchy will be familiar to those with an interest in class studies. Mental labour comes with a high financial value and is carried out by professionals with a distinct body of knowledge that allows them to plan and organise the work of others. Manual labour carries with it a lower financial value and involves 'merely' carrying out tasks in line with what professionals have dictated.[84] It is not difficult to figure out which category nursing and midwifery, historically (and however wrongly), were assigned to: both were regarded as eminently

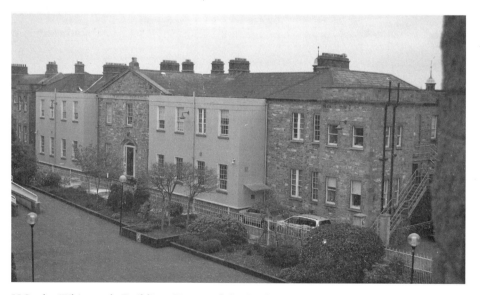

HQ: the Whitworth Building. Home of the INO since 2003. Courtesy Lisa Moyles/ INMO.

practical (manual) and neither had its own distinct body of knowledge. Third-level education brought the potential for change, as the INO could argue for pay parity with allied health professionals – all of whom were also educated to degree level. Benchmarking failed to deliver, but the organisation kept the flame burning. Little did it know that the years ahead were not going to be like those that had gone before. Economic storm clouds were looming, a financial crisis of unprecedented parallels was evolving and soon the INO would find itself struggling, not so much as to win parity with allied health professionals, but merely to maintain the previous decade's hard-won gains.

CHAPTER 12

A Decade Never to be Forgotten, 2009–19

Knowing what will happen next is a critical part of a historian's toolbox; it allows an account to be written about the past, with one eye fixed on the future, and it assists in telling the story in a unique way that the reader is most likely unaware of. As historians sift through a deluge of archival materials, they make choices as to what events make the final cut and what events get placed back in the box. The events that are chosen are generally those that are regarded as important. The reader is spared the false starts, side roads and dead ends that are encountered along the way. The 'chosen' events are those that lead us to where we are today; their geneses are detailed; their paths are followed and their outcomes are weighed up. However, when writing contemporary history, this is more difficult. The historian is robbed of foresight, and like those they write about, is none the wiser as to what will happen next. Contemporary history veers toward a simple description of events, but perhaps that is no bad thing. The story of the sheer scale of what occurred in Ireland as the first decade of the new century closed, and the ramifications for the INO and its members, is a book in itself. The real history of that era is best judged by whichever historian comes next. This is just a taster.

I. Death by a Thousand Cuts

In a period where the INO turned ninety years old, there should have been much to celebrate. A special badge was minted for the occasion and a celebratory party was held. But the organisation's milestone might have been a happier affair were it not for Ireland's looming economic storm. In the early years of the new century, it became clear, at least to some, that Ireland's economic growth was largely based on a property bubble. The state's coffers were lined with the proceeds of a construction boom, and when the housing market collapsed in 2007, income dried up. The impending recession of the world economy and trouble in Ireland's banks would make things worse. Mortgage lending rose exponentially during the property boom, as did loans by banks to the construction industry. Payback of these loans was predicated on the continued rise in property prices, a trend that soon became stuck in reverse. In order to stem the risk of banks defaulting on their liabilities, the state intervened by guaranteeing them. An editorial in the *World of Irish Nursing* struck an incredulous tone:

> The Irish banking system appeared to come to the brink of collapse save for the government's guarantee scheme which now amounts to €485 billion (yes I did say billion) … I think that [the] acceptance of harder times [ahead] rapidly disappeared as people realised that the government had chosen to inflict cutbacks that would lead to real and severe hardship upon the old, the young and those who relied upon the public health service … the state of the economy was a greater priority than the state and wellbeing of Irish society.[1]

The guarantee was not the end of the matter. In a surrendering of Ireland's fiscal sovereignty, the Troika of the International Monetary Fund (IMF), the European Union Central Bank and the European Commission effectively took charge, and in 2010, the state acceded to a €85 billion rescue package. The Irish government, having to live within the limits set, turned to austerity as a corrective measure. Public servants and those depending on the state for services were hit hard. The Celtic Tiger was well and truly over.

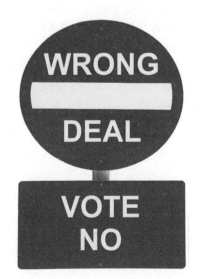

Getting the message across in the *World of Irish Nursing* in 2010. Courtesy INMO.

Cuts affected the INO's industrial and professional gains. In 2009 alone, the country saw a public sector pay freeze and legislation that resulted in a pay cut of between 3 and 10 per cent.[2] A pension levy, representing a further pay cut of 7.5 per cent, was also imposed.[3] The number of places on undergraduate nursing degree programmes was reduced from 1,880 to 1,570; the state floated its intention to discontinue paying college fees for nurses and midwives undertaking part-time degree courses, and plans were afoot to reduce the number of places on post-registration specialist courses.[4] The year 2010 brought with it negotiations on a pay deal, known as the Croke Park Agreement, which hoped to yield extra savings. The agreement emphasised the need for mobility and flexibility among the workforce – referred to as 'doing more with less' by some and as 'unmanaged downsizing' by others. The agreement, in the main, protected employees from redundancy and further pay cuts but incorporated a number of stipulations, including cuts to the number of inpatient beds and a ban on industrial action.[5] Set against the backdrop of an outbreak of the H1N1 virus and a ruthlessly applied ban on recruitment, the INO advised members to reject the agreement, which they did by a majority of 84 per cent.[6] In spite of their dissent, congress's Public Services Committee accepted the deal, meaning that the INO ultimately did too.

The Croke Park Agreement crystallised a period of pessimism in the public services that showed no signs of abating. A universal social charge, a tax by any other name, was introduced for all except those on the smallest incomes in 2011. It was announced that student nurses and midwives, during their 36-week rostered clinical placement, would receive a staggered reduction in their pay, with the payment abolished entirely in 2015. An INO campaign of protest forced a stop to the plan, but only 50 per cent of the original payment rate was restored. It was also announced that new entrants to the public service, including nurses and midwives, would start on the first rung of a salary scale that was 10 per cent lower than those already in post.[7] 'Public sector bashing', as the INO's Dave Hughes referred to it, became an almost fashionable pastime. Hughes outdid himself as a rabble-rouser, waging a vendetta in defence of workers and pushing himself and his audiences to states of near-spontaneous combustion at INO Annual Conferences throughout the recession. Hughes even took a case to the Broadcasting Complaints Commission regarding a remark related to public-service pensions made by a television broadcaster, which he perceived to be misleading.[8]

Late 2012 brought discussions on a successor to the Croke Park Agreement. Considering it more advantageous to try and influence matters rather than grumble about their outcomes, the INO participated. There was a concern that premium pay was under threat from the get-go, and this was poised to be detrimental to the salaries of shift workers such as nurses, midwives, gardaí and prison officers. The INO, sensing this, sought strength in numbers and arranged itself as part of a coalition termed the 24/7 Frontline Services Alliance. As discussions on Croke Park II got under way, the INO spearheaded a show of muscle in helping to convene a 4,000-strong rally of the alliance at the National Basketball Arena in Dublin. Upon realising that members were to suffer cuts to Sunday and evening premium pay, the INO led a walkout from the negotiations on Croke Park II and brought with it the Irish Medical

Organisation, the Civil and Public Services Union and Unite.[9] Dave Hughes
recalled:

> We said, 'No we are not accepting that' … We were going to get huge flak
> from our members and we didn't think it was right anyway so we said, 'We
> are not having it.' So it came to the crunch, [Director of Industrial Relations]
> Phil Ní Sheaghdha, myself, Liam [Doran], [Director of Regulation and Social
> Policy] Edward Mathews were all there and the President [of the INO, Claire
> Mahon,] was there … and I remember Phil and myself saying, 'Liam, we can't
> stay here, if we stay here this is going to be done to us, they are going to do it.
> We have no choice but to walk out, we can't let them do this to us.' So we got
> the other three unions with us and we walked out.[10]

The INO and its bedfellows were now officially out on a limb. While the
organisation's leaders headed to a press conference to explain themselves,
those trade unionists who remained at the negotiating table concluded a pact
to put to their members. The stakes were now running very high, and the INO
and the three other defectors mobilised themselves against the proposed deal
in a manner similar to David versus Goliath. Liam Doran recalled:

> Without being colourful, that was extremely challenging … We were invited
> in for talks … and we went in there on a Friday and it was bizarre. They
> had already made their mind up, they were looking for savings and a major
> part of the savings would be cutting premium pay on Sundays and public
> holidays … They didn't really engage with us … And I want to make it clear,
> the Executive Council [of the organisation] met … [they] are silent heroes to
> a certain extent, and we told them what was going on … We were given the
> direction on the Saturday night, I remember it quite clearly, about 9:30 p.m.
> that if they don't confirm the maintenance of those premiums we were to
> walk. So we went back in about 2:00 p.m. on the Sunday and I got no traction.
> None whatsoever. So then the challenge was would we walk alone or would
> we walk with some others? And there were nineteen unions in there and four
> walked out … all the others stayed in … A hugely challenging time.[11]

The organisation led a campaign of political lobbying and public meetings,
encouraging all union members, including its own, to reject the terms of Croke
Park II. For an organisation that was once mocked and maligned by its fellow
trade unionists, the INO's unwavering stance, coupled with Doran's unrivalled
articulacy and media exposure, influenced a sea change of opinion among

public sector workers. The proposal was subsequently rejected by a sufficient number of trade union members to see it consigned to history. Doran and the INO had assumed the mantel of leaders in public services' trade unionism in Ireland. The majority of the ICTU, at official level, had effectively promoted a set of proposals which were both unpalatable and unfair to their members and rightly found themselves answering some difficult questions. In the end, all public servants benefitted from the INO's actions. Meanwhile, the state retreated to the drawing board.

A new set of proposals, christened the Haddington Road proposals, soon emerged. Its provisions were severe though less penal than their predecessor. Among other things, they entailed a return to a 39-hour week for nurses and midwives, and undid a hard-won gain from 2007. INO Industrial relations Officer, Noreen Muldoon, recalled:

> As far as I am concerned one of the biggest aspects of any piece of work that any union has done was the introduction of the 37.5-hrs week … To me it was the most difficult time that I spent in the organisation … not having it negotiated, having it implemented. It was a huge achievement but it was resisted by an awful lot of the management side and to a lesser extent … people within other unions which made life rather difficult for us … I will never forget it … And now we are back to, a number of years down the road, [a 39-hour week] … I think it is a shame.[12]

The bitter pills did not stop there. In an effort to offset the workforce shortage caused by the recruitment ban, a new Graduate Recruitment Programme was imposed in which newly qualified nurses and midwives would receive a two-year contract on 80 per cent of the first point of qualified nurses'/midwives' salary scale.[13] Sunday premium pay, however, remained untouched. The organisation urged members to accept the new proposal only because it represented the lesser of two evils; the state threatened to legislate for alternative cuts, without negotiation, should Haddington Road collapse. Faced with the frying pan or the fire, INO members chose the former.[14] Of course by then the organisation had a reputation to uphold and was not simply going to take the deal lying down. It urged members to boycott the Graduate Scheme with success. It is thought that just thirty applications were initially received for the scheme,[15] and it was ignominiously dropped in 2014 but not before the damage was done. The reduction in students' pay during their rostered placement combined with the Graduate Scheme left a bitter taste in the mouths of new graduates, and a large number quit the Irish health services entirely. INO Director of Industrial

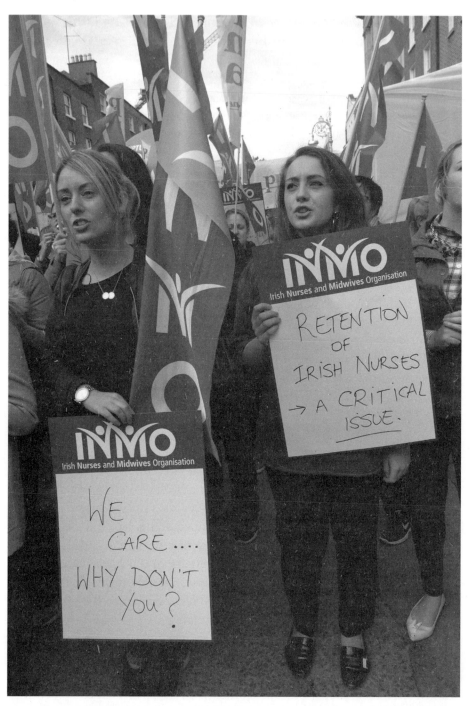

Recently graduated nurses protest over their terms and conditions outside Dáil Éireann.
Courtesy Aiveen Ahern/INMO.

Relations, Phil Ní Sheaghdha, remarked: 'Wherever they are in the world now they, I would imagine, have a very poor memory of how they were treated by the employer and government when they were here.'[16]

The early chapters of this book were written during the most austere years of the recession, and the feeling at the INO's headquarters was that of an organisation that was running merely just to stand still. There is an echo here of times past and of the old saying 'history does not repeat itself, but it often rhymes'. INO members found the wherewithal to contribute large sums to the organisation's Benevolent Fund throughout the austerity of the 1940s and 1950s, and they contributed likewise throughout the recession of the new century. The organisation sent a small team to Africa in 2008 in order to establish an expertise sharing network with nurses in Ireland. The team visited a clinic that lacked electricity and running water and had a ratio of one nurse to 6,500 patients.[17] The organisation subsequently took the decision to sponsor the education, as nurses, of two women in Ethiopia.[18] INO members also raised thousands of euros for the victims, 500 of whom were student nurses, of an earthquake in Haiti in 2010.[19] An influx of foreign nurses to Ireland resulted in the establishment of a vibrant and colourful International Nurses' and

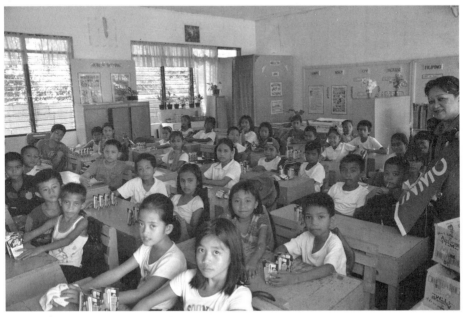

An INMO member, Gina Baldesco, delivering milk and health promotion advice to children during a visit to a school in Tacloban following Typhoon Haiyan. Courtesy INMO.

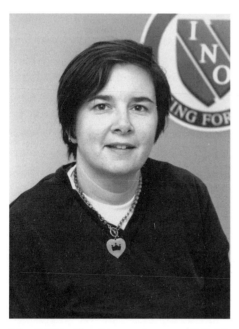

The INO's Clare Treacy. Courtesy INMO.

Midwives' Section within the INO; many were from the Philippines, and the organisation helped send seven members to assist in the aid effort following a devastating typhoon there in 2014.[20]

These activities were manifestations of the organisation's broad and developing concern with social justice; a dedicated Social Policy Division, headed up by former Industrial Relations Officer, Clare Treacy, was formed in 2002. The division campaigned on a range of issues from safeguarding the rights of migrant workers to combatting racism and establishing medically supervised injection facilities for intravenous drug users. The organisation became the first trade union to support the 'Turn Off the Red Light Campaign' in 2011. This movement sought to end prostitution in Ireland by, among other measures, criminalising those who bought sex.[21] Treacy recalled:

> I was approached by the Immigrant Council of Ireland [and they were] trying to get as many organisations and trade unions involved in the campaign. So I got the INO to agree to be involved … It is a horrific industry. As I always say to people if you went into the dole office and you said, 'I can't find work', would the dole office say to you, 'have you considered prostitution?' So to me that was a key campaign that the INO got involved in … This is a crime, it is a crime against women, it is a crime against society … Having sex is not a human right, it is a consensual issue … And I think that literally changed [peoples'] views … a significant number of nurses got involved … I also got some other unions involved … I would be most proud of that.[22]

The campaign was successful, and the purchase of sex was outlawed under the *Criminal Law (Sexual Offences) Act* of 2017.[23] The organisation also threw its weight behind the ultimately successful campaign to permit same-sex marriage in Ireland in 2015.[24]

Nursing pioneer Ethel Bedford Fenwick noted that 'the nurse question was the woman question' in the early 1900s. In so doing, she drew attention to the fact that the issues affecting nurses were manifestations of the issues affecting women more generally. Treacy was elected as Chairperson of the National Women's Council of Ireland in 2010, bringing the INO's concerns and agenda to a larger audience and facilitating mutual interchange between both bodies:

> I tried to bring a gender perspective to it ... I think other unions are guilty of this as well [and] are a bit blind to the gender element. We [tend to think that] we are all at the same start line, but we are not ... Certainly my view is that the workplace is really a little microcosm of society and the same gender inequalities that happen in society are replicated in the workplace.[25]

The organisation's involvement in the Women's Council is fitting, considering the council's genesis in the work of the IHA, of which Marie Mortished was once Chairperson. Treacy divided her time in the organisation's Social Policy Division with a new growth area – fitness to practise. INO members had occasionally been subject to disciplinary measures for professional shortcomings, and midwives, for instance, were reported to the Central Midwives' Board for substandard record-keeping as far back as the 1930s. The 1950 *Nurses Act* provided for the establishment of a committee by An Bord Altranais in order to investigate complaints against nurses and midwives, and if deemed necessary, to remove their names from the register.[26] This, as it happened, was a rather extreme outcome and occurred infrequently. The 1985 *Nurses Act* brought with it a change, with the implementation of less extreme measures such as advising or censuring a nurse or midwife found guilty of professional shortcomings.[27] The fitness to practise process became more formal and litigious in the years that followed, and the number of complaints against nurses and midwives rose.

Treacy again: 'When I took over the role ... I distinctly remember there was one open file on fitness to practise, we had one file and I can remember at my interview I wasn't even asked a question on fitness to practice because it wasn't of any particular importance.'[28] She continued: 'It was an unfortunate nurse that got reported to fitness to practice ... And then for some reason, year on year, it just kept getting bigger and bigger.'[29] In 2014, a total of fifty-six initial complaints against nurses or midwives were received by An Bord Altranais.[30] In 2015, some seventy-five complaints were received.[31] One nurse was suspended without pay and reported to the board for failing to initiate resuscitation on a man the nurse found dead in a hospital chair. The nurse recalled: 'This decision, based on my clinical assessment and the patient's right to die with dignity, was to affect my life and career in a profound and immutable way.'[32] The nurse remembered the expertise and support that the INO offered: '[The organisation's barrister] managed to pose a question that remained unanswered at the end of the inquiry: namely, if I were guilty of professional misconduct, then why were not others on the scene [including a doctor who did not actively disagree with the nurse's judgement] ... not also culpable ... two standards appeared to operate.'[33]

The increasing volume and complexity of complaints levelled at its members resulted in the INO developing significant skill in the fitness to practise arena. The organisation is now an exemplar to other organisations in this regard, and evidence suggests that the majority of those who join the INO, some 85 per cent, do so for the broadly related issue of indemnity.[34] Crucially, the INO has never sought to defend or excuse bad practice and described a range of poor practices at a Dublin nursing home, including staff sleeping on duty, as 'disgraceful and indefensible', when they were aired on Irish national television as part of an undercover investigation into care standards in 2005.[35] The organisation did, however, fear that its members might become 'additional victim[s]' of An Bord Altranais' fitness to practise machinery – especially considering the protracted length of time, with all the associated stress, that it sometimes took for a formal hearing into a complaint to come to fruition: at least eighteen months and sometimes longer.[36] Clare Treacy remarked:

I think it is probably the most horrific thing that you could put a nurse through ... I know there were definitely at least two nurses that died by suicide in and around fitness to practice ... I personally found that extraordinarily difficult ... It was a very difficult thing to know somebody and try to help them, try to represent them and then they died by suicide ... it took its toll on me ... And most nurses, I suppose on one hand appreciated that the INO was representing them but, on the other hand, were acutely embarrassed that they were now the subject of a complaint; be it incompetence, be it drug and alcohol abuse, be it professional misconduct ... I think the key word would be embarrassment ... And that is what you do in the first session with them, try and get over that and work towards ... putting forward as good and robust response as possible with the assistance of legal personnel if necessary.[37]

Working through the Preliminary Proceedings Committee, a group responsible for the initial consideration of complaints, the organisation was able to resolve the majority of complaints before they became the subject of a full hearing.

When public hearings became the norm in 2014, the INO campaigned that some be conducted in private.

Amid reports that the economy was recovering and as the Haddington Road Agreement was approaching its end, the organisation's Director of Industrial Relations, Phil Ní Sheaghdha, took to the stage at the Annual Conference in 2015. Ní Sheaghdha, a formidable negotiator who, according to one colleague, 'wouldn't let a fly land on your nose twice without claiming an allowance for it', suggested that members' terms and conditions be restored as fast as they had been ravaged: 'The pay cuts … were rapid and they were blunt, and you suffered the consequences.'[38] But members would have to make do with a more gradual approach. The third agreement of its kind, the Lansdowne Road Agreement, was bartered just a stone's throw away from the former home of early INO leader Kathleen Nora Price. It provided for a relaxation of the pension levy and a modicum of salary restoration. A final decision as to the acceptance or rejection of the agreement was communal, and fearful of finding itself ostracised from other unions that might accept it, the organisation's Executive Council begrudgingly recommended it to members as a first step in greater things to come. INO members agreed by a margin of 71 per cent in favour in the summer of 2015 as did their fellow trade unionists in congress.[39]

While this represented 'progress' on a scale applicable to all public servants, all the while the INO waged a relentless battle to undo the austerity measures as applied to its members. It skilfully and painstakingly secured the reversal of many of the hardships nurses and midwives were forced to endure. The organisation, working through the Labour Court, secured the restoration of the valuable and hard-won senior staff nurse/midwife scale, which had been removed spuriously as collateral damage with a ban on promotions. This was one of the first cuts to be reversed for any group of public servants. The organisation also secured, for student nurses in their final year, restoration of and an increase in their salary, to 80 per cent of the starting salary of qualified nurses/midwives; students' rostered placement was to qualify for incremental credit, and the INO also won the reinstatement of the only premium removed from nurses and midwives – the evening premium.

The organisation also submitted a compelling case to the Public Sector Pay Commission and drew attention to the sharp drop in the number of nurses and midwives that the recruitment moratorium caused: nursing numbers fell from over 39,000 in 2007 to 35,330 in 2015.[40]

Recruitment and retention were flashpoints, and the INO pressed home details of the global market in which employers competed for labour – the USA alone is estimated to see a shortage of one million nurses by 2020.

Nonetheless, where pay was concerned, the commission did not recommend specific pay increases for nurses and midwives. It did, however, suggest further investigation into occupational sectors where recruitment and retention of staff was problematic,[41] with health being one such area. This was a response with a somewhat familiar ring to it, but members' annoyance had been tempered by the recent announcement, on foot of threatened industrial action, of a funded workforce plan. The plan was ring-fenced for nursing and midwifery, with a commitment to employ an additional 1,200 nurses and midwives, the replacement of all those who left or retired, the offer of permanent full-time jobs to all those on recruitment panels and to all graduating nurses and midwives in 2016 and 2017, devolved authority for recruitment to nurse and midwife managers, increases in the number of student nurses, increases in the number of promotional posts and an improved incentivised scheme to entice nurses/ midwives working abroad to return to Ireland. The organisation's members, in strategically accepting the successor to Lansdowne Road, also put in train an examination of recruitment and retention in nursing and midwifery, with a report due in mid-2018. Crucially, if nurses and midwives receive improved conditions from the process, there can be no knock-on claims from other employment sectors.

II. From Broke to Broken

At the Association of Secondary Teachers, Ireland, convention in the 1980s, one teacher quipped: 'Do you think that, when miners have their conference, they talk about coal?'[42] The suggestion was that some teachers would prefer if their union focussed more on the welfare of teachers as opposed to the welfare of students or the educational system. This line of questioning never permeated the INO, and a recent slogan employed by the organisation, 'Serving Nurses, Midwives *and* Patients since 1919' [emphasis added], points to an organisation that is as concerned with the plight of patients as it is at the plight of members. This concern was amplified during the recession. Compared to Germany's six beds, Ireland had an average of three beds per 1,000 of the population in 2001,[43] and that was before the cuts, which witnessed 570 beds lying idle in 2009.[44] The consequences were harrowing, and the INO invited affected patients to record their experiences on a website it established. One went:

> On August 15, 2008, an MRI scan showed that I had two large aneurysms on the main artery going into my brain … I attended the clinic on November 12 2008 to be told I needed surgery on both. I was told these operations will be

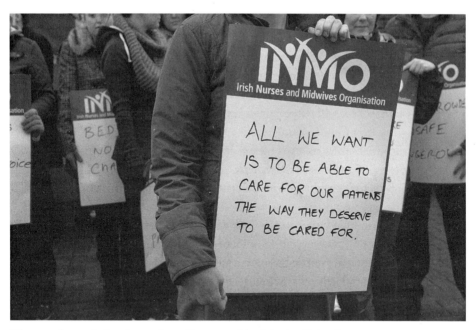

The words speak for themselves. Courtesy Lisa Moyles/INMO.

done before Christmas. GUESS WHAT!!! I am still waiting. Due to cutbacks only emergency operations are being done … I am 46 years of age. I have a good job and three children and I have paid my taxes all my working life. I don't deserve to die because no-one can get a bed.[45]

These sentiments formed part of a suite of concerns for patient welfare. The *Francis Report* of 2013 detailed how the Mid Staffordshire Trust in Britain cut staff numbers with an apparent disregard for patient safety.[46] The quality of care duly plummeted, with poor standards being readily tolerated by those in authority as the overriding focus moved to the trust's targets and finances. The INO was concerned that the report might, one day, find echo in Ireland and convened a national conference on the issue.[47] The organisation also requested that the Health Information and Quality Authority carry out unannounced inspections of hospitals in order to ascertain that standards were being adhered to.[48] Inequalities in the Irish healthcare system also entered the INO's crosshairs. The healthcare system in Ireland witnesses those who can afford to pay gaining rapid access to consultants, diagnostic tests and procedures while those without the same financial means wait for months or years. Dave Hughes recounted:

I came to work for the INO in December '98 and I was at [my] first conference in May of the following year [and] one of the things that surprised me was the absolute abhorrence that nurses speaking at the podium had for private health care. My vision or my view of nurses was that they were largely conservative, middle class people and that it wouldn't even be on their agenda ... So I had to listen very carefully. To put it bluntly, people with very posh accents were totally opposed to private medicine and I couldn't get [it] into my head why they would be. But I realised at the end of that conference it is because they have seen ... that private patients are treated better than public ones and that it matters in terms of access whether you are private or public and they know this ... So they know the difference between private and public delivery and they are instinctively against it.[49]

The INO soon formally adopted a human rights-based approach to health, campaigning for a health service funded by general taxation with a minimum spend of 10 per cent of gross domestic product in which need alone, not the ability to pay, determined access. The organisation impressed this upon the Committee on the Future of Healthcare, established by the state in 2016.[50] The INO also indicated that political consensus would be necessary to bring

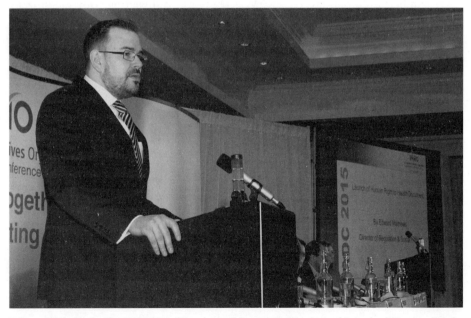

Edward Mathews, the INMO's Director of Social Policy, launching the 'Human Right to Health' document in 2015. Courtesy Lisa Moyles/INMO.

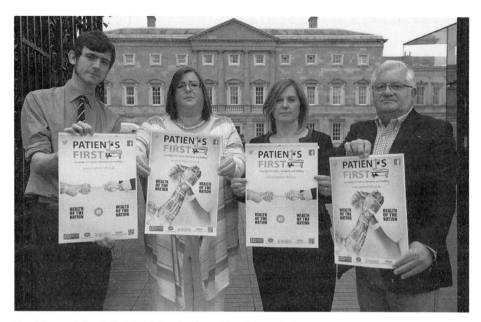

President of the INMO Claire Mahon (third from left) joins representatives of the Irish Medical Organisation, Patient Opinion and the Irish Patients' Association to launch the 'Patients First' campaign in 2014. Mahon trained as a general nurse at the County and City Infirmary Waterford and, before her election to the position of President, was Clinical Nurse Manager, Trauma Services at Waterford Regional Hospital. Courtesy Lisa Moyles/INMO.

about such a change, and significant inroads were made in this regard with the launch of the all-party *Sláintecare Report* in 2017.[51]

The overcrowding of Emergency Departments remained the most visible manifestation of Ireland's ailing health services. The INO had first supplied the state with figures on hospital overcrowding in 1977 and commenced Trolley Watch in 2005, a daily tally of the number of patients in Emergency Departments awaiting admission. The count garners massive exposure, serving as a talking point in media and political circles and has become a de facto barometer of the general health of the hospital services. The organisation attempted to mobilise public opinion behind its patient advocacy drive, and in conjunction with the Irish Patients' Association, Cystic Fibrosis Ireland and the Irish Medical Organisation, launched a campaign known as 'Patients First' in 2014.[52] For all of the INO's efforts, the return has been minimal, and the number of patients on hospital trolleys on 3 January 2018 reached almost 700 – a new high, a new low. Liam Doran remarks:

Remember the passport office dispute a few years ago. A young fellow chained himself to the bloody railings outside the Molesworth Street [passport] Office because he couldn't get a flipping passport. That day there was forty-one people on a trolley [at a Dublin hospital] and no one protested. So it is what it is ... I think Trolley Watch has been an excellent vehicle for the [organisation] in terms of visibility ... But I do accept that twelve years on it is an admission of failure but ... it is not for the want of trying ... The missing link in the chain is the general public and until the general public say ... we ain't having it, and that manifests itself in the ballot box, it won't be solved.[53]

In 2009, the HSE experienced a funding shortfall of over one billion euros,[54] posts that became vacant due to retirement were not to be filled and temporary contracts, held by some 4,000 nurses and midwives, were not to be renewed.[55] The work environment became increasingly challenging, as recalled by one nurse who wrote to the INO:

I'VE [sic] just finished a shift today and the place is beyond horrendous. Two staff were reduced to tears, but this seems to be the norm. Five ambulances

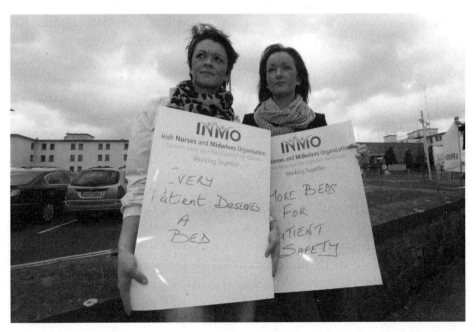

Suzanne Lynch and Anne O'Connell protest outside Limerick Regional Hospital in September 2011. Courtesy Press 22.

were waiting to be triaged when I arrived. There were no cubicles to see newly presenting patients … Patients were out by x-ray on trolleys, outside [the] resuscitation room with no nurse looking after them. Patients with raised troponins were waiting up to three hours to be seen and when I left at 8:30 p.m., there were patients still waiting who had presented to the department at 11:30 a.m. It is disgusting for the night staff coming into that. The place smells awful and is still 10 degrees above boiling … Morale is non-existent at the moment and the nurses are broken![56]

As Sheila Dickson assumed the Presidency of the organisation, she correctly interpreted the sense of desperation: 'I would say to any nurse or midwife who is a member of the INO that they should never feel that nobody cares because we do … I feel we need to reconnect with these people and let them know that they are not alone and that there is help there.'[57] Help soon assumed a tangible form. The INO had provided members with indemnity insurance since 1977, with a medical plan since 1989, and a counselling and legal helpline was soon

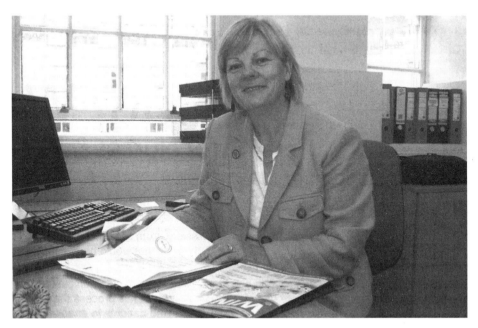

Sheila Dickson trained as a nurse at North Middlesex Hospital, London, and worked in the UK for many years afterwards. She returned home to Co. Kerry to take up a position as a nurse at St Columbanus Home, Killarney. She served as President of the INMO, 2008–12. She was later elected to the Board of the National Women's Council of Ireland. Courtesy INMO.

added to member services. Now, at a cost of tens of thousands of euros, the organisation rolled out a series of 'Tools for Safe Practice' workshops nationwide which guided members in issues related to documentation, priority setting and accountability. Annette Kennedy explained:

> The reason that safe practice and that kind of education came in was that it was a time when government were really taking [our] salaries, our conditions were dis-improving and the union had very little power to change [it] ... [But] our members are still paying their membership ... and I thought we needed something to give them to support them at [that] time ... When we couldn't get an increase in salary, when we couldn't do different things in relation to [industrial relations, then safe practice] had to come in and take precedence with our members to try and support them.[58]

Kennedy retired from the organisation in 2012. Not one to let the grass grow under her feet, in 2017 she was elected President of the ICN – the first Irish nurse/midwife to hold such an accolade. Elizabeth Adams, who had more than proven her worth in driving nurse and midwife prescribing some years earlier, then assumed the helm at the organisation's Professional Development Centre. Adams remarked:

> Now is the time to ensure that nurses and midwives are practising safely and to support them on the frontline to be able to make decisions to ensure safe patient care and to be competent to deliver that effectively ... my current priority is to support those on the frontline to make a clinical judgement in relation to what is safe and what is not safe.[59]

Historically, nurses and midwives lacked the research data to support their claims, but hard facts in relation to staffing levels were now fast adding legitimacy and gravitas to their cause. A seismic paper by Linda Aiken and her team in *The Lancet* in 2014 suggested that an increase in a nurse's workload by just one patient increased the likelihood of an inpatient dying within thirty days of admission by 7 per cent.[60] Aiken's research utilised data from the RN4CAST project, an outgrowth of which had been funded by the INO.[61] RN4CAST studies how the organisational aspects of hospital care impact nurse recruitment and retention and patient outcomes. The INO's involvement was part of a broader strategy to quantify the importance of nursing/midwifery and to have this reflected in the dwindling allocation of financial and human resources. The need for the INO's involvement was self-evident, as one survey at the time found that only one quarter of nurses in Ireland believed that there were enough nurses to provide patients with quality care.[62] In 2014, the internationally recommended ratio of one midwife to every 29.5 births was not in place in any Irish hospital.[63]

External developments provided both hope and guidance. The state of California, USA, passed legislation in the late 1990s cementing specific nurse to patient ratios, even during meal breaks. Judith Kieja, Acting General Secretary of the New South Wales Nurses' and Midwives' Association, addressed the INO's Annual Delegate Conference in 2014 and recounted a militant campaign that witnessed her members actively closing beds, defying a Labour Court order not to strike and ultimately winning a ratio framework for nurse and midwife staffing in New South Wales, Australia, in 2011.[64] INO members took note. But just as members got their blood up, the state intervened and announced a Taskforce on Nurse Staffing, on which the INO was to be represented. The body issued an interim report in late 2015 which recommended that staffing be decided by use of a patient dependency tool.[65] Whilst not trying to dampen expectations, the Working Party on General Nursing recommended similarly in 1980, as did the *Report of the Commission on Nursing* in 1997. Yet the piloting of a dependency tool, in three hospitals in 2016, shows some progress – however slow.

III. Buildings, Bills and Bills

For all the challenges the recession brought some opportunities. The heads of a new Nurses and Midwives Bill were published in 2008, and the INO seized the opportunity to influence the ensuing legislation. The organisation's initial concerns over the bill revolved around whether nursing/midwifery were being treated as the poor cousins of the medical profession. It had been widely touted that the legislation would formally necessitate nurses and midwives to maintain their professional competence. Yet the bill appears to have lacked the same commitment to continuing professional development as the *Medical Practitioners Act* of 2007, and the INO feared that the financial burden of continuing education would fall entirely on its members.[66] Negotiations led to an agreement whereby employers would assist in this regard.[67] In preparation for the formal requirement for nurses and midwives to maintain their professional competence, the INO then made a shrewd and strategic move. The former Richmond Hospital, one of Dublin's most iconic buildings, came on the market in 2013. Just a stone's throw from the organisation's headquarters at the Whitworth Hospital, the building caught the attention of the organisation's personnel. Liam Doran explained:

[The staff in the Professional Development Centre] were saying we could do more if we had more space … We looked at a couple of buildings on the South Circular Road that could be college-type buildings [but] one day we were coming to work and the 'For Sale' sign was on the window [of the Richmond] … Elizabeth [Adams] came into me … she looked at me and I looked at her like, 'Did you see it?', 'Yeah, did you see it?', 'Yeah I saw it, we will have to try for this.' So I rang the President [Claire Mahon] and Claire was, 'Go for it' … So that was it, and we have it … I want it to be our building but I also want it to be a building that will serve the community … So it is very timely and as we hit our centenary I think it will leave the organisation structurally in a position where we can look forward with confidence knowing we can hopefully deliver the strands of services that members would reasonably expect, want and require as practising nurses and midwives.[68]

Elizabeth Adams oversaw renovations to the building, and the former hospital now serves as the organisation's Education and Event Centre. The Richmond was formally opened in 2018 with fitting fanfare. The organisation's slogan for the building, 'Shaped by the Past, Shaping the Future', was appropriate. The Richmond was the venue for the INO's first ever refresher course for nurses in February 1938. A photograph of the event survives that shows some eighty nurses and their lecturers standing on the steps that lead to the hospital's entrance; the same steps that the organisation's members ascend today to undertake the organisation's continuing education courses. But let's not get too syrupy and sentimental; other important business remains.

The era of self-regulation for the professions was over, and impending legislative change meant that An Bord Altranais was to have a non-nursing/midwifery majority – undoing years of the INO's efforts to increase such representation. Just eight members of the twenty-three member-board were to be nurses or midwives democratically elected by the professions.[69] The organisation largely resigned itself to the development but requested the further democratisation of the board, with the representation of all branches of nursing and the heightened recognition of midwifery in the impending legislation. The Commission on Nursing had helped get the ball rolling in this regard and with good reason. Over the years, midwifery had been subsumed by nursing. Legislation referred to midwifery and midwives under the title nursing and nurses, respectively, and midwifery education was seen by many as merely a finishing school for nurses.[70] This was matched in discourse, and one nurse recalled her time in a maternity hospital: 'In the height of labour I never heard anybody shouting for a midwife, it was always, nurse, nurse.'[71] The new

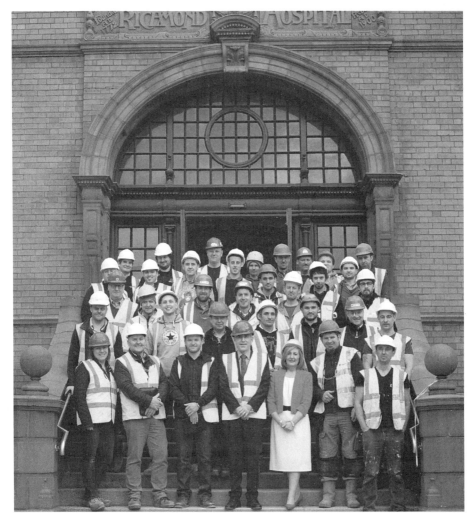

Transformation nearly complete: work progressing on the refurbishment to the Richmond in 2017. Liam Doran is front and centre with Elizabeth Adams to his right. Courtesy Lisa Moyles/INMO.

act was titled the *Nurses and Midwives Act* of 2011, but it was the INO that lead the way. An undergraduate degree course in midwifery commenced in Ireland in 2006, and in order to reflect future graduates and members who might not necessarily be nurses, the Irish Nurses' Organisation became the Irish Nurses' and Midwives' Organisation (INMO) on 1 January 2010. Midwives now had a place in the organisation's title, some eighty-five years after having been removed from it.

In the act's early stages, much of the INMO's concerns about the proposed legislation related to safe standards of care, and the organisation wished that the board be given the power to inspect hospitals and devise the requirements needed in order to ensure that nurses/midwives could practice safely.[72] The organisation was attempting to put safe practice on a legislative footing and clearly saw the new act and An Bord Altranais as the vehicles through which to advance its aim. In a letter to the board's Chief Executive Officer in 2009, Liam Doran asked:

> Will An Bord Altranais please indicate what a nurse or midwife should do when he/she has repeatedly made known their concerns, about standards of care, to the appropriate authorities, eg, their employer, and these concerns, both verbal and in writing, have been totally ignored? ... There are currently large numbers of nurses and midwives working in locations which, in the view of those nurses and midwives, is unsafe and which, following independent third party examination, have been found to involve high risk to patients ... What should these nurses and midwives now do in order to adhere to their Code of Professional Conduct?[73]

If tensions between the INMO and An Bord Altranais were rising, they were about to get a whole lot worse. In late 2014, the board announced that it was increasing its annual retention fee by 50 per cent. The pot was long past bubbling and was about to boil over; history explains why. In the late 1980s An Bord Altranais entered a situation of dire financial straits. The information technology infrastructure necessary for the board to establish a live register of nurses and midwives at the time was priced at £300,000,[74] and to add to the board's woes, in 1988, it experienced a cost overrun on a computers' symposium it convened, contributing to reports that it was 'technically bankrupt'.[75] In response, the board took a decision to increase nurses' and midwives' annual retention fee from £25 to £33. The INO reacted angrily as the fee rise did not reflect increases in its members' salaries or in the consumer price index.[76] The board was not for turning, however, and warned registrants that a failure to pay would render them liable to have their names removed from the register.[77]

The ultimate agreement reached was a compromise whereby nurses and midwives would pay an annual retention fee of £31, and the INO would be kept abreast of any future plans to alter the fee. The organisation was facing Hobson's choice as the state refused to clear An Bord Altranais' debts and warned the board that if it did not become self-financing it faced replacement with a board of civil servants.[78] This was unpalatable to the INO, who, after many years battling, was slowly winning increases in the number of nurses/ midwives at board level: the first nurse President of the Board, Johanna Barlow, was only elected in 1979.

The 1989 fee dispute, occurring at the tail end of a period of punishing austerity measures, was less about money than it was about the board's apparent detachment from the realities of practicing nurses and midwives. P.J. Madden wrote a scathing letter to An Bord Altranais in 1988 and referenced ongoing short-staffing and what he perceived as the board's failure to take a 'public stance in defence of overworked nurses ... and their professional obligations to provide optimum levels of care'.[79] The board, however, denied that it had a 'clearly-defined role' and asserted that it was not responsible for the delivery of services – this role being that of the Department of Health's and individual hospitals.[80] It appears that the board had a better understanding of its parameters than of its potential. The board's architect, Noël Browne, implied a wide-ranging role for An Bord Altranais when he created it in the late 1940s: 'There is nothing to stop this Board making recommendations to me in regard to anything,' he noted while drafting the 1950 *Nurses Act*.[81] Nor was the board necessarily driving wide-ranging or radical change in other areas of nursing

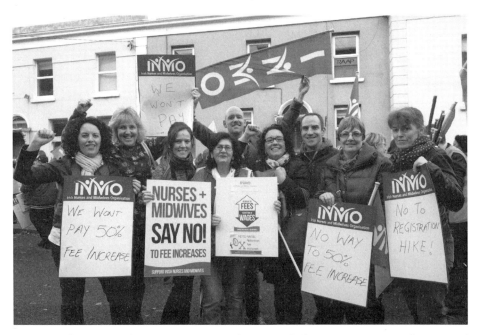

A group of nurses/midwives protesting at the NMBI's decision to increase their annual retention fee. Courtesy Lisa Moyles/INMO.

and midwifery. If judged by the brevity of its submission to the Commission on Nursing, a 16-page document composed almost entirely of bullet points, An Bord Altranais' aspirations for the professions were modest to say the least.[82]

All of this helped set the mood for what was coming. The board imposed a small fee hike, from €85 to €88 in 2010, which, on the promise of an era of glasnost between both bodies, the INMO acceded to.[83] No sooner had members of the organisation amended their direct debits than the fee had risen to €100, and in late 2014, a rise to a bill of €150 was touted. This represented a 70 per cent rise in retention fees in just two years. It also represented a tipping point. The INMO showed dogged resolve and advised its members to pay the

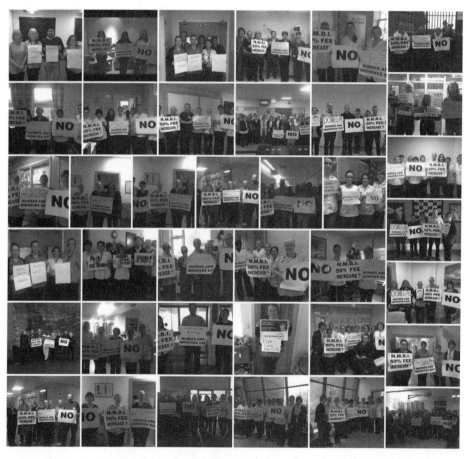

Images from the INMO's 'thunderclap' protest against increase in its members' annual retention fee in 2015. Hundreds of images, like these, of protesting nurses and midwives were rolled out via social media. Courtesy INMO.

existing €100 fee only. In conjunction with other nurses'/midwives' unions, it arranged a 2,000-strong protest rally at the board's headquarters, during which a petition of protest was delivered. The organisation also issued members with badges denoting that they had paid the €100 fee as an emblem of solidarity. In its early days, the INMO communicated with members through paper periodicals. Later came telephones, but technological developments meant that the fee debacle was the first to witness, on a grand scale, the employment of social media as an ally. These platforms took their place alongside the INMO's by then unparalleled print and media presence, which was worth over €6 million by 2010.[84]

At the heart of the INMO's stance on rising retention fees were fears over where the increases would end. Implementing the many provisions of the new *Nurses and Midwives Act* looked set to be costly, and the state was not in a giving mood. The debacle also had echoes of its forerunning dispute in the 1980s. At the request of An Bord Altranais, the Commission on Nursing enshrined the protection of the public as one of the board's explicit concerns.[85] Considering the widespread cuts at the time and all of the associated concerns for patient welfare, nurses and midwives understood the term 'protection' in its broadest sense and anticipated a meaningful statement on the topic by the board; Emergency Departments, if judged by trolley numbers, were now operating almost daily in what a government minister had once called a 'national emergency'. But nurses and midwives were to be left waiting, and over 60,000 of them received a letter in November 2014 from the President of the board, by then known as the Nursing and Midwifery Board of Ireland (NMBI), that went:

> While many of you think we should intervene in local disputes about staffing etc, it is only relating to [regulation, registration, education and standard-setting] that the Board has a role ... I would ask you all, irrespective of how unhappy you feel about it, to pay [the increased fee] as without registration you unfortunately will not be allowed to work.[86]

The board was clearly not for turning and was arguably living up to the fears that some had expressed when it had first been touted back in the late 1940s. One speaker in the Senate in 1949, Mrs Concannon, winced when she heard of the coming about of An Bord Altranais: 'We asked for bread and while we were not given a stone we were given something as hard – a board.'[87] Many nurses and midwives, spooked at the prospect of finding themselves unable to work, defied the INMO's direction and paid the increased fee. In mid-January

2015, the board issued a statement that 'daily payments [were] now in their thousands'.[88] The statement appears to have come across as somewhat gloating if not downright smug and backfired, with at least 10,000 nurses and midwives refusing to pay.[89] They effectively dug their heels in and rowed in behind the INMO's position. A stand-off of very serious proportions ensued. The NMBI's future operations were in doubt if it could not meet its costs through nurses' and midwives' fees; likewise, many nurses' and midwives' jobs were in doubt as, without paying the fee, they were unable to work.

The Minister for Health and Children, Leo Varadkar, recognised the dispute's severity and urged dialogue between the INMO and the board.[90] The outcome was a success for the INMO, and following a special meeting of the board in early March 2015, it was decided that the fee would remain at €100. The win gave the INMO a much-needed shot in the arm, particularly after seven years of recession. Indeed, the €100 annual fee was enshrined into subsequent national pay policies. After the fact, revelations of costly niceties of the board's staff emerged, such as business class flights.[91] During the debacle, nurses and midwives also expressed a view that the board largely had two functions – to issue them with a yearly fee and to discipline them.[92] Revelations that it had spent €2.3 million in fitness to practice-related legal fees in 2014, twice that of the previous year and one third of its total income from nurses'/midwives' fees, did little to allay that view.[93] Soon after an external report described the NMBI as 'dysfunctional', as failing in many of its responsibilities and as having a financial situation that was of 'serious concern'.[94] Madeline Spiers, a member of the board and past President of the INMO, recalled:

The history of An Bord Altranais, as provided for in the 1985 *Nurses Act*, to its transition under the 2011 *Nurses and Midwives Act* and subsequent emergence as the Nursing and Midwifery Board of Ireland, is one of missed opportunities rooted in its abject failure to understand its core objectives: the protection of the public and the need to ensure the integrity of the nursing and midwifery professions. I say this as a vindication of the nurses and midwives who spoke truth to power and the INMO who raised concerns over the failure of the NMBI to discharge its statutory responsibilities over many years. I was elected by nurses and midwives to the board of the NMBI in 2012. I was selected to speak on their behalf, to inform the board of their clinical governance concerns and to speak up regarding concerns about the quality and quantum of care they could safely give to their patients. Once elected, I was shocked at how remote the board's Executive was to nurses and midwives, to their concerns and to issues regarding public safety. We seemed to spend most of our time on fitness to practice issues, occasionally reading briefs on cases running to thousands of pages. This alone often occupied ten to fifteen hours of my time each week with millions of euros being spent on legal fees. From the beginning of my term, I sensed the intention to increase nurses' and midwives' retention fees in order to meet the costs of implementing the 2011 *Nurses and Midwives Act*. I supported the initial increase in the fee to €100; however, I was unhappy with the contempt that I perceived registrants and the unions were viewed by the NMBI; it seemed that the full financial burden of implementing the Act was to be carried by nurses and midwives. I feared that if the increase demanded of the registrants succeeded it would increase year on year, and could end up at a bill of over €400 a year in the very near future. The whole debacle caused a breach of trust and forced a boycott of the retention fee by the main nursing unions. I fully supported this stance and declined to pay my own fee in solidarity. From inside the headquarters of the NMBI, I watched the union protest on the street outside and my heart lifted to see such solidarity and support. Nurses and midwives, it seems to me, have to fight for everything; everything comes at a cost. I recall leaving the building to walk in solidarity with them and it felt right. We would not be bullied and several thousand nurses and midwives not paying the fee acted as a political reality check. We eventually turned the tide with the board rescinding its decision for a myriad of reasons, not least, that the health system cannot function without us.'[95]

History teaches a valuable lesson from this debacle. Faced with the removal of thousands of nurses and midwives from the register, the NMBI, arguably an agent of the state, 'concern[ed] for the potential impact on the provision of health care', backed down.[96] Just like the INO's threat of mass resignations in 1978 that yielded a significant dividend, it shows that the prospect of a removal or withdrawal of nursing/midwifery labour is one of the most potent weapons in nurses' and midwives' armoury. Could this be on the horizon? Pay parity with allied health professionals remains the INMO's Holy Grail and Doran concludes: 'My view is [that] the time is going to come where we have to do it all again if we want to get [to] where we believe we deserve to be ... The work is never finished ... I believe anyone who comes after me, should never lose sight, that is the goal, parity.'[97] But while the goal may be clear, the means for achieving it are not. To add yet another potential complication to nurses' and midwives' relationship with strike action, the state was about to deliver another curveball.

Conclusion, Epilogue …
and Over to You

Martina Harkin-Kelly, nurse educator, struck a chord with INMO members in 2016 during her campaign to become the organisation's President when she remarked: 'Well behaved women rarely make history.' Whether or not Harkin-Kelly was referring to militancy is unclear, but a touted ban on strikes in essential services, put forward by Leo Varadkar during his successful campaign to become Taoiseach in 2017, indicates a harder stance by the state and the potential of complicating matters further still for the INMO.[1] Measures such as that referred to by Varadkar are usually instituted in occupational sectors where it is regarded as irresponsible or unethical to withdraw one's labour, but in the case of nursing and midwifery, the measure raises as many questions about responsibility and ethics as it seeks to (at least supposedly) address. The INMO convened one national strike in its 100-year existence. That strike was engineered to have as little impact on patient welfare as possible, and nurses and midwives worked for nothing to ensure that this was the case. Does this smack of irresponsibility? And now to ethics. Is it ethical to remove a worker's right to strike? What effect would such a course of action have? When all other industrial relations' avenues have been exhausted and failed, does it condemn a nurse or midwife to tolerate the status quo indefinitely? If so, what kind of relationship would this foster between employer and employee? Would it be a helpful relationship that is conducive to getting the job done?

Those who seek to impose such measures might also ponder whether they are in any credible position to act as ethical arbiters. The state has, through its actions and inactions, arguably, engineered a health service with some of the longest waiting lists in Europe, with hundreds of patients languishing on hospital trolleys each day and with a critically underdeveloped primary care system. They expound the merits of an equitable public health service on Monday whilst turning the sod on a private hospital on Tuesday. Are these people in a position to lead on ethics, to dictate what is ethical or otherwise and to cast themselves as moral saviours of some sort? As former President of the INMO, Madeline Spiers once noted: 'hypocrisy is the homage vice pays to virtue'.[2]

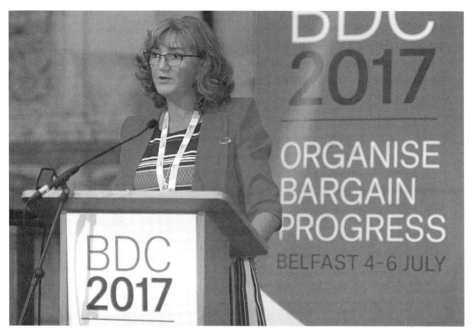

Martina Harkin-Kelly speaking at the Biennial Delegate Conference of ICTU in Belfast in 2017. Harkin-Kelly is from Glenmaquin, Co. Donegal. She trained as a nurse at Sligo General Hospital in the 1980s and later specialised in ophthalmic nursing before moving into the field of nurse education. Courtesy Lisa Moyles/INMO.

As the state was treating hard-pressed workers to its musings on strike action, the INMO unveiled a new leader: Phil Ní Sheaghdha. Ní Sheaghdha graduated from her position as the INMO's Director of Industrial Relations to General Secretary in 2018. A native Irish speaker from Kerry (sound familiar?), she was one of the last nurses to enter training at the Charitable Infirmary, Jervis Street, Dublin. Upon qualification, she was unable to find a job amid the health service cuts that characterised the 1980s. She emigrated and returned to Ireland in the 1990s with a new perspective: '[The] thing I noticed [most] was the nursing role was very subservient.'[3] She described one occasion wherein she witnessed a consultant who, having clearly mistaken a colleague for a lackey, asked a nurse to fetch some x-rays. The incident was a tipping point, and after a word in the doctor's ear, Ní Sheaghdha helped implement a number of changes in her workplace aimed at improving patient care and advancing the nursing perspective in matters of policy and practice. She soon became a nurse representative and in 1998 landed a position as Industrial Relations Officer with the INO.

On the cusp of her assuming leadership of the organisation, I put a question to Ní Sheaghdha regarding militancy. In answering, she paints a picture of herself as a rebel with a cause or, in her own words, 'not militant for the sake of militancy'.[4] Ní Sheaghdha describes the current negotiations on salaries and staffing levels and indicates a keenness to exhaust policy and procedural avenues prior to countenancing an industrial dispute:

> I think in nursing trade unionism the essential services we provide is [a] very important element of contingency planning. I believe that we have gained more, and maintain more control over a dispute, when the contingency is properly and carefully conducted ... This has worked well, and better in fact, than an all-out strike in many locations as, in an 'all-out', the hospital can easily replace [strikers] with agency and other staff ... whereas when the emergency service is provided as part of the contingency, the strike committee ... can have greater control ... we are controlling what [care] we give and that prevents a huge amount of scab labour being brought in ... This forces management to take us more seriously and seek to arrive at a realistic settlement as quickly as possible ... When you don't provide emergency services, or don't articulate that you will, you provoke the old debate about [whether] emergency services have the right to strike and this leads to threats of government introducing legislation to prevent emergency services taking action.[5]

Ní Sheaghdha sees a prohibition on strike action as a measure that could not be introduced easily. While acknowledging that the right to strike was not absolute, a recent ruling by the European Court of Human Rights suggested that the right to collectively bargain went hand in glove with the right to withdraw one's labour.[6] This considered, she continues: 'I think we have to be cautious about how we exercise the right to strike but we have to maintain the right to do so. I would argue that it is part and parcel of the collective bargaining process because, as one commentator put it, collective bargaining without the right to strike is more aptly described as "collective begging".'[7] Her admission provides a bookend of sorts: the greatest threat facing the INMO upon its establishment was concerns over the possibility that the organisation may take strike action.

Now, one hundred years later, serious issues may arise if the right to strike is threatened. We have travelled a long way, only to end up back at the same destination: the thorny issue of striking. But this time we have arrived by a different road. What we once shunned we now cling to. Why is that? It's because nurses and midwives are jaded and jaundiced of the praise, pious platitudes and promises. It's because they find themselves run ragged on hospital wards, in units and in the community. It's because activity levels and expectations continue to increase but are not matched by a corollary increase in staff numbers. Most importantly, it's because they see the feckless risks to patient safety that cost-savings and all those who fumble in that greasy till have created. And they toss and turn on this.

And now over to you. I know that as a solitary nurse or midwife you feel that you cannot do anything: that the system is too big, too unwieldy and too disinterested to change. But nobody is asking you to go it alone. The twenty nurses and midwives who founded the INMO one hundred years ago did so with nothing but enthusiasm, pluck and hope. Those twenty pioneers now number 40,000. True, in the broad swathes of time and in the social, economic and religious ebb and flow, that hope waxed and waned. Progress, on occasions, was glacial. But when judging the INMO's success, bear in mind that nurses and midwives had the odds stacked squarely against them. Hospitals pleaded the poor mouth, the founding members were chastised by their colleagues and matrons looked down their noses at the sheer thought of a nurses'/midwives' trade union. Politicians strung us along for years – broken promises, long-fingered claims and a hefty serving of condescension and 'couldn't care less' that would become an almost stock response to claims.

And don't get me started on employers. Some calculated nurses' annual leave based on the length of lunar months, as opposed to typical calendar months, as lunar months are slightly shorter. Unfortunately (or perhaps conveniently), and in spite of all their ingenuity, winter and all it brings continues to take the same wise guys by surprise each year. And don't forget the Catholic Church. One Ward Sister at a Dublin hospital obsessed that the wheels on hospital beds must face in a particular direction. Each morning, before getting down to work, the sister would kneel and pray, and if any misplaced wheel caught her attention, would say: 'In the name of the Father and of the Son … "Nurse straighten those wheels" … Amen.'[8] But the blending of religiosity with practice was far less important than the blending of religiosity with principles and, once internalised, this led to a pious, non-monetary devotion to duty by nurses and midwives that complicated matters further still. And there's more. The long-lived apprenticeship model of education meant that nurses and midwives could not lay claim to professional standing in order to further their status. They inhabited a no-man's-land wherein they were expected to adhere to professional standards but were simultaneously denied the formal educational structures and rewards commensurate with those same standards.

And I'm not finished yet. Why would a nurse or midwife who could not remain in her job after marriage bother investing herself in a struggle for better conditions? The state engineered an industrial relations-disinterested workforce whose apathy and resultant slow progress was completely understandable. To add insult to injury, the state believed it acceptable to pay women less than men and stubbornly clung to this trend until women's organisations and accession to the EEC dragged Ireland to a more enlightened position. All the while, those unions that represented men sat back and reaped the benefits of the patriarchal dividend. And this work continues. The next time a pay commission comes up less than adequate, don't ponder whether it's the fault of the dwindling honey bee population, of global warming or of the disappearance of the curlew. It is to do with the fact that nurses and midwives are mainly women, and their work, vital as it is, is gender-coded and thus automatically accorded a low value. Of course we will never be able to prove this, but anyone who wants to refute it might start by publishing the deliberations of the first Benchmarking body, if they can find them. And all of that before we even get to strikes. Those unions that represented workers in non-essential services were able to shut up shop in a dispute and wait for employers to capitulate. But it is not like that in nursing and midwifery. But you've read enough about strikes, right?

So remind yourself that those twenty pioneers who founded the INMO had to weather the perfect storm. But they persisted. In many ways we do not need this book to tell us that. In spite of the challenges, the fruits of the INMO's labours are all around us. The organisation has enhanced and enriched almost every aspect of nurses' and midwives' professional lives. Who drove the issue of salary standardisation? Who doggedly fought for a reduction in working hours? Who commandeered a pension scheme? Who established a Benevolent Fund while that scheme was being hammered out? Who led nurses and midwives into conciliation and arbitration? Who steered nurses and midwives back to the negotiating table in order to engage with national wage agreements? Who fought a relentless campaign to improve post-registration education for nurses and midwives – even going so far as to provide this education itself? Who was party to the establishment of the ground-breaking Commission on the Status of Women? Who, in the main, forced the state's hand into establishing the equally ground-breaking Commission on Nursing? Who then forced the state's hand into seeing that the findings of that commission, including the establishment of undergraduate degree education, were implemented? Who is the only union in Ireland aligned with the ICN and in a position to exert its influence at global level? Who is, almost single-handedly, driving the patient safety agenda in Ireland? The INMO.

And those are just the achievements that make the headlines. What about all the nurses and midwives who are represented in confidence, as individuals or in smaller groups, with issues as diverse as bullying, study leave or salary increments? It has taken time, enthusiasm and energy to get us this far, and it is going to take the same to get us further still. This is where you come in. The INMO is not a monolith. It is not just a building in Dublin; it is not the emblem on your lanyard or pen torch; it is not the journal that arrives in your letter box every few weeks. The INMO is you. Remember that trade unionism is far too important to be left to trade unionists alone. The rallying cry that Louie Bennett sent INMO members from the podium as she closed the organisation's first Annual Meeting is as valid today as it was in 1920. She told assembled nurses and midwives:

> We are still only an infant. It is the first business of an infant to grow. We have grown and grown lusty. We have kicked and crowed. Very soon our fumbling attempts to grapple with the evils that affect the lives of Nurses and of the people at large will become stronger and more assured. We can claim to have done good work already. We can be sure of doing very much more if the Nurses and Midwives of Ireland will all give freely in enthusiasm, in thought … and in patient hard work.[9]

So enough now of words. Let there be action.

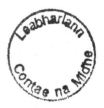

Endnotes

INTRODUCTION

1   E.H. Carr, *What is History?* (2nd edn, London: Penguin, 1987), p. 132.

CHAPTER 1

1   J. Dunsmore Clarkson, *Labour and Nationalism in Ireland* (New York: AMS Press, 1970), p. 102.

2   In 1770, two men were whipped from Newgate Prison (near Christchurch Cathedral) to College Green, Dublin for engaging in trade union activity. See A. Boyd, *The Rise of the Irish Trade Unions* (Tralee: Anvil Books, 1972), p. 12.

3   J. Wallace, P. Gunnigle, G. McMahon and M. O'Sullivan, *Industrial Relations in Ireland* (4th edn, Dublin: Gill and Macmillan, 2013), p. 25.

4   Boyd, *The Rise of the Irish Trade Unions*, p. 32. Violence against employers was treated with the utmost gravity. In 1816, a plot to blow up the residence of a textile manufacturer in dispute with his employees resulted in those found guilty being hanged; see J.W. Boyle, *The Irish Labor Movement in the Nineteenth Century* (Washington: The Catholic University of America, 1988), p. 15.

5   H. Pelling, *A History of British Trade Unionism* (3rd edn, Harmondsworth: Penguin, 1976), p. 101.

6   E. O'Connor, *A Labour History of Ireland: 1824–2000* (Dublin: University College Dublin Press, 2011), pp. 50–62.

7   Unskilled labourers numbered some 45,000 and earned approximately eighteen shillings per week, in contrast to skilled labourers who could earn up to two pounds per week; see P. Yeates, *Lockout, Dublin 1913* (Dublin: Gill and Macmillan, 2000), p. 31.

8   Ibid., p. 107.

9   'To the Masters of Dublin, an Open Letter', *Irish Times*, 7 October 1913.

10 *Irish Opinion*, January 1918, cited in T. Moriarty, *Work in Progress: Episodes from the History of Irish Women's Trade Unionism* (Dublin and Belfast: The Irish Labour History Society and UNISON, 1994), p. 20.

11 Yeates, *Lockout*, p. 152.

12 Delia Larkin worked as a nurse in Liverpool prior to her move to Ireland. See A. Buckley, 'Delia Larkin and the founding of the Irish Women Workers' Union' (Dublin: Trinity College, 1996), p. 2.

13 *Irish Worker*, September 1913, cited in Yeates, *Lockout*, p. 152.

14 E. O'Connor, 'Dawn Chorus: The Origins of Trade Unionism in Vocational Education, 1899–1930', in J. Logan (ed.), *Teachers' Union: The TUI and its Forerunners in Irish Education, 1899–1994* (Dublin: A. & A. Farmar, 1999), p. 46.

15   P. Rouse and M. Duncan, *Handling Change: A History of the Irish Bank Officials' Association* (Cork: The Collins Press, 2012), p. 37.

16   'Irish Nurses' Union, Branch of Irish Women Workers' Union', *Irish Citizen*, August 1919.

17   The commentary referred to proposals to establish a trade union for nurses in England, but its sentiments were just as applicable in Ireland. See 'The Nurses' Trade Union', *British Journal of Nursing*, LXII, 1650 (15 November 1919), p. 302.

18   D. Ferriter, *The Transformation of Ireland, 1900–2000* (London: Profile Books, 2005), p. 214.

19   'The Needs of Nurses', *Irish Times*, 28 February 1919.

20   Ibid.

21   Ibid.

22   Ibid.

23   'The Unthroning of the Nurse', *Irish Citizen*, March 1919.

24   'Nurses of Ireland Plead for Reform', *Weekly Irish Times*, 8 March 1919.

25   'International Council of Nurses', *British Journal of Nursing*, 101, 2222 (October 1953), p. 122.

26   C. Black, *King's Nurse – Beggar's Nurse* (London: Hurst and Blackett, 1939), p. 42.

27   'Who's Who in the Irish Hospital World', *Irish Nursing and Hospital World*, hereafter referred to as *INHW*, 1, 2 (15 September 1931), p. 7.

28   J. Hallam, *Nursing the Image: Media, Culture and Professional Identity* (London: Routledge, 2000), p. 20.

29   P. Yeates, *A City in Wartime: Dublin, 1914–18* (Dublin: Gill and Macmillan, 2011), p. 139; O. Walsh, *Anglican Women in Dublin: Philanthropy, Politics and Education in the Early Twentieth Century* (Dublin: University College Dublin Press, 2005), p. 200.

30   S. Horgan Ryan, 'Irish Military Nursing in the Great War', in G.M. Fealy (ed.), *Care to Remember: Nursing and Midwifery in Ireland* (Cork: Mercier Press, 2005), pp. 89–101.

31   Ibid., p. 96.

32   D. Fitzpatrick, 'Strikes in Ireland, 1914–21', *Saothar*, 6 (1980), pp. 26–39.

33   F. Devine, *Organising History: A Centenary of SIPTU* (Dublin: Gill and Macmillan, 2009), p. 14.

34   E. O'Connor, 'War and Syndicalism, 1914–23', in D. Nevin (ed.), *Trade Union Century* (Cork: Mercier Press, 1994), p. 57.

35   Ibid. For a more comprehensive analysis of syndicalism in Ireland, see E. O'Connor, *Syndicalism in Ireland: 1917–23* (Cork: Cork University Press, 1988).

36   A plaque in the foyer of that hospital commemorates O'Farrell's place in history. Her gravestone in Glasnevin Cemetery, Dublin reads: 'When duty called on the field of battle she went, under orders, the foe to meet bearing sadly, unfearingly, proudly, the flag of surrender but not defeat.'

37   For a comprehensive history of Cumann na mBan, see C. McCarthy, *Cumann na mBan and the Irish Revolution* (Cork: The Collins Press, 2007).

38   She was later released having gone on hunger strike; see B. Dirrane, R. O'Connor and J. Mahon, *A Woman of Aran* (Dublin: Blackwater Press, 1997), pp. 37–40.

39   S. McGann, A. Crowther and R. Dougall, *A History of the Royal College of Nursing, 1916–90: A Voice for Nurses* (Manchester: Manchester University Press, 2009), p. 27.

40   The campaigns are synopsised here but are much more masterfully arranged and analysed by Mary Cullen in her contribution to vol. VII of *A New History of Ireland*. See M. Cullen,

'Women, Emancipation, and Politics, 1860–1984', in J.R. Hill (ed.), *A New History of Ireland, vol. VII, 1921–84* (Oxford: Oxford University Press, 2003), pp. 826–91.

41 For a comprehensive analysis of the achievement of women's suffrage in Ireland, see R. Cullen Owens, *Smashing Times: A History of the Irish Women's Suffrage Movement, 1889–1922* (Dublin: Attic Press, 1984).

42 R. Cullen Owens, *Louie Bennett* (Cork: Cork University Press, 2001), p. 25.

43 For a comprehensive analysis of the *Irish Citizen* newspaper, see L. Ryan, *Irish Feminism and the Vote: An Anthology of the Irish Citizen Newspaper, 1912–20* (Dublin: Folens, 1996).

44 P. Scanlan, *The Irish Nurse, A Study of Nursing in Ireland: History and Education, 1718–1981* (Manorhamilton: Drumlin Publications, 1991), p. 78.

45 'District Midwives' Union', *Irish Independent*, 29 January 1919.

46 C. Hart, *Behind the Mask: Nurses, their Unions and Nursing Policy* (London: Baillière Tindall, 1994), pp. 21–2.

47 'District Midwives' Union', *Irish Independent*, 29 January 1919.

48 'Dispensary Midwives' Union', *Freeman's Journal*, 19 February 1919.

49 'Irish Midwives in Meeting', *Leitrim Observer*, 3 May 1919.

50 'Nurse' was the term reserved for female asylum attendants. It was 1921 before the General Nursing Council (Ireland) established a supplementary division in its register for mental nurses. Admission to this division was contingent on passing the exam of the Medico-Psychological Association or on being considered a bona fide nurse with at least three years' experience; see A. Sheridan, 'Psychiatric Nursing Practice: A Historical Overview', in J. Morrissey, B. Keogh and L. Doyle (eds), *Psychiatric/Mental Health Nursing: An Irish Perspective* (Dublin: Gill and Macmillan, 2008), pp. 3–15; A.J. Sheridan, 'The Impact of Political Transition on Psychiatric Nursing – A Case Study of Twentieth-Century Ireland', *Nursing Inquiry*, 13, 4 (2006), pp. 289–99.

51 For a short account of the strike, see D. Ó Drisceoil, *Peadar O'Donnell* (Cork: Cork University Press, 2001), pp. 12–13. See also P. Hegarty, *Peadar O'Donnell* (Cork: Mercier Press, 1999), pp. 48–52.

52 'Monaghan and Cavan Asylum', *Northern Standard*, 18 January 1919.

53 Ibid.

54 'Remarkable Sequel to Asylum Strike', *Irish Times*, 30 January 1919.

55 'Asylum Staff Mutiny', *Irish Independent*, 31 January 1919.

56 'Asylum Strike', *Anglo-Celt*, 15 February 1919.

57 D. Bates, 'Keepers to Nurses? A History of the Irish Asylum Workers' Trade Union, 1917–24' (Dublin: University College Dublin, 2010), p. 22.

58 Hegarty, *Peadar O'Donnell*, p. 52.

59 For a comprehensive account of the influenza epidemic, see C. Foley, *The Last Irish Plague: The Great Flu Epidemic in Ireland, 1918–19* (Dublin: Irish Academic Press, 2011).

60 D. Coakley, *Baggot Street: A Short History of the Royal City of Dublin Hospital* (Dublin: Royal City of Dublin Hospital, 1995), p. 55.

61 Foley, *The Last Irish Plague*, p. 145.

62 At the annual meeting of the Nurses' Insurance Society of Ireland in 1919, some 138 nurses claimed insurance benefits for having contracted influenza; see 'Nurses' Insurance Society of Ireland', *Weekly Irish Times*, 2 August 1919.

63 *Midwives (Ireland) Act (1918)*; *Nurses Registration (Ireland) Act (1919)*.

64   Rouse and Duncan, *Handling Change*, pp. 19–20.

65   T.J. O'Connell, *A History of the Irish National Teachers Organisation, 1868–1968* (Dublin: Irish National Teachers' Organisation, 1970), p. 12; J. Cunningham, *Unlikely Radicals: Irish Post-Primary Teachers and the ASTI, 1909–2009* (Cork: Cork University Press, 2009), pp. 44–7.

CHAPTER 2

1   P.G. Forster, *The Esperanto Movement* (The Hague: Mouton Publishers, 1982), p. 188.

2   'Irish Woman Workers' Union', *Irish Citizen*, February 1920. The National Union of Trained Nurses (NUTN) was already in existence in England when the INU was conceived. However, in spite of its title, the NUTN was not a trade union; see 'National Union of Trained Nurses, The N.U.T.N and the P.U.T.N', *British Journal of Nursing*, LXV, 1683 (3 July 1920), p. 12.

3   See 'The 1910 Union of Midwives', *British Journal of Nursing Supplement*, XLIV, 1143 (26 February 1910), pp. 179–80.

4   A.M. Rafferty and G. Boschma, 'The Essential Idea', in B.L. Brush and J.E. Lynaugh (eds), *Nurses of all Nations: A History of the International Council of Nurses, 1899–1999* (Philadelphia: Lippincott, Williams and Wilkins, 1999), p. 61.

5   The Independent Labour Party and Labour Research Department, *Trade Unions in Soviet Russia* (London: The Independent Labour Party and Labour Research Department, 1920), p. 37.

6   For further information on MacCallum and the Professional Union of Trained Nurses, see 'The Passing of a Great Spirit', *British Journal of Nursing*, LXXIV, 1896 (July 1926), pp. 155–6. There was a friendly reciprocity between both unions and a mutual membership agreement was bartered, whereby members of the INU working in England could avail of the services offered by the Professional Union of Trained Nurses and vice versa.

7   Little is known of the Irish Nurses' Association's past. For the most comprehensive account, see S. McGann, *The Battle of the Nurses* (London: Scutari Press, 1992), pp. 130–59.

8   Ibid., p. 138. See also P. O'Morain, *The Irish Association of Directors of Nursing and Midwifery, 1904–2004: A History* (Dublin: The Irish Association of Directors of Nursing and Midwifery, 2004), p. 7.

9   'Unionateness' is understood as the degree to which an organisation subscribes to trade union principles; see R.M. Blackburn, *Union Character and Social Class: A Study of White Collar Unionism* (London: Batsford, 1967), pp. 18–19.

10   'How Should Nurses Continue to Organise?' *Irish Nurses' Union Gazette*, hereafter referred to as *INU Gazette*, 13 (May 1925), p. 4.

11   M. Jones, *These Obstreperous Lassies: A History of the Irish Women Workers' Union* (Dublin: Gill and Macmillan, 1988), pp. 25–6; *Report of the Provisional Committee to the First Annual Conference of the INU*, 1920 (Irish Nurses' and Midwives' Organisation Archives, hereafter referred to as INMO Archives, Dublin, Archives Box).

12   Jones, *These Obstreperous Lassies*, pp. 38–9.

13   Ibid., p. 40.

14   Bennett has been the subject of two biographies to date. See R.M. Fox, *Louie Bennett: Her Life and Times* (Dublin: The Talbot Press, 1958); Cullen Owens, *Louie Bennett*.

15   A. Frazier, *Hollywood Irish: John Ford, Abbey Actors and the Irish Revival in Hollywood* (Dublin: The Lilliput Press, 2011), pp. 101–2; F. McGarry, *The Abbey Rebels of 1916* (Dublin: Gill and Macmillan, 2015), p. 112.

16   'Saturday's Child Has Far to Go'. Unpublished Manuscript and Field Notes in the Shields Family Archive (James Hardiman Library Archives, Galway, T13/A/512, T13/A/511(1)).

17   P. Ó Duigneáin, *Linda Kearns: A Revolutionary Irish Woman* (Manorhamilton: Drumlin, 2002), pp. 52, 169.

18   C. Callan, 'RJP Mortished (1891–1957)', *Saothar*, 32 (2007), pp. 45–8.

19   Ibid., p. 46; Cullen Owens, *Louie Bennett*, p. 127. Ronald Mortished read a tribute to Bennett, broadcast on national radio, on the occasion of her death; see Jones, *These Obstreperous Lassies*, p. 233.

20   Minutes of meeting of IWWU, 15 April 1920 (Irish Labour History Society Archives, hereafter referred to as ILHS Archives, Dublin, IWWU Minutes Book: 1060/2/V7A).

21   McGarry, *The Abbey Rebels of 1916*, pp. 151, 160, 173, 176.

22   E. O'Connor, 'Syndicalism, Industrial Unionism, and Nationalism in Ireland', in S. Hirsch and L. van der Walt (eds), *Anarchism and Syndicalism in the Colonial and Post-Colonial World, 1870–1940* (Leiden: Brill, 2010), p. 214.

23   J. Connolly, *Socialism Made Easy* (Dublin: The Plough Book Service, 1971), p. 32.

24   Minutes of meeting of IWWU, 4 December 1919 (ILHS Archives, Dublin, IWWU Minutes Book: 1060/2/V7A).

25   'The Irish Nurses Union', *Irish Citizen*, January 1920.

26   Ibid.

27   'Mrs Mortished's Resignation', *Irish Nurses' and Midwives' Union Members' Circular*, hereafter referred to as *INMU Members' Circular*, 6 (July 1921), p. 2.

28   Minutes of meeting of IWWU, 11 and 25 September 1919 (ILHS Archives, Dublin, IWWU Minutes Book: 1060/1/V7A).

29   *Sunday Independent*, 23 November 1919.

30   'An Open Letter from Miss Bennett, IWWW', *INU Gazette*, 14 (October 1925), p. 2.

31   'Report of Annual Council Meeting, May 7 and 8 1926', *INU Gazette*, 16 (July 1926), p. 1.

32   'Annual Report, May 1927', *INU Gazette*, 19 (July 1927), p. 4.

33   Department of Industry and Commerce, *Census of Population 1926, vol. II, Occupations* (Dublin: The Stationery Office, 1928), p. 11.

34   D. Nevin, 'Decades of Dissension and Divisions, 1923–59', in Nevin (ed.), *Trade Union Century*, p. 87.

35   *Irish Independent*, 1 March 1919.

36   Letter from Kathleen Nora Price to Annie Smithson, 19 February 1925 (INMO Archives, Dublin, Archives Box).

37   'Irish Nurses, Meeting in Dublin, A Proposed Trade Union', *Irish Times*, 1 March 1919.

38   M. Carney, 'Nurses as Managers: A History of Nursing Management in Ireland and England', in Fealy (ed.), *Care to Remember*, pp. 185–97; S. Horgan Ryan, 'The development of nursing in Ireland, 1898–1920' (Cork: University College Cork, 2004), pp. 85–6.

39   'Trade Union for Irish Nurses', *Evening Telegraph*, 8 March 1919.

40   'Adelaide Hospital Dublin. Readjustment', *Irish Times*, 21 March 1919; 'Adelaide Hospital Dublin. Readjustment', *Irish Times*, 22 March 1919; 'Adelaide Hospital Dublin. Readjustment', *Irish Times*, 28 March 1919.

41   'Adelaide Hospital Dublin. Readjustment', *Irish Times*, 8 March 1919.

42   'An Irish Nurses' Union', *Irish Independent*, 25 February 1919.

43   'Irish Nurses' Organisation', *Irish Independent*, 27 February 1919.

44   *Irish Independent*, 27 February 1919.

45   'Reliance on Male Effort', *Irish Independent*, 1 March 1919.

46   The piece noted 'The Irish hospital nurse is expected to do more dirty, rough work than any self-respecting lodging-house "slavey" would consent to do for the same wages, and she has to pay a heavy fee for the privilege'; see J. Brennan, 'The Irish Hospital Nurse – Slave and "Lady"', *Bean na h-Éireann* (August 1909), pp. 13–14.

47   K. Steele, *Women, Press, and Politics During the Irish Revival* (New York: Syracuse University Press, 2007), p. 110.

48   M. Ó hÓgartaigh, 'Irish Nurses, Emerging States and Trade Unions, 1918–39', *Saothar*, 37 (2012), p. 60.

49   Horgan Ryan, 'The development of nursing in Ireland', pp. 45–6.

50   C. McCarthy, *Trade Unions in Ireland, 1894–1960* (Dublin: Institute of Public Administration, 1977), p. 93.

51   'Report of Annual Council Meeting, 1927', *INU Gazette*, 19 (July 1927), p. 1.

52   Letter from [name withheld] to Marie Mortished dated 27 November 1920 (INMO Archives, Dublin, Archives Box).

53   'Nurses' Union, Meeting to Form a Galway Branch', *Connacht Tribune*, 16 October 1926.

54   'Irish Nurses, Meeting in Dublin, A Proposed Trade Union'.

55   'Nurses' Working Hours', *Freeman's Journal*, 17 November 1920.

56   It is doubtful if this Association was a branch of the Irish Nurses' Association. Rather, it appears to have been a standalone and short-lived (albeit militant) entity.

57   Minutes of meeting of Macroom Board of Guardians, 13 February 1920 (Cork City and County Archives, Cork, Book: BG115A19).

58   Minutes of meeting of Macroom Board of Guardians, 8 April 1922 (Cork City and County Archives, Cork, Book: BG115A21).

59   'Irish Nurses, Meeting in Dublin, A Proposed Trade Union'.

60   Ibid.

61   O'Connor, *A Labour History of Ireland: 1824–2000*, p. 75.

62   O'Connor, *War and Syndicalism: 1914–23*, p. 57.

63   'An Irish Nurses' Union'.

64   *Irish Independent*, 1 March 1919.

65   'Irish Nurses, Meeting in Dublin, A Proposed Trade Union'.

66   Accompaniment notes to the First Annual Conference of the INU, 1920 (INMO Archives, Dublin, Archives Box).

67   'Irish Nurses' Union', *Irish Citizen*, August 1919.

68   'The Irish Nurses' Union, a Manure Cart for Midwives', *British Journal of Nursing*, LXIV, 1667 (13 March 1920), p. 164.

69   Ibid.

70   Ibid.

71   Minutes of meeting of IWWU, 8 December 1921 (ILHS Archives, Dublin, IWWU Minutes Book: 1060/3).

72 'Dublin Union Hospital', *INMU Members' Circular*, 5 (December 1920), p. 3. There was a North and South Dublin Union Hospital, but the INU's documentation rarely made explicit to which one it was referring.

73 Ibid.

74 'Rights of the Nurse', *Freeman's Journal*, 1 April 1919.

75 Ibid.

76 'Irish Nurses' Association', *British Journal of Nursing*, LXII, 1615 (15 March 1919), p. 172.

77 'In Bondage Never! Pathetic Ireland Asked Albinia Broderick [*sic*] to Turn her Back on Comfort and Tradition', *Kerryman*, 2 January 1965.

78 See 'In Bondage Never, A Profile of Albinia Broderick [*sic*], the Rebel Born to Wealth and Title', *Kerryman*, 26 December 1964; K. Ó Céirín and C. Ó Céirín, *Women of Ireland* (Kinvara: Tir Eolas, 1996), pp. 28–9; A. Wickham, 'The Nursing Radicalism of the Honourable Albinia Brodrick, 1861–1955', *Nursing History Review*, 15 (2007), pp. 51–64; P. Ó Loingsigh, *Gobnait Ní Bhruadair* (Baile Átha Cliath: Coiscéim, 1997). The latter source is written in Irish, and I would like to thank Pádraig Mac Fhearghusa for supplying me with portions of the original English manuscript.

79 'The Status of Irish Nurses', *British Journal of Nursing*, LXII, 1616 (22 March 1919), p. 192.

80 Ibid., p. 194.

81 Yeates, *Lockout*, p. xxvi.

CHAPTER 3

1 T. Brown, *Ireland: A Social and Cultural History, 1922–2002* (2nd edn, London: Harper Perennial, 2004), p. 5.

2 O'Morain, *The Irish Association of Directors of Nursing and Midwifery*, p. 33.

3 'Private Midwives' Fees', *INMU Members' Circular*, 5 (December 1920), p. 4.

4 'Irish Nurses' Union, Meeting of Waterford Branch', *Munster Express*, 28 April 1923.

5 'Report on District Midwives' Claim', *INMU Members' Circular*, 5 (December 1920), p. 3.

6 'Nenagh Board of Guardians', *Nenagh Guardian*, 3 January 1920.

7 Midwife Annie Lyons had almost one year's service and earned £40 per year in the Nenagh district while 'Nurse' Nolan, with fifteen years' service, earned £15 per year for her work in the Ballina district; see Ibid.

8 Ibid.

9 Ibid.

10 When the INU wrote to the Loughrea Board of Guardians, County Galway, requesting a salary increase for a dispensary midwife, one of the board members noted that she had 'a good private practice' and no increase was awarded; see 'Guardians and Irish', *Connacht Tribune*, 24 July 1920.

11 Minutes of meeting of Macroom Board of Guardians, 12 January 1922 (Cork City and County Archives, Cork, Book: BG115A21).

12 The midwife noted: 'During the year ended 30th September 1928, I attended 68 ticket cases with an average visit to each nine times, or making a total of 612 [visits] … so that it will be easily seen I am not left very much time for private practice'; see 'Kildare Board of Health, Nurse's Application', *Kildare Observer*, 24 November 1928.

13   Ibid.

14   'Rights of Officials', *Connaught Telegraph*, 15 January 1921.

15   Ibid.

16   'Irish Nurses' Union: What it has Done for Midwives'. Promotional Leaflet 8, 1925 (INMO Archives, Dublin, Archives Box).

17   'Report on District Midwives' Claim', p. 4.

18   'Cavan Health Board', *Anglo Celt*, 1 September 1928.

19   Ibid.

20   'Nurse News', *Weekly Irish Times*, 17 July 1920.

21   'Appointment of Jubilee Nurse as Midwife in Sneem, Co. Kerry', *INU Gazette*, 25 (December 1928), p. 3.

22   'Guardians and Irish'.

23   For a more comprehensive description of these events, see R. Barrington, *Health, Medicine and Politics in Ireland, 1900–70* (Dublin: Institute of Public Administration, 1987), pp. 91–5.

24   Accompaniment notes to the First Annual Conference of the INU, 1920.

25   'Irish Nurses and Corporation', *Irish Independent*, 1 September 1920.

26   Commission of Inquiry into Local Government (Military Archives, Dublin, Bureau of Military History, No. 1413).

27   'Leitrim County Home', *Leitrim Observer*, 7 June 1924.

28   'The Irish Nurses' Union, a Manure Cart for Midwives', p. 164.

29   Ibid.

30   'Irish Nurses' Union: What it has Done for Midwives'.

31   'Leitrim County Home'.

32   *Midwives (Ireland) Act (1918)* Section 2 (1).

33   Ibid., Section 1 (2).

34   'Leitrim County Home'.

35   *Midwives (Ireland) Act (1918)* Section 1 (2).

36   Minutes of meeting of Central Midwives' Board of Ireland, 19 February 1925 (Nursing and Midwifery Board of Ireland Archives, hereafter referred to as NMBI Archives, Dublin, P220/207).

37   'Further Progress on the Midwives' Badge', *INU Gazette*, 19 (July 1927), p. 4.

38   Minutes of meeting of Central Midwives' Board of Ireland, 19 February 1925.

39   'Irish Nurses' Union: What it has Done for Midwives'.

40   'Handywomen', *INU Gazette*, 13 (May 1925), p. 2.

41   'Union Activities: The Fight Against Unqualified Women', *INU Gazette*, 21 (January 1928), p. 3.

42   'Action Against Handywomen', *INMU Members' Circular*, 12 (August 1924), p. 1.

43   A very small number of women, about 5 per cent of applicants, applied to have their names placed on the Roll of Midwives under the 'bona fide' stipulations in the *1918 Midwives (Ireland) Act*; see E.A. McMahon, 'The regulation of midwives with special reference to aspects of the regulation of midwives in Ireland, 1918–50' (Dublin, University College Dublin, 2000), pp. 60, 71.

44   'Deputation to the Coombe Hospital Re Handywomen', *INU Gazette*, 14 (October 1925), p. 5.

45   N. Leap and B. Hunter, *The Midwife's Tale* (London: Scarlet Press, 1993), p. 27.

46   Ibid., p. 23.

47   Ibid., pp. 19–20.

48   'Cavan Health Board, Nurses' Union and Handywomen', *Anglo Celt*, 1 March 1930.

49   Ibid.

50   *Midwives Act (1931)* Section 3–4.

51   L. Earner-Byrne, *Mother and Child: Maternity and Child Welfare in Dublin, 1922–60* (Manchester: Manchester University Press, 2007), pp. 37–9.

52   'The Irish District Nurse – 85 Years Ago', *World of Irish Nursing*, hereafter referred to as *WIN*, 20, 6 (December 1991), p. 21.

53   An excerpt from Max Millard's biography; see http://www.medicine.tcd.ie/alumni/assets/pdf/Dr-Max-Solomon-Millard.pdf (pp. 109–10). Date accessed: 1 August 2013.

54   'Cavan Co. Council', *Anglo Celt*, 23 October 1926.

55   Barrington, *Health, Medicine and Politics in Ireland*, pp. 102–5.

56   Census return for 1926 show that of the 2,051 doctors in Ireland, 208 were female and 1,843 were male; see Department of Industry and Commerce, *Census of Population 1926, vol. II, Occupations*, p. 11.

57   'The Position of Trained Nurses in Co. Hospitals and Homes', *INU Gazette*, 13 (May 1925), p. 6.

58   'Report of Trade Union Congress, Held at Cork, in August 1920', *INMU Members' Circular*, 5 (December 1920), p. 1.

59   'Who's Who in the Irish Hospital World', p. 7.

60   'National Children's Hospital', *Irish Times*, 1 June 1920.

61   Ibid. Needlework was not necessarily a pastime. Fealy suggests that it was expected of nurses, even in their time off-duty, for their hospital's 'advantage'; see G.M. Fealy, 'A history of the provision and reform of general nurse education and training in Ireland, 1879–1994, vol. 1' (Dublin: University College Dublin, 2002), p. 215.

62   'Nurses' Hours of Duty', *Irish Times*, 3 June 1920.

63   'Our Own Affairs', *INHW*, 1, 2 (15 September 1931), p. 31.

64   'Nurses' Working Hours', *Irish Times*, 10 June 1920.

65   Ibid.

66   'Report of the First Meeting of the Joint Session and Sectional Committees Elected at the Annual Conference in September', *INMU Members' Circular*, 5 (December 1920), p. 2. There is no evidence that a distinct badge for midwives was ever minted.

67   'The Union's Name', *INU Gazette*, 13 (May 1925), p. 5.

68   'Report of Annual Council Meeting, 1927', p. 1.

69   'Editorial', *INU Gazette*, 23 (July 1928), p. 1.

70   'Cavan Health Board', *Anglo Celt*, 29 June 1935.

71   Ibid.

72   'On Poaching', *INU Gazette*, 17 (November 1926), p. 3.

73   'Annual Council', *INU Gazette*, 27 (July 1929), p. 2.

74   'From our Broadcasting Station. Loyalty', *INU Gazette*, 29 (January 1930), p. 1.

75   Minutes of meeting of Irish Nurses' Union Executive, hereafter referred to as INU Executive, 26 September 1934 (INMO Archives, Dublin, Archives Box).

76   'Nursing Appointments in Kerry', *Irish Press*, 25 November 1932.

77   'Dispensary Midwives', *INU Gazette*, 18 (April 1927), p. 3.
78   Minutes of meeting of INU Executive, 13 December 1932 (INMO Archives, Dublin, Archives Box).
79   Minutes of meeting of INU Executive, 28 February 1933 (INMO Archives, Dublin, Archives Box).

CHAPTER 4

1   J.J. Lee, *Ireland, 1912–85: Politics and Society* (Cambridge: Cambridge University Press, 1989), pp. 108–9.
2   R. Roberts, 'Trade Union Organisation in Ireland', *Journal of the Statistical and Social Inquiry Society of Ireland*, XX, 2 (1958/59), pp. 93–111.
3   Brown, *Ireland: A Social and Cultural History: 1922–2002*, p. 92.
4   McGann, *The Battle of the Nurses*, p. 155.
5   Cullen, 'Women, Emancipation, and Politics', p. 868.
6   'The International Council of Nurses', *INU Gazette*, 13 (May 1925), p. 7.
7   Reference for Annie Smithson from Edinburgh Royal Infirmary, see M. Bashford-Synnott, 'Annie M.P. Smithson: romantic novelist/revolutionary nurse, a literary biography' (Dublin: University College Dublin, 2000), no pagination.
8   Letter from Kathleen Nora Price to Annie Smithson, 19 February 1925.
9   'Editorial', *INU Gazette*, 23 (July 1928), p. 1; Letter from Kathleen Nora Price to Louie Bennett, 14 May 1928 (INMO Archives, Dublin, Archives Box).
10   Letter from Kathleen Nora Price to Louie Bennett, 14 May 1928.
11   Minutes of meeting of IWWU, 23 August 1923 (ILHS Archives, Dublin, IWWU Minutes Book: 1060/4).
12   Minutes of meeting of IWWU, ?4 October 1923 (ILHS Archives, Dublin, IWWU Minutes Book: 1060/4).
13   Minutes of meeting of IWWU, 10 April 1924 (ILHS Archives, Dublin, IWWU Minutes Book: 1060/4).
14   'Extracts from the Secretary's Report to the Half-Yearly Meeting of the Joint Executives of Nurses and Midwives Membership', *INMU Members' Circular*, 6 (July 1921), p. 2.
15   M.E. Daly, 'Women and Trade Unions', in Nevin (ed.), *Trade Union Century*, p. 107.
16   Minutes of meeting of Irish Nurses' Organisation Executive, hereafter referred to as INO Executive, 3 February 1941 (INMO Archives, Dublin, Archives Box).
17   'Report of Annual Council Meeting, 1928', *INU Gazette*, 23 (July 1928), p. 4.
18   Minutes of meeting of IWWU, 23 May 1928 (ILHS Archives, Dublin, IWWU Minutes Book: 1060/5).
19   Letter from Louie Bennett to Kathleen Nora Price, 26 May 1928 (INMO Archives, Dublin, Archives Box).
20   Letter from Kathleen Nora Price to the Labour Party and Trade Union Congress, 1 June 1928 (INMO Archives, Dublin, Archives Box).
21   'Report of Annual Council Meeting, 1927', p. 1.
22   'Irish Nurses' Union Annual Council Meeting', *INU Gazette*, 31 (June 1930), p. 6.
23   Ibid.

24   Minutes of meeting of INU Executive, 15 November 1932 (INMO Archives, Dublin, Archives Box).

25   Minutes of meeting of INU Executive, 9 May 1933 (INMO Archives, Dublin, Archives Box).

26   Irish Nurses' Organisation, *Irish Nurses' Organisation Souvenir Book* (Dublin: Irish Nurses' Organisation, 1947), p. 19.

27   *Report of the Provisional Committee to the First Annual Conference of the INU*, 1920.

28   'Nurses' Campaign for Improvements', *Irish Press*, 1 December 1937.

29   Minutes of meeting of INU Executive, 13 February 1935 (INMO Archives, Dublin, Archives Box).

30   Ibid.

31   Minutes of meeting of INU Executive, 27 February 1935 (INMO Archives, Dublin, Archives Box).

32   Minutes of meeting of INU Executive, 7 May 1935 (INMO Archives, Dublin, Archives Box).

33   'Mrs. Mortished's Resignation', p. 2.

34   Liam Price was a barrister, antiquarian, historian and district court judge in County Wicklow; see C. Corlett and M. Weaver (eds), *The Price Notebooks, vol. I* (Dublin: Dúchas, 2002).

35   L. Price, *Dr Dorothy Price: An Account of Twenty Years' Fight Against Tuberculosis in Ireland* (For private circulation only, 1957); A. Mac Lellan, *Dorothy Stopford Price: Rebel Doctor* (Sallins: Irish Academic Press, 2014).

36   Price's socialist activities are detailed in a Department of Justice file on communist activities in Saorstát Éireann; see Note from the Department of Justice regarding the Friends of Soviet Russia, 19 March 1930 (The National Archives of Ireland, Dublin, File on Communist Activities, 1929–30: S5074A).

37   Letter from Kathleen Nora Price to Louie Bennett, 14 May 1928.

38   For an account of the trip, see Dublin Trades Union and Labour Council, *Report of Irish Labour Delegation to Union of Socialist Soviet Republics* (Dublin: Dublin Trades Union and Labour Council, 1929).

39   Minutes of meeting of INU Executive,18 June 1936 (INMO Archives, Dublin, Archives Box).

40   Minutes of meeting of INO Executive, 15 December 1936 (INMO Archives, Dublin, Archives Box).

41   'The Irish Nurses' Organisation', *Irish Nurses' Journal*, hereafter referred to as *INJ*, I, 3 (July 1936), p. 23.

42   'Syllabus for Midwifery Course', *INU Gazette*, 24 (October 1928), pp. 1–2.

43   The course comprised instructions in: 'Storeroom and larder management' and 'extermination of household pests'; see Ibid., p. 1.

44   Minutes of meeting of INO Executive, 1 October 1936 (INMO Archives, Dublin, Archives Box).

45   'Annual Report, 1928/29', *INU Gazette*, 27 (July 1929), p. 7.

46   'The Annual Report, 1929/30', *INU Gazette*, 31 (June 1930), p. 2.

47   'Secretary's Report, 1935/36', *INJ*, I, 1 (May 1936), p. 3.

48   'Hospital Nurses and Dispensary Midwives', *Nenagh Guardian*, 23 October 1937.

49   Ibid.

50   'Nurses to Strike?', *Irish Press*, 25 January 1937.

51   Ibid.

52   'Mental Hospital Staff to Strike', *Irish Independent*, 26 January 1937.

53   'Ardee Hospital Dispute', *Irish Press*, 28 January 1937.

54   Letter from [name withheld] to Annie Black, Registrar, General Nursing Council, 3 March 1937 (NMBI Archives, Dublin, P220/504). Black responded that it was not within the board's jurisdiction to get involved in such a matter; see Letter from Annie Black, Registrar, General Nursing Council to [name withheld], 16 March 1937 (NMBI Archives, Dublin, P220/504).

55   'Grievances of Nurses', *Irish Press*, 30 January 1937.

56   'Strikers Back at Work', *Irish Press*, 4 June 1937.

57   'The Irish Nurses' Organisation', *Irish Times*, 1 May 1940.

58   'Housing for Dispensary Midwives', *Irish Nurses' Magazine*, hereafter referred to as *INM*, 13, 59 (April 1946), p. 6.

59   *Local Government Act (1925)* Section 42.

60   'Our Own Affairs, A Pension Fund for Nurses', *INHW*, 1, 3 (1 October 1931), p. 2.

61   'The Pension Fund and Benevolent Scheme for Nurses', *INU Gazette*, 31 (June 1930), p. 7.

62   Minutes of meeting of INU Executive, 30 September 1931 (INMO Archives, Dublin, Archives Box).

63   Minutes of meeting of INU Executive, 1 March 1932 (INMO Archives, Dublin, Archives Box).

64   Minutes of meeting of INU Executive, 6 October 1931; minutes of meeting of INU Executive, 3 November 1931 (INMO Archives, Dublin, Archives Box).

65   'Our Own Affairs', *INHW*, 2, 16 (15 April 1932), p. 1.

66   'Pensions for Nurses', *Irish Independent*, 10 April 1931.

67   *INU Gazette*, 33 (January 1931), p. 5.

68   'News from G.H.Q's', *INHW*, 1, 4 (15 October 1931), p. 11.

69   M. Coleman, *The Irish Sweep: A History of the Irish Hospitals Sweepstake, 1930–87* (Dublin: University College Dublin Press, 2009), p. 35.

70   Ibid., pp. 35–6.

71   'Drawing the Counterfoils in the November Handicap Sweep', *INHW*, 1, 7 (1 December 1931), p. 18.

72   'Fortune Finders', *INHW*, 2, 15 (1 April 1932), p. 6.

73   'Annual Report, 1932/33', *INU Gazette*, I, 1 (June 1933), p. 3.

74   'My Day', *INJ*, 2, 8 (December 1937), p. 60.

75   Other benefactors included nurses who contracted tuberculosis, nurses recuperating following surgery and one nurse who was 'crippled with rheumatism'; see Leaflet Regarding INO Benevolent Fund, 1939 (INMO Archives, Dublin, Archives Box).

76   Minutes of meeting of INU Executive, 9 June 1941 (INMO Archives, Dublin, Archives Box).

77   The post of Parliamentary Secretary is similar to today's post of Junior Minister.

78   'Still Pressing for a Pensions Scheme', *INHW*, 3, 8 (1 July 1933), p. 1.

79   'Stating the Case for a Pensions Scheme', *INHW*, 3, 9 (1 August 1933), pp. 10–11.

80   'Are We Nearing the Goal?', *INHW*, 3, 9 (1 August 1933), p. 1.

81 'The Present Position of the Proposed Pensions Scheme for Nurses and Midwives', *INHW*, 4, 3 (1 March 1934), p. 1.

82 'Pressing the Claim for a National Pensions Scheme', *INHW* (1 April 1934), pp. 1–2.

83 'Diary of the Month', *INHW*, 6, 7 (July 1936), p. 1.

84 'Who's Who in the Hospital World', *INHW*, 1, 6 (15 November 1931), p. 4.

85 The 1936 census indicates that there were 1,621 midwives and 5,534 'sick nurses' in Ireland. That same year, INO membership was 937, meaning that just 13 per cent of nurses and midwives were members of the organisation; Department of Industry and Commerce, *Census of Population 1936, vol. II, Occupations* (Dublin: The Stationery Office, 1940), p. 79.

86 'Diary of the Month, Nurses and Pensions', *INHW*, 7, 5 (May 1937), p. 2.

87 Minutes of meeting of INU Executive, 14 March 1933 (INMO Archives, Dublin, Archives Box).

88 'Suggested Amalgamation with the Irish Nurses' Association', *INU Gazette*, 34 (March 1931), p. 2.

89 'Our Own Affairs', *INHW*, 1, 10 (15 January 1932), p. 1.

90 'Fun Without Money', *INHW*, 7, 7 (July 1937), p. 10.

91 Ibid.

92 Coleman, *The Irish Sweep*, p. 54.

93 'The Present Position of the Proposed Pensions Scheme for Nurses and Midwives', p. 3.

94 R. Cullen Owens, *A Social History of Women in Ireland, 1870–1970* (Dublin: Gill and Macmillan, 2005), p. 238.

95 E. O'Leary, 'The Irish National Teachers' Organisation and the Marriage Bar for Women National Teachers, 1933–58', *Saothar*, 12 (1987), p. 48.

96 *Local Government Act (1941)* Section 21.

97 'What Our Readers Think, Careers After Marriage', *INHW*, 1, 5 (1 November 1931), p. 40.

98 Jones, *These Obstreperous Lassies*, p. 235.

99 *INM*, 3, 12 (April 1939), p. 8.

100 'Noble Work Ill Paid', *Evening Herald*, 12 December 1947.

101 The Census of Population of 1926 notes the presence of 5,266 female 'sick nurses', of whom 523 were married, 546 were widows and 4,197 were single; see Department of Industry and Commerce, *Census of Population 1926, vol. V, Part II, Ages and Conjugal Conditions*, p. 36. This number excludes midwives who, up to the 1930s, were frequently married mothers. This was a prerequisite to them being 'taken seriously' by pregnant women; see McMahon, 'The regulation of midwives', p. 12.

102 The Census of Population of 1936 notes the presence of 5,454 female 'sick nurses' of whom 263 were married, 193 were widows and 4,998 were single; see Department of Industry and Commerce, *Census of Population 1936, Vol. V, Part II, Ages and Conjugal Conditions*, p. 41. This figure is exclusive of midwives.

103 'Pension Scheme for Saorstat [*sic*] Nurses', *INHW*, 5, 13 (March 1936), p. 7.

104 Expectations of marriage did not only impinge on pension arrangements in nursing; such expectations were a factor in women's employment in general. Research by Kaim-Caudle and Byrne, which analysed pension arrangements in a number of manufacturing industries in Ireland in the 1960s, showed that pension coverage was higher for men than women owing to higher withdrawal rates among women workers – most probably due

to marriage. That research also showed that, unlike male workers, the majority of whom entered pension schemes at age twenty-five or younger, some employers barred women from entering pension schemes 'until they reach the age at which their expectation of marriage begins to decline'; see P.R. Kaim-Caudle and J.G. Byrne, *Irish Pension Schemes, 1969* (Dublin: Economic and Social Research Institute, 1971), p. 12.

105 'Pension Scheme for Saorstat [*sic*] Nurses', p. 6.

CHAPTER 5

1 'My Day', pp. 60–1.
2 A. Smithson, *Myself – and Others* (Dublin: The Talbot Press, 1944), pp. 113, 120.
3 Letter from unknown sender to unknown recipient, 27 April 1922 (Military Archives, Dublin, Annie MP Smithson Papers, Lot No: 46, A/1035).
4 Smithson, *Myself – and Others*, p. 269. Smithson's experience during the Civil War was fictionalised in her novel '*The Marriage of Nurse Harding*'.
5 Ibid., pp. 288–9.
6 Ferriter, *The Transformation of Ireland*, p. 383.
7 'Mayo Branch', *INM*, 11, 9 (January 1941), p. 6.
8 'Exodus of Nurses to Britain', *Irish Independent*, 12 January 1944.
9 'Deputation to Department of Supplies', *INM*, 13, 41 (September 1944), p. 3.
10 'Department of Supplies', *INM*, 12, 19 (November 1942), p. 3.
11 'I Can't Manage Without a Bike', *INM*, 13, 52 (August 1945), p. 9.
12 'The Problem of Nurses' Hours and Salaries', *Sunday Independent*, 11 January 1942.
13 'A Nurses' Lot is Not a Happy One', *Sunday Independent*, 4 January 1942.
14 Ibid.
15 'Trust Nothing, Men of Ireland, But the Deep Resolve of Your Own Hearts', *INM*, 13, 53 (September/October 1945), p. 3.
16 'Hints to Doctors', *Sunday Independent*, 18 January 1942.
17 'Trinity College Meeting, See Florence and Die: Wanted – a Gale-in-the-Night Nursing Reform', *INM*, 13, 37 (May 1944), pp. 6–9.
18 See http://www.medicine.tcd.ie/alumni/assets/pdf/Dr-Max-Solomon-Millard.pdf (p. 103). Date accessed: 1 August 2013.
19 H. Moore, J.A. Glynn, M. Tierney, J.P. Shanley, M.M. MacKen, J. Kay Jamieson, A.M. Smithson, R.C Nicolls and P.J. Gannon, 'The Nursing Profession and its Needs', *Studies*, 31, 123 (September 1942), pp. 273–95.
20 Remarks by William Norton TD, Dáil Éireann Debate, vol. 91, No. 11, 3 November 1943.
21 'Richmond, Whitworth and Hardwicke Hospitals, Proposed Syllabus for Post-Graduate Nurses', *INJ*, 2, 10 (February 1938), p. 79.
22 'Secretary's Report, 1938/39', *INM*, 10, 2 (June 1939), p. 7.
23 'Annual General Meeting, 1953', *INM*, 20, 3 (March 1953), p. 1; 'A Meeting of the Executive Council Followed', *INM*, 19, 5 (May 1952), pp. 2–3.
24 'Secretary's Report, 1936–37', *INJ*, 2, 2 (June 1937), p. 12.
25 'The Irish Nurses' Organisation', *INM*, 12, 27 (July 1943), p. 3.
26 'Organisation Work', *INM*, 11, 12 (April 1941), p. 8.
27 'Sunlight and Cancer', *INJ*, 1, 5 (September 1936), p. 38.

28   'Cancer Not Contagious', *INJ*, 3, 7 (November 1938), p. 5.

29   'Swallowed a Nail, 8,000 Miles to Get it Out', *INJ*, 1, 5 (September 1936), p. 38.

30   Moore et al., 'The Nursing Profession and its Needs', p. 289.

31   'The Irish Nurses' Organisation', *INM*, 12, 22 (February 1943), p. 2; 'The Irish Nurses' Organisation', *INM*, 13, 66 (December 1946), p. 6.

32   For an engaging feminist account of women's travails at Trinity College, see S.M. Parkes (ed.), *A Danger to the Men? A History of Women in Trinity College Dublin: 1904–2004* (Dublin: The Lilliput Press, 2004).

33   Smithson is buried in Dublin's Whitechurch Cemetery – a distinctive white headstone marks her grave. 1948 also witnessed the death of the organisation's first nurse President, Mrs McCarry.

34   'Social Page', *INM*, 17, 5 (May 1950), p. 14.

35   'A Social Review', *INM*, 14, 8 (August 1947), p. 1.

36   For an account of the Home, see Ó Duigneáin, *Linda Kearns*, pp. 156–65.

37   'Correspondence', *INM*, 13, 39 (July 1944), p. 12; 'Convalescent Home Appointment', *INM*, 13, 40 (August 1944), p. 1; 'A Matter for Explanation', *INM*, 13, 41 (September 1944), p. 1; 'Correspondence', *INM*, 13, 41 (September 1944), p.11.

38   See especially A. Smithson (ed.), *In Times of Peril: Leaves from the Diary of Nurse Linda Kearns from Easter Week 1916 to Mountjoy 1921* (Dublin: The Talbot Press, 1922).

39   See 'The Sentence on Nurse Kearns', *Irish Independent*, 2 April 1921.

40   Letter from Marie Mortished to David Lloyd George, 13 April 1921 (The National Archives, Kew, England, CO 904/44/9).

41   'Correspondence', *INM*, 13, 39 (July 1944), p. 12.

42   'Secretary's Report, 1936/37', p. 12.

43   'Secretary's Report, 1939/40', *INM*, 11, 2 (June 1940), p. 3.

44   'Annual Meeting, General Secretary's Report', *INM*, 13, 62 (July 1946), p. 3; 'General Secretary's Report, 1946/47', *INM*, 14, 6 (June 1947), p. 1.

45   Owing to the small number of 'mental nurses' in INO membership, the census category 'mental attendants' was not factored into the density calculation; see Central Statistics Office, *Census of Population 1946, vol. II, Occupations* (Dublin: The Stationery Office, 1953), p. 12.

46   R. Dingwall, A.M. Rafferty and C. Webster, *An Introduction to the Social History of Nursing* (London: Routledge, 1988), p. 104.

47   Ministry of Health, *First Report of Nurses' Salaries Committee, Salaries and Emoluments of Female Nurses in Hospitals* (London: His Majesty's Stationery Office, 1943).

48   Ibid., p. 24.

49   This was the same entity as the aforementioned College of Nursing. It was granted Royal Charter in 1928.

50   'Editorial', *INM*, 12, 24 (April 1943), p. 1.

51   The centre of the badge was silver and on a blue border was inscribed the organisation's name and the emblems of the four provinces of Ireland.

52   'Spring is Here, Spring is Here, Fifty Thousand Robins Can't Be Wrong', *INM*, 13, 47 (March 1945), p. 3.

53   'Twelve Straight Tips How to Kill an Association', *INM*, 19, 9 (October 1952), p. 7.

54   'Nurse's Remuneration', *Irish Independent*, 24 September 1930.

55   Hospital nurses in Ireland were paid £60–£85 per year, while their counterparts in England were paid £120–£140 per year. Ward sisters in Ireland were paid £75–£80 per year, while their counterparts in England were paid £130–£200 per year; see 'The Cause and its Consequences', *INM*, 12, 29 (September 1943), pp. 1–2.

56   'Nurses' Grievances', *INM*, 13, 37 (May 1944), p. 1.

57   'Correspondence', *INM*, 13, 38 (June 1944), p. 11.

58   'Nurses' Salaries, Statistical Summary of Grievances', *INM*, 13, 44 (December 1944), pp. 11–12.

59   'Nurses' Salaries, Secretary's Views on the Increases', *INM*, 13, 45 (January 1945), p. 10.

60   'Reporting Progress', *INM*, 13, 45 (January 1945), p. 3.

61   M.E. Baly, *Nursing and Social Change* (3rd edn, London: Routledge, 1995), p. 204.

62   Emoluments had a value of £88 in 1945.

63   O'Connor, *A Labour History of Ireland: 1824–2000*, p. 154.

64   'Memorandum to Minister for Health', *INM*, 18, 5 (May 1951), p. 3.

65   Wallace et al., *Industrial Relations in Ireland*, p. 279.

66   'Circ. P143/46', *INM*, 13, 66 (December 1946), pp. 3–4.

67   Ibid., p. 4.

68   *Drogheda Independent*, April 1946, cited in 'Meath Infirmary Committee: No Nurses Available', *INM*, 13, 60 (May 1946), p. 10.

69   'The Irish Nurses' Organsiation [*sic*]', *INM*, 14, 4 (April 1947), p. 4.

70   K.C. Kearns, *Ireland's Arctic Siege: The Big Freeze of 1947* (Dublin: Gill and Macmillan, 2011), pp. 143–4.

71   'The Protection of the Nurse's Health', *INM*, 10, 1 (May 1939), pp. 6–7.

72   'Pension Scheme Circular', *INM*, 3, 12 (April 1939), p. 2.

73   'Conditions for Nurses Condemned', *Sunday Independent*, 1 February 1942.

74   Remarks by Senator Thomas Farren, Seanad Éireann Debate, vol. 20, No. 15, 20 November 1935.

75   'Annual Meeting', *INM*, 13, 61 (June 1946), p. 4.

76   Ibid.

77   'Executive Council Resolutions to be Submitted to the Annual General Meeting – May 6, 1948', *INM*, 15, 4 (April 1948), p. 5.

78   'Pension Scheme, Organiser's Formidable Task', *INM*, 13, 35 (March 1944), p. 2.

79   This figure does not include midwives; see Central Statistics Office, *Census of Population 1946, vol. V Part II, Ages, Orphanhood and Conjugal Conditions* (Dublin: The Stationery Office, 1950), p. 37.

80   Provincial Town Organiser's Report Book, Entry of July 1956, County Hospital, Kildare (INMO Archives, Dublin, Archives Box).

81   'Some Superstitions Related to Midwifery in the Midlands', *INJ*, 2, 2 (June 1937), p. 14.

82   Among other insights the page offered were: 'In Kerry it is not considered right to leave a mother and newly born babe alone for even a minute, in case [it would be swapped for a] changeling'; see 'Our Folklore Page', *INJ*, 3, 3 (July 1938), p. 7.

83   'What Westportites Say', *INM*, 10, 8 (December 1939), p. 3.

84   *INM*, 11, 6 (October 1940), p. 7.

85   'Wedding Bells', *INM*, 11, 7 (November 1940), p. 1.

86   'Midwifery in a Country District 38 Years Ago', *INJ*, 2, 8 (December 1937), p. 59.

87   'Address by Dr James Ryan', *INM*, 20, 7 (July 1953), p. 1.

88   'The Cause and its Consequences', p. 1.

89   Quote from an address by Rev Hubert Fee, Honorary President of the Limerick Branch of the INO; see 'Irish Nurses Deserving of Better Treatment', *Limerick Leader*, 4 June 1949.

90   'Two Pictures', *INM*, 13, 36 (April 1944), p. 1.

91   *Trade Union Act (1941)* Section 7.

92   Ibid., Section 6; F. Von Prondzynski and W. Richards, *European Employment and Industrial Relations Glossary: Ireland* (London: Sweet and Maxwell, 1994), pp. 82–3.

93   'Trade Union Act, 1941', *INM*, 12, 14 (June 1942), p. 4.

94   Ibid.

95   Ibid.

96   'Disorganisation is Degradation', *INM*, 13, 42 (October 1944), p. 1.

97   'News from the Branches', *INM*, 17, 3 (March 1950), p. 9.

98   'Correspondence', *INM*, 13, 48 (April 1945), p. 11.

99   For a comprehensive account of the strike, see E. McCormick, *The INTO and the 1946 Teachers' Strike* (Dublin: The Irish National Teachers' Organisation, 1996).

100   Irish Nurses' Organisation, *Irish Nurses' Organisation Souvenir Book*.

CHAPTER 6

1   W. Beveridge, *Social Insurance and Allied Services* (London: His Majesty's Stationery Office, 1942).

2   Barrington, *Health, Medicine and Politics in Ireland*, pp. 168–74.

3   Ibid., p. 187.

4   Ibid., p. 139; 'Refresher Courses for Public Health Nurses', *INM*, 14, 6 (June 1947), pp. 12–13; 'Refresher Courses for Public Health Nurses', *INM*, 14, 8 (August 1947), p. 5.

5   'The Health Bill, 1947', *INM*, 14, 10 (November 1947), p. 1.

6   Ibid., p. 2.

7   *Health Act (1947)* Section 21–8.

8   Earner-Byrne, *Mother and Child*, pp. 139–40; Barrington, *Health, Medicine and Politics in Ireland*, pp. 218–19).

9   'Towards Vocationalism?', *INM*, 18, 6 (June 1951), p. 2.

10   'Address Given by the Minister for Health at the Annual General Meeting, 1948', *INM*, 15, 6 (June 1948), p. 1.

11   'Nurses Resign, Trouble at County Infirmary', *Limerick Leader*, 6 February 1950.

12   'Irish Nurses' Organisation, Mallow Chest Hospital', *INM*, 18, 2 (February 1951), p. 3.

13   'Chest Hospital, Mallow Nurses' Home', *INM*, 18, 3 (March 1951), p. 8.

14   *Cork Examiner*, January 1950, cited in Ibid. See also 'Nurses' Home – Mallow Chest Hospital', *INM*, 18, 4 (April 1951), p. 14.

15   N. Browne, *Against the Tide* (Dublin: Gill and Macmillan, 1986), pp. 67–9.

16   'Address Given by the Minister for Health at the Annual General Meeting, 1948', p. 1.

17   'Nurses' Home, County Surgical Hospital, Cavan', *INM*, 18, 4 (April 1951), p. 15.

18   Provincial Town Organiser's Report Book, Entry of 20 September 1956, District Hospital, Boyle, Co. Roscommon (INMO Archives, Dublin, Archives Box).

19 Provincial Town Organiser's Report Book, Entry of 10 June 1955, County Home, Mullingar, Co. Westmeath (INMO Archives, Dublin, Archives Box).
20 'Important', *INM*, 15, 7 (July 1948), p. 15.
21 For a short piece on Reidy's appointment, see 'Appointment of Nursing Officer in the Department of Health', *INM*, 16, 8 (August 1949), p. 13.
22 'General Secretary's Annual Report 1950', *INM*, 18, 7 (July 1951), p. 3.
23 Pius XI, *Quadragesimo Anno* (Rome: 1931).
24 J.H. Whyte, *Church and State in Modern Ireland, 1923–79* (2nd edn, Dublin: Gill and Macmillan, 1980), p. 160.
25 A. Kelly, 'Catholic Action and the Development of the Irish Welfare State in the 1930s and 1940s', *Archivium Hibernicum*, 53 (1999), pp. 107–17.
26 'If Only', *INM*, 18, 2 (February 1951), p. 4.
27 'Why Should You Be a Member of the Irish Nurses' Organisation?' *INM*, 21, 10 (November 1954), p. 10.
28 'Social Security', *INM*, 17, 2 (February 1950), p. 1.
29 'Towards Vocationalism?', pp. 1–2.
30 Leinster House, on Dublin's Kildare Street, is the home of Ireland's parliament.
31 *Irish Ecclesiastical Record*, cited in 'The National Health Service in England', *INM*, 17, 5 (May 1950), p. 10.
32 'The White Paper on Improved and Extended Health Services', *INM*, 19, 11 (December 1952), p. 2.
33 *Health Act (1953)*.
34 'Health Bill, 1953', *INM*, 20, 4 (April 1953), p. 2. Note that this commentary closely mirrored that of certain influential clerics, such as social ethicist Fr James Kavanagh, who also viewed proposed changes to healthcare provision as a financial burden on taxpayers; see Earner-Byrne, *Mother and Child*, p. 135.
35 Correspondence from Thomas O'Higgins, Minister for Health, reproduced in the INO's journal indicates that, in 1944, voluntary hospitals received £246,954 of sweepstake funding while State-run hospitals received £123,834. By 1953 the allocations were £2,194,057 and £2,155,230, respectively; see 'Voluntary Hospital Correspondence', *INM*, 22, 1 (January 1955), p. 3.
36 'Voluntary Hospital Nursing Personnel', *INM*, 23, 3 (March 1954), p. 4.
37 'Meath Hospital', *INM*, 20, 5 (May 1953), p. 3.
38 'Meath Hospital', *INM*, 20, 11 (December 1953), p. 4; 'Superannuation for Nurses and Hospital Staffs in Ireland', *INM*, 24, 12 (December 1957), pp. 8–10.
39 'Co. Board of Health', *Connaught Telegraph*, 22 February 1930.
40 *Report of the Provisional Committee to the First Annual Conference of the INU, 1920*. Doyle remained a supporter of the union until her retirement from the Charles Street Dispensary, Dublin in 1947.
41 'Nuns as Nurses', *Freeman's Journal*, 27 September 1917.
42 'Dublin Hospitals' Staff', *Irish Independent*, 12 September 1919.
43 Minutes of meeting of IWWU, 13 November 1919 (ILHS Archives, Dublin, IWWU Minutes Book: 1060/2/V7A).
44 'Letter to the Editor, Irish Nurses' and Midwives' Union', *Clare Champion*, 11 February 1922.

45   Letters from [name withheld] to the General Nursing Council, 10 May 1922; 17 June 1922;
      1 November 1922 and Letters from the General Nursing Council to [name withheld], 11
      May 1922; 24 October 1922; 5 December 1922 (NMBI Archives, Dublin, P220/445).

46   'Clare Health Board, Nuns and Night Nursing', *Clare Champion*, 4 February 1922.

47   'News and Topics of the Month', *INHW*, 5, 3 (March/April 1935), p. 20.

48   Undated note regarding Sisters of Mercy and the Dublin Union Hospitals (Dublin
      Diocesan Archives, Dublin, Hospitals [General] Box, Unnamed File). It is not made
      explicit whether the note referred to the North or South Dublin Union.

49   'Union Nurses, Question of Continuous Night Duty Raised', *INHW*, 4, 3 (1 March 1934),
      p. 25.

50   'Clare Health Board, Nuns and Night Nursing'.

51   'Letter to the Editor, the Irish Nurses' and Midwives' Union'.

52   'Claims of Nurses', *Irish Independent*, 4 May 1933.

53   Letter from Annie Smithson to Archbishop Byrne's Secretary, 6 June 1933 (Dublin
      Diocesan Archives, Dublin, Irish Nurses' Union File).

54   Letter from Annie Smithson to Archbishop Byrne undated but probably *c.* mid-to-late
      1930s (Dublin Diocesan Archives, Dublin, Irish Nurses' Union File).

55   Browne, *Against the Tide*, p. 145.

56   Smithson, *Myself – and Others*, p. 100.

57   Bashford-Synnott, 'Annie M.P. Smithson: romantic novelist/revolutionary nurse', p. 53.

58   'An S.O.S.', *INM*, 3, 10 (February 1939), p. 2.

59   'County Home and Hospital, Killarney', *INJ*, 2, 2 (June 1937), p. 14.

60   'Holy Year, 1950', *INM*, 17, 9 (September/October 1950), p. 6.

61   'Irish Guild of Catholic Nurses', *INM*, 21, 9 (October 1954), p. 8.

62   The proposed affiliation never transpired; see 'Public Health Nurses' Section', *INM*, 25, 3
      (March 1958), p. 9.

63   Irish Nurses' Organisation, *Irish Nurses' Organisation Souvenir Book*, p. 19. The historic
      meaning of the word 'sectarianism' was confirmed as 'adherence or excessive attachment
      to a particular sect or party, esp. in religion'; see W. Little, H.W. Fowler and J. Coulson,
      The Shorter Oxford English Dictionary on Historical Principles (London: Oxford University
      Press, 1944), p. 1,827.

64   Ferriter, *The Transformation of Ireland*, p. 408.

65   T. Inglis, *Moral Monopoly: The Rise and Fall of the Catholic Church in Modern Ireland* (2nd
      edn, Dublin: University College Dublin Press, 1998), pp. 72–3.

66   M. Hazard, *Sixty Years A Nurse* (London: Harper Element, 2015), p. 2.

67   Letter from Z.M. Goodall to R.J. Fenney, 28 April 1953 (The National Archives, Kew,
      England, An Bord Altranais File, DV12/47).

68   Inglis, *Moral Monopoly*, p. 91.

69   *Catholic Herald*, cited in 'Moral Disease – Seen Through the Eyes of a Young Hospital
      Nurse', *INJ*, 3, 7 (November 1938), pp. 3–4.

70   Ibid., p. 3.

71   Ibid., p. 4.

72   'World Greets Papal Decision on Painless Childbirth', *INM*, 23, 3 (March 1956), pp. 6–7.

73   Ibid., p. 6.

74   Hegarty tragically lost his life in a plane crash at Tuskar Rock, County Wexford, in 1968.

75   'Medical Ethics for Nurses II: The Commandments', *INM*, 24, 6 (June 1957), p. 9.

76   'Medical Ethics for Nurses II: The Commandments', *INM*, 24, 8 (August 1957), p. 8.

77   Paul VI, *Humanae Vitae* (Rome:1968).

78   'Correspondence', *INJ*, 2, 2 (February 1969), p. 12.

79   'Contraception', *WIN*, 3, 9 (September 1974), pp. 157–62.

80   Ibid., pp, 157, 162.

81   'Contraception and Abortion', *WIN*, 3, 4 (April 1974), p. 56.

82   *Health (Family Planning) Act (1979)* Section 4.

83   'Health (Family Planning) Bill 1978', *WIN*, 8, 3–7 (March/April/May/June/July 1979), p. 1.

84   *The Irish Nurses' Organisation and National Council of Nurses of Ireland, Policy Document on Family Planning, 1979* (INMO Archives, Dublin, INO Policy/Discussion Documents Folder).

85   Earner-Byrne, *Mother and Child*, p. 42.

86   'Medical Ethics For Nurses II: The Commandments', *INM*, 24, 5 (May 1957), p. 8.

87   'Medical Ethics for Nurses II: The Commandments', *INM*, 24, 9 (September 1957), p. 10.

88   'Medical Ethics For Nurses II: The Commandments', *INM*, 24, 5 (May 1957), p. 9.

89   'Campaign for Pro-Life Amendment to the Constitution', *WIN*, 10, 7–8 (July/August 1981), p. 2.

90   Hazard, *Sixty Years A Nurse*, pp. 182–4.

91   'Resolutions Adopted at the 1982 AGM', *WIN*, 11, 10–12 (October/November/December 1982), p. 7.

92   For a comprehensive analysis of the referendum, see B. Girvin, 'Social Change and Moral Politics: The Irish Constitutional Referendum, 1983', *Political Studies*, XXXIV (1986), pp. 61–81.

93   'Campaign for Pro-Life Amendment to the Constitution', p. 2.

94   *Irish Nursing News*, 1, 12 (May 1981), p. 1; *Irish Nursing News*, 2, 1 (August 1981), p. 3.

95   *Nurses Act (1950)*. An Bord Altranais translates to 'The Nursing Board'. For a history of An Bord Altranais, see J. Robins, *Nursing and Midwifery in Ireland in the Twentieth Century: 50 Years of An Bord Altranais (The Nursing Board), 1950–2000* (Dublin: An Bord Altranais, 2000).

96   An Bord Altranais, *Code for Nurses* (Dublin: An Bord Altranais, 1985), p. 6.

97   Inglis, *Moral Monopoly*, p. 21.

98   *The Irish Nurses' Organisation and National Council of Nurses of Ireland, Policy Document on Nurses' Involvement in Tubal Ligation, 1985* (INMO Archives, Dublin, INO Policy/Discussion Documents Folder).

99   'Contraception, Enabling Choice Through Education', *WIN*, 9, 5 (June 2001), pp. 23–4.

100   'Fifty Years of the Pill', *WIN*, 18, 8 (September 2010), p. 44.

101   I would like to acknowledge Kathleen Craughwell for bringing this (and many other pieces of valuable information) to my attention.

102   Motions for Debate at the Annual Delegate Conference of the Irish Nurses' and Midwives' Organisation, 2012 (INMO Library, Dublin).

103   T. Flannery, *The Death of Religious Life* (Dublin: The Columba Press, 1997), p. 62.

104   'The Nursing Profession and Vocational Organisation', *INM*, 15, 5 (May 1948), p. 1.

105   'Our Sister Tutors', *INM*, 29, 5 (May 1962), p. 1.

106   Letter from [name withheld] to James Keogh, CEO, An Bord Altranais, 2 January 1978 (NMBI Archives, Dublin, P220/495).
107   Oral history interview conducted with Lenore Mrkwicka on 29 May 2013.
108   Oral history interview conducted with anonymous respondent No. 1 on 18 February 2013.
109   'Nurses' Strike Notice, County Infirmary Position', *Limerick Leader*, 13 February 1950.
110   C. Clear, *Nuns in Nineteenth-Century Ireland* (Dublin: Gill and Macmillan, 1987), p. 131.
111   The newspaper source does not indicate which county board.
112   'County Home Nurses and their Apartments', *Connaught Telegraph*, 18 January 1930.
113   Ibid.
114   Ibid.
115   'Medical Ethics for Nurses II: The Commandments', *INM*, 24, 6 (June 1957), p. 9.
116   For a good explanation of the Encyclical, see J. Molony, *The Worker Question: A New Historical Perspective on Rerum Novarum* (Dublin: Gill and Macmillan, 1991).
117   'The Black List', *INM*, 13, 42 (October 1944), p. 9.
118   Ibid.
119   This grade actually formed a number of sections along regional/provincial lines.
120   'Outdoor Nursing Officers', *INM*, 17, 8 (August 1950), p. 12; 'Memorandum to Minister for Health, Public Health Nurses', *INM*, 18, 5 (May 1951), p. 2; 'Revised Salary Scales, Public Health Nurses', *INM*, 19, 9 (October 1952), p. 6. In practice, public health nurses' roles encompassed education regarding maternity and child welfare, infection control and the provision of vaccinations.
121   'Executive Council Meets, Public Health Nurses', *INM*, 20, 7 (July 1953), p. 9.
122   'Reply from the Minister for Health, Public Health Nurses', *INM*, 26, 1 (January 1959), p. 4.
123   'Thirty-Fifth Annual Report, June 1955, Jubilee Nurses' Section', *INM*, 22, 8 (September 1955), p. 8.
124   'Notes on a Lecture Given by the Master, National Maternity Hospital, to the Midwives Attending the Post-Graduate Course at that Hospital', *INM*, 12, 7 (November 1941), p. 7.
125   *Health Act (1953)* Section 17.
126   'Thirty-Sixth Annual Report, June 1956, Dispensary Midwives' Section', *INM*, 23, 7 (July 1956), p. 3; 'Thirty-Seventh Annual Report, 1956/57, Dispensary Midwives' Section', *INM*, 24, 10 (October 1957), p. 14.
127   'General Secretary's Report, Membership', *INM*, 15, 6 (June 1948), p. 1; 'General Secretary's Annual Report, 1950, Membership', *INM*, 18, 7 (July 1951), p. 6.
128   *Health Act (1947)* Section 98; *Health Act (1953)* Section 41.
129   '38th Annual Report, 1957/58, National Health Council', *INM*, 25, 6 (June 1958), p. 1.
130   *Health Act (1953)* Section 41.
131   '38th Annual Report, 1957/58, National Health Council', p. 1.
132   Jones, *These Obstreperous Lassies*, p. 219.
133   Letter from Dr F. O'Donnell, Mercer's Hospital, to Archbishop Byrne, 20 November 1930 (Dublin Diocesan Archives, Dublin, Archbishop Byrne, Holles Street Hospital, Jervis Street Hospital and Other Hospitals File).

CHAPTER 7

1 The grave is in the cemetery's Sheltering Hills section, not far from the main gate and security cabin.

2 Lee, *Ireland, 1912–85*, p. 354.

3 O'Connor, *A Labour History of Ireland: 1824–2000*, p. 221.

4 Trade union membership rose from 310,000 to 410,000 between 1960–72; see Ibid., p. 225.

5 I would like to thank Therese Bradley, Ena's niece, for supplying me with this description of her aunt.

6 International Labour Office, *Employment and Conditions of Work of Nurses* (Geneva: International Labour Office, 1960).

7 The decimalisation of results by the ILO seems unusual in the era of pounds, shillings and pence. It appears to have been methodologically necessary, as the survey was conducted in a number of countries with a number of different currencies, and because the methodology of calculating nurses' hourly remuneration involved dividing their yearly remuneration by the number of hours they worked per year; see Ibid., p. 98.

8 'Annual General Meeting, 1960, President's Address', *INM*, 27, 7 (July 1960), p. 3.

9 *Industrial Relations Act (1946)* Section 10–24.

10 For a more detailed description of the Labour Court, see B. Hillery, 'Industrial Relations: Compromise and Conflict', in D. Nevin (ed.), *Trade Unions and Change in Irish Society* (Dublin: Mercier Press, 1980), pp. 39–52.

11 Mental nurses had access to the Labour Court.

12 C. McCarthy, *Elements in a Theory of Industrial Relations* (Dublin: Irish Academic Press, 1984), p. 35.

13 B. Cox and J. Hughes, 'Industrial Relations in the Public Sector', in *Industrial Relations in Ireland, Contemporary Issues and Developments* (Dublin: Department of Industrial Relations, University College Dublin, 1987), p. 81.

14 Barrington, *Health, Medicine and Politics in Ireland*, p. 259.

15 'Annual General Meeting, 1961, Address by the Minister for Health at the Annual General Meeting of the Irish Nurses' Organisation at Jury's Hotel, Dublin, on Wednesday, 31 May 1961', *INM*, 28, 7 (July 1961), pp. 9–10.

16 Oral history interview conducted with Kathleen Craughwell, 9 May 2013.

17 'Salary Negotiations', *INM*, 28, 8 (August 1961), p. 1.

18 'Correspondence', *INM*, 28, 10 (October 1961), p. 3.

19 'Annual Report, Working Hours for Trained Staff', *INM*, 29, 6 (June 1962), p. 8.

20 'Dublin Branch Protest Meeting', *INM*, 28, 10 (October 1961), p. 6.

21 Oral history interview conducted with Kathleen Craughwell, 9 May 2013.

22 'Final Offer', *INM*, 28, 11 (November 1961), pp. 1, 3.

23 Ibid., p. 1.

24 'Nurses to Vote on Resignation', *Irish Times*, 6 July 1961.

25 '300 Nurses Vote for Strike', *Irish Press*, 30 September 1961.

26 The E.S.B, or Electricity Supply Board, was Ireland's largest electricity supply company at the time.

27 'They are Unfair to Nurses', *Sunday Independent*, 25 May 1969.

28 'Correspondence Re: A New Salary Structure for Voluntary Hospitals', *Irish Nurse*, hereafter referred to as *IN*, 1, 6 (January 1964), pp. 173–4.
29 The Irish Congress of Trade Unions came into being when the historical split between the Congress of Irish Unions and the Irish Trade Union Congress (ITUC) was mended in 1959 with the amalgamation of both bodies under the title of the ICTU.
30 'The Federation of Professional Associations', *IN*, 5, 6 (January 1967), p. 96.
31 'Professional Men Get Organised', *Irish Times*, 5 November 1966.
32 'Conciliation and Arbitration', *INM*, 30, 1 (January 1963), p. 1.
33 'Presidential Address to the 1963 Annual General Meeting, Arbitration', *INM*, 30, 7 (July 1963), p. 5.
34 McCarthy, *Elements in a Theory of Industrial Relations*, p. 35.
35 The act notes: 'It shall not be lawful for a member of the Garda Síochána to be or become a member of any trade union ... of which the objects or one of the objects are or is to control or influence the pay, pensions, or conditions of service'; see *Garda Síochána Act (1924)* Section 13.
36 Ibid., Section 14.
37 'Arbitration – Its Importance to the Nursing Profession', *IN*, 1, 1 (August 1963), p. 5.
38 Ibid., pp. 8–9.
39 'Arbitration Award', *IN*, 3, 7 (February 1965), pp. 111–13.
40 International Labour Office, *Employment and Conditions of Work of Nurses*, p. 167.
41 'Working Hours', *IN*, 5, 2 (September 1966), p. 19.
42 International Labour Office, *Employment and Conditions of Work of Nurses*, p. 32.
43 'Texans Appreciate Irish Nurses', *INM*, 30, 5 (June 1963), p. 11.
44 'Nursing in the USA', *IN*, 1, 3 (October 1963), pp. 67–9.
45 'Branch Notes, Wicklow', *INM*, 30, 2 (February 1963), p. 11.
46 'Recommendations to the Hospitals' Commission', *INM*, 29, 9 (September 1962), p. 4.
47 P.R. Kaim-Caudle, 1964, cited in 'Superannuation-Voluntary Hospitals', *IN*, 3, 11 (June 1965), p. 187.
48 Ibid.
49 'Address to Public Health Nurses', *IN*, 4, 5 (December 1965), pp. 319–20.
50 'Inside Politics, The O'Malley Mission', *Irish Times*, 9 July 1966.
51 Government of Ireland, *The Health Services and their Further Development* (Dublin: The Stationery Office, 1966), pp. 47, 65.
52 Ibid., pp. 58–60. Health service spending rose from £5.7 million in 1948 to £17.7 million in 1961 and £61.5 million in 1971, that is, from 1.7 per cent to 3.7 per cent of the gross national product; see B. Hensey, *The Health Services of Ireland* (4th edn, Dublin: Institute of Public Administration, 1988), pp. 178–9.
53 Government of Ireland, *Outline of the Future Hospital System: Report of the Consultative Council on the General Hospital Services* (Dublin: The Stationery Office, 1968).
54 Ibid., p. 86.
55 M. Ó hÓgartaigh, 'Flower Power and "Mental Grooviness": Nurses and Midwives in Ireland in the Early Twentieth Century', in B. Whelan (ed.), *Women and Paid Work in Ireland, 1500–1930* (Dublin: Four Courts Press, 2000), p. 138.
56 'The Pro's Lament', *INJ*, 3, 6 (October 1938), p. 7.
57 'The Nursing Profession, Need for Changed Conditions', *Irish Independent*, 15 March 1919.

58   A. Hennigan and N. Kenny, 'Anna Hennigan, Interview Part 3', *Oral History @UCC*, accessed 30 December 2017: http://www.oralhistoryucc.com/items/show/22.

59   'A New Experiment', *INM*, 23, 3 (March 1956), pp. 1, 3.

60   'Modern Trends in Nursing Education', *IN*, 1, 5 (December 1963), p. 135.

61   Ibid., p. 136.

62   Scanlan, *The Irish Nurse*, p. 283.

63   'Priorities for Nurses', *Sunday Independent*, 14 September 1969.

64   'Protest by Angry Nurses in Galway', *Connacht Tribune 1st edn*, 25 September 1965.

65   Ibid.

66   Ibid.

67   'Object to Dismissal of Nurses', *Irish Press*, 19 October 1965.

68   'Four Nurses Discharged: Councillors Back Hospital Decision', *Connacht Tribune 1st edn*, 9 October 1965.

69   'Let Me Say Firmly, I am Against Sacred Cows', *IN*, 4, 4 (November 1965), p. 287.

70   'View of the Minister for Health on the Improvement of Conditions for Student Nurses', *IN*, 4, 11 (June 1966), pp. 431–2.

71   Oral history interview conducted with Maureen McCann, 16 April 2013.

72   Oral history interview conducted with Lenore Mrkwicka, 29 May 2013.

73   Government of Ireland, *Outline of the Future Hospital System*, p. 26.

74   'Commission on Relief of Poor and Insane', *INU Gazette*, 14 (October 1925), p. 7.

75   'Training of Nurses', *Irish Independent*, 16 March 1968.

76   'Key Resolutions Relating to Education Adopted by the Annual General Meeting 1967', *IN*, 6, 3 (October 1967), p. 263.

77   *Nurses Act (1950)* Section 54–5.

78   'Post-Basic Education', *INJ*, 1, 10 (October 1968), p. 7.

79   'Higher Education for Nurses', *INM*, 12, 25 (May 1943), p. 6.

80   Oral history interview conducted with Kathleen Craughwell, 9 May 2013.

81   Ibid.

82   'Correspondence', *INM*, 18, 1 (January 1951), p. 6.

83   E. Prendergast and H. Sheridan, *Jubilee Nurse: Voluntary District Nursing in Ireland, 1890–1974* (Dublin: Wolfhound Press, 2012), p. 43.

84   'Direct Visual Repair of Atrial Septal Defect Under Hypothermia', *INM*, 25, 4 (April 1958), pp. 12–16.

85   'Modern Trends in Nursing Education', p. 137.

86   Scanlan, *The Irish Nurse*, p. 155.

87   Ibid., p. 156.

88   'New Trends in Nursing Education', *INM*, 22, 6 (June 1955), p. 10.

89   'Intensive Care Unit', *IN*, 5, 12 (July 1967), pp. 211–14.

90   'Intensive Care and Cardiac Resuscitation', *INJ*, 1, 6 (June 1968), pp. 23–6.

91   Ministry of Health, *Report of the Committee on Senior Nursing Staff Structure* (London: HMSO, 1966).

92   'Executive Council Meets, Cork: Ward Sisters Posts', *INM*, 28, 3 (March 1961), p. 11.

93   'Ward and Departmental Sisters', *INM*, 29, 3 (March 1962), p. 8.

94   'Post-Basic Education', p. 7.

95   'New Year Campaign, Education', *INJ*, 3, 1 (January 1970), p. 4.

96	Minutes of meeting of INO Executive, 4 February 1937 (INMO Archives, Dublin, Archives Box).

97	Scanlan, *The Irish Nurse*, pp. 254–5.

98	'Executive Council Meets, Ward and Departmental Sisters Section', *INM*, 29, 2 (February 1962), p. 11.

99	Oral history interview conducted with P.J. Madden, 18 February 2013.

100	M. Gowan, 1944, cited in Scanlan, *The Irish Nurse*, p. 277.

101	International Labour Office, *Employment and Conditions of Work of Nurses*, p. 58.

102	'Future Challenges in the Nursing World', *INM*, 29, 7 (July 1962), p. 4.

103	Ibid., p. 5.

104	Oral history interview conducted with Kathleen Craughwell, 9 May 2013.

105	'Training and Use of the Nursing Auxiliary in the Ward Situation', *IN*, 4, 9 (April 1966), pp. 399–402.

106	'Protest to the Minister for Health, The Establishment of Human Rights in the Nursing World', *IN*, 6, 5 (December 1967), p. 298.

107	'Job Satisfaction', *IN*, 4, 6 (January 1966), p. 331.

108	See 'Correspondence', *WIN*, 4, 1 (January 1975), p. 10 in which it was alleged that SENs were working as matrons in welfare homes and were acting up as registered nurses in psychiatric hospitals in England.

109	*Local Government Act (1941)* Section 21.

110	'Nurses Bill, 1961', *INM*, 28, 10 (October 1961), p. 9.

111	Ibid.

112	G.K. Bixler and R.W. Bixler, 'The Professional Status of Nursing', *American Journal of Nursing*, 59, 8 (August 1959), pp. 1142–7.

113	Ibid., p. 1146.

114	'The Nurses Bill, 1949', *INM*, 16, 9 (September–October 1949), p. 5.

115	M. Bostridge, *Florence Nightingale, The Woman and Her Legend* (London: Viking, 2008), p. 454.

116	'Mercer's Hospital Dublin, Post Graduate Course for Nurses', *INM*, 3, 12 (April 1939), p. 9.

117	'Future Challenges in the Nursing World', p. 6.

118	Evidence suggests that O'Farrell ran for election to the organisation's Midwives' Committee in 1925; see 'Ballot Paper for Election of Officers and Executive Committees of the Irish Nurses' Union for the year 1925' (INMO Archives, Dublin, Archives Box). Evidence also suggests that O'Farrell attended the organisation's tenth Annual Council Meeting in 1930 to represent Dublin midwives; see 'Annual Council Meeting, 1930', *INU Gazette*, 31 (June 1930), p. 1.

119	Oral history interview conducted with Anne Cody, 12 August 2013.

120	Irish Nurses' Organisation, *INO Annual Report and Accounts, 1967/68* (Dublin: Irish Nurses' Organisation, 1968), no pagination.

121	Address by Margrethe Kruse to INO members delivered at the Mater Hospital Dublin, 10 September 1969 (INMO Archives, Dublin, Archives Box).

CHAPTER 8

1   'The Victors', *WIN*, 2, 4 (April 1973), pp. 73, 76.

2   J. Levine, 1995, cited in L. Connolly, *The Irish Women's Movement From Revolution to Devolution* (Dublin: The Lilliput Press, 2003), p. 119.

3   'Look Your Best–1', *IN*, 1, 4 (November 1963), p. 110.

4   'Look Your Best–3', *IN*, 1, 6 (January 1964), p. 170.

5   *IN*, 4, 12 (July 1966), no pagination.

6   See H. Tweedy, *A Link in the Chain: the Story of the Irish Housewives' Association, 1942–92* (Dublin: Attic Press, 1992), pp. 75, 114.

7   Irish Housewives' Association, *The Irish Housewife: The Irish Housewives' Association Yearbook* (Dublin: Irish Housewives' Association, 1948), p. 95.

8   Ibid., foreword, no pagination.

9   Letter from Louie Bennett to Kathleen Nora Price, 26 May 1928.

10   Jones, *These Obstreperous Lassies*, p. 44.

11   'Nurses Make History in the Labour Court, What a Victory for the Fighting Four', *Sunday Independent*, 27 February 1972.

12   Ferriter, *The Transformation of Ireland*, pp. 466–7.

13   Census returns for 1946 show that of 8,703 female 'sick nurses', a category that does not include midwives or mental attendants, 8,014 were single, 425 were married and 264 were widows; see Central Statistics Office, *Census of Population 1946, vol. V, Part II, Ages, Orphanhood and Conjugal Conditions*, p. 37. Census returns for 1951 show that of 8,379 female 'nurses and midwives', a category that does not include mental nurses or nurses in training, 7,355 were single, 685 were married and 339 were widows; see Central Statistics Office, *Census of Population 1951, vol. II, Part II, Ages and Conjugal Conditions* (Dublin: The Stationery Office, 1954), p. 46. Census returns for 1961 show that of 8,405 female 'nurses and midwives', a category that does not include mental nurses and nurses in training, 7,494 were single, 643 were married and 268 were widows; see Central Statistics Office, *Census of Population 1961, vol. V, Occupations* (Dublin: The Stationery Office, 1964), p. 42. Census returns for 1966 show that of 8,797 female 'nurses and midwives', a category that does not include mental nurses and nurses in training, 7,765 were single, 756 were married and 276 were widows; see Central Statistics Office, *Census of Population 1966, vol. V, Occupations and Industries* (Dublin: The Stationery Office, 1969), p. 46.

14   Oral history interview conducted with Annette Kennedy on 29 July 2016.

15   Oral history interview conducted with Lenore Mrkwicka on 29 May 2013.

16   'Engagements', *INJ*, 3, 9 (September 1970), p. 21.

17   Hallam, *Nursing the Image*, pp. 22, 69.

18   *INJ*, 3, 11 (November 1970), no pagination.

19   *INJ*, 3, 5 (May 1970), no pagination.

20   'Lighter Side of the War', *INM*, 12, 26 (June 1943), p. 7.

21   Marriage gratuities were paid in order to compensate women who had to retire on marriage. 'Nurses in Dispute', *Irish Press*, 2 March 1970.

22   'Managers Informed of INO Resolutions', *INJ*, 1, 9 (September 1968), p. 11.

23   'Correspondence Page', *INJ*, 3, 10 (October 1969), p. 20.

24   O'Leary, 'The Irish National Teachers' Organisation and the Marriage Bar', p. 51.

25   Government of Ireland, *Report of the Commission on the Status of Women* (Dublin: Stationery Office, 1972), p. 7.

26   Ibid., p. 110.

27   Oral history interview conducted with Noreen Muldoon, 23 August 2013.

28   'Resolutions Adopted at the AGM, 1971', *WIN*, 1, 1 (January 1972), p. 9.

29   'Referendum on Resolution Re Permanent Posts for Married Women', *WIN*, 1, 4 (April 1972), p. 76.

30   'Where are all the Single Nurses?', *Kerryman*, 10 July 1971.

31   'Referendum on Resolution Re Permanent Posts for Married Women', p. 76.

32   'The AGM Annual Dinner', *WIN*, 1, 12 (December 1972), p. 243.

33   Letter from Anonymous to James Keogh, CEO, An Bord Altranais, 10 October 1977 (NMBI Archives, Dublin, P220/495).

34   'Difficult Exchequer Situation and Rising Expectations', *WIN*, 12, 11/12 (November/ December 1983), p. 10.

35   'Fullest Use of Job-Sharing Urged', *WIN*, 3, 1 (March/April 1995), p. 8.

36   'Tenth Round', *IN*, 5, 6 (January 1967), p. 91.

37   Ferriter, *The Transformation of Ireland*, p. 570.

38   'Tenth Round', p. 91.

39   *INHW*, 2, 24 (15 August 1932), p. 2.

40   'News from G.H.Q's', *INHW*, 3, 7 (1 June 1933), p. 11; 'News from G.H.Q's', *INHW*, 5, 6 (July 1935), p. 10.

41   Letter from Ruth Nicolls to Archbishop Byrne,16 August 1939 (Dublin Diocesan Archives, Dublin, Irish Guild of Catholic Nurses File).

42   'Why Our Nurses Are Leaving', *Irish Times*, 12 August 1969.

43   *Anti-Discrimination (Pay) Act (1974)* Section 2.

44   'New Horizons', *WIN*, 1, 11 (November 1974), p. 6.

45   Census returns for 1971 show that of 16,590 female 'nurses', a category that appears to include mental nurses and midwives, although this is not made explicit, 13,915 were single, 2,270 were married and 405 were widows; see Central Statistics Office, *Census of Population 1971, vol. V, Occupations and Industries* (Dublin: The Stationery Office, 1975), p. 34. Census returns for 1981 show that of 26,938 female 'nurses', a category that appears to include mental nurses and midwives, 16,922 were single, 9,445 were married and 571 were widows; see Central Statistics Office, *Census of Population 1981, vol. 7, Occupations* (Dublin: The Stationery Office, 1986), p. 214. Census returns for 1986 show that of 28,914 female 'nurses', a category that appears to include mental nurses and midwives, 15,467 were single, 12,928 were married and 519 were widows; see Central Statistics Office, *Census of Population 1986, vol. 7, Occupations* (Dublin: The Stationery Office, 1993), p. 238. See also C. Ó Gráda, *A Rocky Road, The Irish Economy Since the 1920s* (Manchester: Manchester University Press, 1997), pp. 204–5.

46   The Fighting Fund was originally established in 1964 in order to meet the costs of the organisation's participation in conciliation and arbitration. It appears to have been diverted to fund the publicity campaign in 1970.

47   'AGM 1977 Motions for Debate', *WIN*, 6, 9 (September 1977), p. 8; Irish Nurses' Organisation, *INO Annual Report and Accounts, 1977/78* (Dublin: Irish Nurses' Organisation, 1978), p. 16.

48 'Extraordinary General Meeting', *INJ*, 3, 4 (April 1970), p. 8.

49 Ibid., p. 9.

50 'News from the Branches, Athy, Baltinglass, Carlow', *INJ*, 3, 6 (June 1970), p. 9.

51 'INO Noticeboard, Wexford Stand-By and On-Call Allowance-Ambulance Duty', *WIN*, 1, 12 (December 1972), p. 248.

52 'Mary McCabe, Nurses' Leader', *Irish Independent*, 22 May 1970.

53 'Nurses' Protest March', *Kerryman*, 4 July 1970.

54 'Galway Protest March and Rally', *INJ*, 3, 8 (August 1970), p. 14.

55 'Summary of Address by Mr Erskine Childers, Tánaiste and Minister for Health, to the Annual General Meeting of the Irish Nurses' Organisation', *INJ*, 3, 11 (November 1970), p. 16.

56 'Nurses Refuse Meals in Pay Row', *Irish Press*, 20 October 1970.

57 'Summary of Address by Mr Erskine Childers', p. 16.

58 'No Need for Strikes, Says Nursing "Union"', *Irish Independent*, 14 June 1975.

59 'Nurses in Dispute'.

60 'Resolutions for Submission to the 1974 AGM', *WIN*, 3, 9 (September 1974), p. 156.

61 'Union Support for Strikes by Nurses', *Irish Times*, 12 December 1969.

62 Ibid.

63 Ibid.

64 'Nurses and Strike Action', *Irish Independent*, 30 October 1975.

65 'A Concept of Professionalism, Accountability and Responsibility', *WIN*, 4, 11 (November 1975), p. 1.

66 Oral history interview conducted with Anne Cody, 12 August 2013.

67 'Stand Up and Be Counted', *INJ*, 3, 8 (August 1970), pp. 5, 7.

68 'Your Organisation's Approach … the Only Rational One', *WIN*, 1, 11 (November 1974), p. 13.

69 'A Concept of Professionalism, Accountability and Responsibility'.

70 Ibid., pp. 1–2.

71 Ibid., p. 1.

72 'Resolutions Submitted for the 1975 AGM', *WIN*, 4, 10 (October 1975), p. 6.

73 'Integrity and Openness', *WIN*, 4, 11 (November 1975), p. 4.

74 'Obituaries, Miss Louie Bennett', *INM*, 24, 1 (January 1957), p. 13.

75 'Spirit of Christmas', *WIN*, 4, 12 (December 1975), p. 8.

76 'Presidential Address, AGM 1976, Manpower Planning', *WIN*, 5, 11/12 (November/December 1976), p. 2.

77 'Extraordinary General Meeting', p. 9.

78 'News from Branches, Galway', *INJ*, 4, 6 (June 1971), p. 7.

79 A. Hennigan and N. Kenny, 'Anna Hennigan, Interview Part 3'.

80 'Annual General Meeting, Preparation for the Future', *INJ*, 3, 10 (October 1970), p. 7.

81 'Resolutions Adopted at the AGM, 1971', p. 8. Note that An Bord Altranais denied that it ever 'officially laid down' a ratio of 1:100 clinical instructors to student nurses; see 'Correspondence', *WIN*, 1, 7 (July 1972), p. 141.

82 'Our Greatest Need', *INJ*, 4, 6 (June 1971), p. 5.

83 S. Byrne, *The Final Journey, An Autobiography* (Kiltimagh: Evelyn and Phil Byrne, 2005), p. 35. This is a fascinating and poignant book and is well worth reading.

84 Oral history interview conducted with Annette Kennedy, 29 July 2016.

85 'Resolutions Adopted by the AGM', *INJ*, 1, 7 (July 1968), p. 21.

86 Council Directive 77/453/EEC, 27 June 1977.

87 'EEC Directives', *WIN*, 8, 3/7 (March/July 1979), p. 7.

88 Council Directive 77/453/EEC.

89 'EEC Directives', *WIN*, 9, 7/8 (July/August 1980), p. 3.

90 'Letters, EEC Directives', *WIN*, 11, 2/3 (February/March 1982), p. 5.

91 'Correspondence', *WIN*, 1, 7 (July 1972), p. 141.

92 E. Hanrahan, *A Social Study of the Training and Career Aspirations of Final Year Student Nurses* (Dublin: Irish Matrons' Association, 1971), pp. 99, 115–16.

93 'INO News, News from the North-Western Region, New General Training Hospital', *WIN*, 4, 10 (October 1975), p. 4.

94 J. Adams, M. Carney and T. Kearns, *RCSI, Faculty of Nursing and Midwifery, 40th Anniversary History: 1974–2014* (Dublin: Royal College of Surgeons in Ireland, 2014), p. 18.

95 Ibid., pp. 31–2.

96 'Comment', *WIN*, 2, 11 (November 1973), p. 203.

97 *Health Act (1970)*.

98 'Kerry Open Air Rally', *INJ*, 3, 9 (September 1970), p. 7.

99 'Our Greatest Need', p. 5.

100 'New Mayor for Galway', *WIN*, 4, 8 (August 1975), p. 1.

101 Scanlan, *The Irish Nurse*, p. 174.

102 'Militant New Blood on Wards', *Irish Press*, 18 September 1979.

103 Government of Ireland, *Report of the Commission on the Status of Women*, p. 189.

104 Ibid., p. 190.

105 'INO Nominees on Health Boards', *INJ*, 4, 2/3 (February/March 1971), pp. 11–13.

106 Government of Ireland, *Report of the Commission on the Status of Women*, p. 198.

107 'Health Act, 1970', *INJ*, 3, 6 (June 1970), p. 7.

108 'Comhairle Na nOspidéal', *WIN*, 1, 8 (August 1972), p. 165.

109 'Nurses Keep a Watch', *Irish Independent*, 5 April 1971.

110 Irish Nurses' Organisation, *Submission to the Commission on Nursing* (Dublin: Irish Nurses' Organisation, 1997), p. 19.

111 'News from the Branches, Cavan', *WIN*, 1, 5 (May 1972), p. 97.

112 M.A. Wren, *Unhealthy State: Anatomy of a Sick Society* (Dublin: New Island, 2003), p. 205.

113 'Integrity and Openness, Concept of Professionalism', p. 5.

114 R.B. Finnegan and J.L. Wiles, *Women and Public Policy in Ireland, A Documentary History: 1922–97* (Dublin: Irish Academic Press, 2005), pp. 390–1.

115 'Congratulations', *WIN*, 5, 3 (March 1976), p. 9; 'Nurses Prove their Point', *Irish Independent*, 7 October 1977.

116 'National Council of Nurses', *INM*, 18, 8 (August/September 1951), p. 7.

117 H. Henry, *A History of the Irish Guild of Catholic Nurses: Seventy-Five Years of Service, 1922–97* (Dublin: Irish Guild of Catholic Nurses, 1998), pp. 88–90, 97.

118 'The National Florence Nightingale Committee of Ireland', *WIN*, 5, 1/2 (January/February 1976), p. 9; 'International and National Nursing Links', *WIN*, 4, 10 (October 1975), pp. 8–9.

119 'Executive Council in Action, National Council of Nurses of Ireland', *WIN*, 5, 3 (March 1976), p. 8.

120 'Executive Council Recommends Restructuring of NCN', *WIN*, 4, 10 (October 1975), p. 2.

121 'Incorporation of the National Council of Nurses into the INO', *WIN*, 7, 5 (May 1978), p. 3.

CHAPTER 9

1 Irish Nurses' Organisation, *INO Annual Report and Accounts, 1968/69* (Dublin: Irish Nurses' Organisation, 1969), p. 2; Irish Nurses' Organisation, *INO Annual Report and Accounts, 1977/78*, p. 5.

2 Oral history interview conducted with Maureen McCann, 16 April 2013.

3 Ibid.

4 Ibid.

5 P.J. Madden, 'The unionateness of the Irish Nurses' Organisation: The formation of a working trade union for nurses, 1978–90' (Keele: University of Keele, 1991), p. 48.

6 'Need for Solidarity', *WIN*, 7, 11/12 (November/December 1978), p. 1.

7 Ibid.

8 D. Keogh, 'Ireland, 1972–84', in Hill (ed.), *A New History of Ireland, vol. VII, 1921–84*, p. 367.

9 D. Ferriter, *Ambiguous Republic: Ireland in the 1970s* (London: Profile Books, 2012), pp. 512–24.

10 R. F. Foster, *Luck and the Irish: A Brief History of Change, c. 1970–2000* (London: Penguin, 2007), p. 23.

11 Madden, 'The unionateness of the Irish Nurses' Organisation', p. 35.

12 'Resolutions Adopted at the Annual General Meeting 1978', *WIN*, 7, 11/12 (November/December 1978), p. 5.

13 The RCN became a trade union in 1977 but maintained its aversion to striking until 1995.

14 'Motions and Resolutions for Submission to the 1978 Annual General Meeting', *WIN*, 7, 8 (September 1978), p. 6; Madden, 'The unionateness of the Irish Nurses' Organisation', Appendix D.

15 Madden, 'The unionateness of the Irish Nurses' Organisation', p. 48.

16 'Motions and Resolutions for Submission to the 1978 Annual General Meeting', p. 6.

17 '4,000 Nurses Storm Dáil Seeking Cure for their Grievances', *Irish Independent*, 23 November 1978.

18 'Campaign for Better Pay', *WIN*, 8, 1/2 (January/February 1979), p. 1.

19 'Executive Council 77–79', *WIN*, 8, 3/4/5/6/7 (March/April/May/June/July 1979), p. 2.

20 In 1979, there were 963 junior managerial nursing staff such as ward sisters, 642 senior managerial nursing staff such as matrons and 9,119 staff nurses or staff midwives; see Department of Health, *Report of the Working Party on General Nursing* (Dublin: The Stationery Office, 1980), p. 23. Note that these figures exclude 5,500 psychiatric nurses and 975 nurses engaged in the care of the 'mentally handicapped'.

21 Oral history interview conducted with Kathleen Craughwell, 9 May 2013.

22 Some interviewees, who were otherwise content to be named, requested that their description of the Executive Council as the 'blue-rinse brigade' be anonymised.

23 Interviewee's name withheld.
24 Oral history interview conducted with Maureen McCann, 16 April 2013.
25 Oral history interview conducted with Kathleen Craughwell, 9 May 2013.
26 Ibid.
27 J. McGowan, *Attitude Survey of Irish Nurses* (Dublin: Institute of Public Administration, 1979), pp. 66–7.
28 Oral history interview conducted with Lenore Mrkwicka, 29 May 2013.
29 Oral history interview conducted with Maureen McCann, 16 April 2013.
30 Ibid.
31 'Nurses in Bid to Take Over Association', *Irish Press*, 27 August 1979.
32 Oral history interview conducted with Maureen McCann, 16 April 2013.
33 'Profile', *WIN*, 1, 3 (March 1972), p. 54.
34 'Nurses Hire a Hard Talker', *Sunday Independent*, 31 July 1977; Irish Nurses' Organisation, *INO Annual Report and Accounts, 1977/78*, p. 5.
35 Letter from Christina Meehan to James Keogh, CEO, An Bord Altranais, 11 January 1980 and letters from James Keogh, CEO, An Bord Altranais to Christina Meehan, 5 February 1980; 25 February 1980 (NMBI Archives, Dublin, P220/501).
36 'Motions for Submission to the AGM 1981', *WIN*, 10, 9 (September 1981), p. 5.
37 'Code of Ethics', *WIN*, 13, 1/2 (January/February 1984), p. 8.
38 'Nurses Reject Increase of £20 a week and £700 in Back Money', *Irish Independent*, 8 October 1979.
39 'Nurses and Librarians', *Irish Independent*, 11 October 1979; 'Librarians Reply to Nurses', *Irish Independent*, 15 October 1979.
40 'Extraordinary General Meeting', *WIN*, 9, 5/6 (May/June 1980), p. 1.
41 Oral history interview conducted with P.J. Madden, 24 February 2014.
42 Discussion Document on 'Future Developments'. Submitted by INO Executive Council to 1980 Annual General Meeting of the INO (The National Archives, Kew, England, Irish Nurses' Organisation File, DT16/306).
43 Memorandum and Articles of Association of the Irish Nurses' Organisation, 1983 (INMO Archives, Dublin, Archives Box).
44 Discussion Document on 'Future Developments'.
45 Oral history interview conducted with Dave Hughes, 10 November 2016.
46 Madden, 'The unionateness of the Irish Nurses' Organisation', pp. 52–3.
47 'Nurses' Union of Ireland', *WIN*, 17, 5 (September/October 1988), p. 3.
48 Oral history interview conducted with P.J. Madden, 24 February 2014.
49 Madden, 'The unionateness of the Irish Nurses' Organisation', p. 53.
50 Ibid., p. 57.
51 Oral history interview conducted with Liam Doran, 24 February 2014.
52 South Eastern Health Board, *The History of the South Eastern Health Board, 1971–2004* (Kilkenny: The Health Service Executive, 2005), p. 19.
53 P. O'Morain, *The Health of the Nation: The Irish Healthcare System, 1957–2007* (Dublin: Gill and Macmillan, 2007), p. 139.
54 Ibid., p. 140.
55 Deloitte and Touche, *Value for Money Audit of the Irish Health System, Main Report* (Dublin: The Department of Health and Children, 2001), p. 56.

56   'Irish Nurses Organisation in Dispute with NWHB', *Leitrim Observer*, 8 May 1982.

57   'Information', *WIN*, 17, 4 (July/August 1988), p. 13.

58   'Nurses Try to Sleep it Out', *Irish Independent*, 20 April 1988.

59   'Nurses Win Battle on Wage Cut', *Irish Press*, 7 April 1988.

60   'Health Cuts Dangerous to Patients Warns Union', *Irish Independent*, 9 February 1985.

61   'Paid Sick Leave', *WIN*, 13, 4/5 (March/April 1984), p. 3.

62   'Conditions in County Hospitals and Homes', *INU Gazette*, 17 (November 1926), p. 1.

63   'Diary of the Month, Overcrowded Hospital', *INHW*, 6, 12 (December 1936), p. 2.

64   'Irish Nurses Want Bigger Salaries and Staffs – Better Hours', *Sunday Independent*, 18 April 1943.

65   'News from Branches, Galway', p. 7.

66   Irish Nurses' Organisation, *INO Annual Report and Accounts, 1976/77* (Dublin: Irish Nurses' Organisation, 1977), p. 8.

67   'Resolutions Adopted at the 1976 Annual General Meeting', *WIN*, 5, 11/12 (November/December 1976), p. 3; 'Executive Council in Action', *WIN*, 6, 5 (May 1977), p. 3.

68   'INO News Reports from Regions and Branches, Kilkenny', *WIN*, 7, 5 (May 1978), p. 5.

69   The nurse's poem was written in response to a poignant poem found amongst a patient's belongings after she had died. The patient's poem concerned her feelings of depersonalisation amid the hustle and bustle of the hospital routine; see 'A Nurse's Reply', *WIN*, 9, 7/8 (July/August 1980), p. 7.

70   'Nurses Vote Confront Dr Woods Cuts in Services', *Connacht Tribune*, 22 October 1982.

71   'Letters Page', *WIN*, 13, 4/5 (March/April 1984), p. 10.

72   Department of Health, *Report of the Working Party on General Nursing*.

73   'Address by the Minister for Health Dr Michael Woods', *WIN*, 9, 11/12 (November/December 1980), p. 8.

74   Department of Health, *Report of the Working Party on General Nursing*, p. 47.

75   'Are We Losing Touch with the Nuts and Bolts of Our Profession?', *WIN*, 7, 9 (November 1999), p. 17.

76   'Chronic Overcrowding', *WIN*, 11, 6/7 (June/July 1982), p. 5.

77   'Branch Representatives' Annual Meeting', *WIN*, 11, 8/9 (August/September 1982), p. 5.

78   B. Tierney, *Stress in Irish Nursing* (Dublin: An Bord Altranais, 1988).

79   Ibid., p. 40.

80   Ibid., p. 79.

81   'Little by Little', *WIN*, 16, 5 (September/October 1987), p. 3.

82   An Bord Altranais, *The Code of Professional Conduct for Each Nurse and Midwife* (Dublin: An Bord Altranais, 1988), no pagination.

83   'We Are Protesting Not for Us But for the Patients', *Irish Times*, 19 July 1989.

84   Ibid.

85   Oral history interview conducted with Kathleen Craughwell, 9 May 2013.

86   Wren, *Unhealthy State*, p. 235.

87   'Protest Stoppage at Hospital in Crisis', *Irish Press*, 18 July 1989.

88   'Patient Care Study to Aid Staffing', *Irish Independent*, 22 August 1989.

89   Oral history interview conducted with P.J. Madden, 18 February 2013.

90   Ibid.

91   Oral history interview conducted with P.J. Madden, 24 February 2014.

92   The INO offered indemnity insurance since as early as 1977.

93   'Unions Warn of All-Out Hospital Picket', *Irish Independent*, 5 June 1979.

94   'Anger Over Strike Breaking Move', *Connaught Telegraph*, 20 April 1983.

95   'Nun Grabbed and Abused on Mercy Mission', *Connaught Telegraph*, 14 December 1983.

96   Oral history interview conducted with P.J. Madden, 18 February 2013.

97   'Four Nurses Discharged: Councillors Back Hospital Decision'.

98   Letter from [name withheld] to James Keogh, CEO, An Bord Altranais, 2 January 1978.

99   Interviewee's name withheld.

100   Oral history interview conducted with Noreen Muldoon, 23 August 2013.

101   Oral history interview conducted with Kathleen Craughwell, 9 May 2013.

102   Oral history interview conducted with anonymous respondent No. 3, 11 March 2013.

103   Oral history interview conducted with P.J. Madden, 24 February 2014.

CHAPTER 10

1   'Angels in the Wings', *IN*, 1, 3 (October 1963), p. 62.

2   C. Hart, *Nurses and Politics: The Impact of Power and Practice* (Basingstoke: Palgrave Macmillan, 2004), p. 87.

3   Oral history interview conducted with Lenore Mrkwicka, 29 May 2013.

4   Government of Ireland, *Programme for Competitiveness and Work* (Dublin: The Stationery Office, 1994).

5   Ibid., p. 81.

6   There were and still are a number of divisions of the Register of Nurses. For instance, midwives, psychiatric nurses, 'mental handicap' nurses, sick children's nurses and nurse tutors had their own individual division on the register, separate to general nurses. It was and still is possible to be registered in more than one division.

7   'Industrial Relations', *WIN*, 2, 5 (September/October 1994), pp. 16–17.

8   Ibid., p. 17.

9   'New Offer May Be Put to Nurses As Labour Relations Commission Intervenes in Dispute', *WIN*, 4, 2 (March/April 1996), p. 6.

10   Oral history interview conducted with Liam Doran, 24 February 2014.

11   'Message Heard Loud and Clear', *WIN*, 4, 3 (May/June 1996), p. 6.

12   The adjudication process examined the abolition of the lower salary for newly qualified nurses, increases in salary for managerial grades, issues regarding special location and dual qualified allowances, early retirement and pay parity for nurse teachers and college lecturers; see 'Significantly Improved Pay Deal Expected to Emerge from Adjudication Process', *WIN*, 4, 4 (July/August 1996), p. 8.

13   Revised Proposals for Agreement on the Pay and Conditions of Nurses as Provided for in the Agreement on Pay Incorporated in the Programme for Competitiveness at Work (INMO Archives, Dublin, Archives Box).

14   'Ballot on Pay Represents Important Milestone in Salary Negotiations for Irish Nurses', *WIN*, 4, 6 (November/December 1996), p. 6.

15   Irish Nurses' Organisation, *Submission to the Commission on Nursing*, p. 20.

16   'Sixteen Years of Negotiation', *WIN*, 5, 1 (February 1997), p. 7.

17   'INO Gears Up for Lengthy Dispute', *WIN*, 5, 1 (February 1997), p. 6.

18   Labour Court Recommendation 15450 (7 March 1997).

19   Ibid.

20   Oral history interview conducted with P.J. Madden, 18 February 2013.

21   Oral history interview conducted with Anne Cody, 12 August 2013.

22   14,457 INO members voted. A total of 10,005 or 69 per cent voted to accept the Labour Court's recommendations and 4,542 or 31 per cent voted to reject the recommendations; see 'Nurses Move Back from the Brink', *WIN*, 5, 2 (March 1997), p. 6.

23   Irish Nurses' Organisation, *Submission to the Commission on Nursing*.

24   Ibid., Part II, p. 1.

25   'Acceptance of Commission's Report Rests on Pay Related Issues', *WIN*, 6, 6 (July/August 1998), p. 6.

26   Discussion Document on 'The Maintenance of Essential Services in Dispute Situations'. Submitted by INO Executive Council to 1998 Annual Delegate Conference of the INO (INMO Archives, Dublin, Archives Box).

27   'INO Draws Up Plan of Action for Industrial Disputes', *WIN*, 6, 5 (June 1998), p. 14.

28   'Into the Future with New Direction', *WIN*, 6, 7 (September 1998), p. 5.

29   Oral history interview conducted with P.J. Madden, 24 February 2014.

30   Government of Ireland, *Report of the Commission on Nursing* (Dublin: The Stationery Office, 1998).

31   Ibid., p. 112.

32   Ibid., p. 113.

33   Ibid., p. 135.

34   Ibid., p. 7.

35   Labour Court Recommendation 16083 (9 February 1999).

36   Labour Court Recommendation 16084 (9 February 1999).

37   'A Glass Half Full or a Glass Half Empty', *WIN*, 7, 2 (March 1999), p. 5.

38   Oral history interview conducted with Liam Doran, 24 February 2014.

39   See especially 'Nurses' Leader Has Issued 27 Strike Threats', *Irish Daily Mail*, 11 May 2013. The same edition referred to Doran as 'Action man' with another headline reading: 'A nurses' strike? Here we go again'.

40   Oral history interview conducted with Liam Doran, 24 February 2014.

41   Ibid.

42   'We Will Wait No Longer for Our Fair Share – Cody', *WIN*, 7, 5 (June 1999), p. 11.

43   Oral history interview conducted with Dave Hughes, 10 November 2016.

44   Ibid.

45   Ibid.

46   Brown, *Ireland, A Social and Cultural History: 1922–2002*, p. 381.

47   Ibid., p. 376.

48   'Hairshirt Haughey's £15,000 Top Tailor Bill', *Irish Independent*, 7 October 1999.

49   'Out to Lunch … On the Nation', *Irish Independent*, 20 October 1999.

50   'Cowen is Public Enemy No 1 as Thousands Take to the Streets in Defiance', *Irish Independent*, 22 October 1999.

51   Labour Court Recommendation 16261 (31 August 1999).

52   Oral history interview conducted with Dave Hughes, 10 November 2016.

53   'Government Cannot Afford to Back Down', *Irish Independent*, 23 September 1999.
54   Irish Nurses' Organisation, *Annual Report 1999* (Dublin: Irish Nurses' Organisation, 2000), p. 19.
55   'Pay Crisis Looms After Ballots of Nurses and Gardaí', *Irish Independent*, 12 October 1999; among those who voted, 82 per cent of the SIPTU members, 89 per cent of the IMPACT members and 89 per cent of PNA members endorsed the strike.
56   Stallknecht served as President of the Danish Nurses' Organisation for twenty-eight years, from 1968–96, and served as President of the International Council of Nurses from 1997–2001.
57   Oral history interview conducted with Anne Cody, 12 August 2013.
58   'Nurses are Threatening Foundation of Progress', *Irish Independent*, 18 October 1999.
59   Oral history interview conducted with Liam Doran, 24 February 2014.
60   'Not Too Late', *Irish Independent*, 15 October 1999.
61   J. Bessant, '"Good Women and Good Nurses": Conflicting Identities in the Victorian Nurses' Strikes, 1985–86', *Labour History*, 63 (November 1992), p. 170.
62   'Nurses' Pay Claim', *Irish Times*, 15 October 1999.
63   'A Jab of Fair Play that Hardly Hurts at All', *Irish Times*, 23 October 1999.
64   'Strike Could Change Public's Attitude to Nursing Forever', *Irish Times*, 23 October 1999.
65   'Stab Story was a Watershed', *Sunday Independent*, 24 October 1999.
66   'INO Claims Cover At Crumlin Children's Hospital Is Adequate', *Irish Times*, 23 October 1999.
67   Oral history interview conducted with Liam Doran, 24 February 2014.
68   Accompaniment notes to the First Annual Conference of the INU, 1920.
69   Oral history interview conducted with anonymous respondent No. 1, 18 February 2013.
70   Oral history interview conducted with Liam Doran, 24 February 2014.
71   'Concern Over Threat To Life', *Sunday Tribune*, 24 October 1999.
72   'Helpful Nurses "Told To Co-Operate Less"', *Sunday Independent*, 24 October 1999.
73   'Baby Comes First At Holles Street', *Irish Times*, 21 October 1999.
74   'Simmering Anger As Stress Levels Rise', *Irish Independent*, 22 October 1999.
75   'A Spirited Show Of Force', *Irish Independent*, 22 October 1999.
76   G.D. Brown, A.M. Greaney, M.E. Kelly-Fitzgibbon and J. McCarthy, 'The 1999 Irish Nurses' Strike: Nursing Versions of the Strike and Self-Identity in a General Hospital', *Journal of Advanced Nursing*, 56, 2 (October 2006), p. 204.
77   Oral history interview conducted with Anne Cody, 12 August 2013.
78   'A Jab of Fair Play that Hardly Hurts at All'.
79   Oral history interview conducted with anonymous respondent No. 3, 11 March 2013.
80   Ibid.
81   Oral history interview conducted with P.J. Madden, 18 February 2013.
82   Oral history interview conducted with Anne Cody, 12 August 2013.
83   An Bord Altranais, *The Code of Professional Conduct for Each Nurse and Midwife*, no pagination.
84   An Bord Altranais, *Annual Report 1983* (Dublin: An Bord Altranais, 1984), p. 13. The board dismissed the claim against all of the nurses who had been involved in the industrial dispute the following year.
85   An Bord Altranais, *Report for the Year 1998* (Dublin: An Bord Altranais, 1999), p. 14.

86   An Bord Altranais, *Annual Report for the Year 1999* (Dublin: An Bord Altranais, 2000), p. 18. In order to control for possible delays, sixteen applications for inquiries into the fitness to practise of nurses were considered in 2000; see An Bord Altranais, *Annual Report for the Year 2000* (Dublin: An Bord Altranais, 2001) p. 25.

87   Oral history interview conducted with Dave Hughes, 10 November 2016.

88   Ibid.

89   'Huge Poll Backing For Nurses' Strike', *Sunday Independent*, 24 October 1999.

90   'Relatives Asked to Make Beds and Meals', *Irish Independent*, 23 October 1999.

91   Oral history interview conducted with Noreen Muldoon, 23 August 2013.

92   Oral history interview conducted with Clare Treacy, 22 November 2017.

93   Oral history interview conducted with Lenore Mrkwicka, 29 May 2013.

94   Oral history interview conducted with Liam Doran, 24 February 2014.

95   Oral history interview conducted with Noreen Muldoon, 23 August 2013.

96   Oral history interview conducted with Dave Hughes, 10 November 2016.

97   Oral history interview conducted with Liam Doran, 24 February 2014.

98   Oral history interview conducted with Liam Doran, 28 July 2016.

99   Oral history interview conducted with Dave Hughes, 10 November 2016.

100   Labour Court Recommendation 16330 (27 October 1999).

101   Oral history interview conducted with Noreen Muldoon, 23 August 2013.

102   Oral history interview conducted with Anne Cody, 12 August 2013.

103   'Quotes of the Week', *Sunday Independent*, 31 October 1999.

104   Oral history interview conducted with Liam Doran, 24 February 2014.

105   'The Irish Nurses' Union, a Manure Cart for Midwives', p. 164.

106   Oral history interview conducted with Noreen Muldoon, 23 August 2013.

107   'Nurses in West View Proposals with Disbelief', *Irish Times*, 29 October 1999.

108   Oral history interview conducted with Anne Cody, 12 August 2013.

109   Irish Nurses' Organisation, *Policy Document on the Maintenance of Essential Services in Dispute Situations* (Dublin: Irish Nurses' Organisation, 2002).

110   'Horoscopes, Your Guide to the Stars', *WIN*, 2, 1 (January/February 1994), p. 33.

111   Personal correspondence with Anne McGowan.

112   Personal correspondence with Madeline Spiers.

113   Personal correspondence with Teresa Hayes.

CHAPTER 11

1   Oral history interview conducted with Dave Hughes, 10 November 2016.

2   Irish Nurses' Organisation, *Submission to the Commission on Nursing*, pp. 13–15, 32–8.

3   Government of Ireland, *Report of the Commission on Nursing*, pp. 143–4.

4   Irish Nurses' Organisation, *Submission to the Commission on Nursing*, p. 8.

5   Government of Ireland, *Report of the Commission on Nursing*, pp. 57–8.

6   An Bord Altranais, *Review of Scope of Practice for Nursing and Midwifery* (Dublin: An Bord Altranais, 2000).

7   'Course Funding Aims to Boost Specialisation', *WIN*, 9, 5 (June 2001), p. 6.

8   'Message From A Trolley', *WIN*, 14, 3 (March 2006), p. 18.

9   'A&E Crisis Now A National Emergency, Says Harney', *Irish Independent*, 29 March 2006.

10   'State Of Emergency', *WIN*, 12, 11 (December 2004), p. 21.

11   'A Long and Arduous Road', *WIN*, 13, 3 (March 2005), p. 18.

12   'ANPs – An Advancing Solution', *WIN*, 12, 11 (December 2004), p. 22.

13   'Advanced Role in Colorectal Screening', *WIN*, 20, 1 (February 2012), pp. 27–8.

14   'Milestone for Midwife-led Unit', *WIN*, 17, 6 (June 2009), pp. 46–7.

15   An Bord Altranais and the National Council for the Professional Development of Nursing
     and Midwifery, *Review of Nurses and Midwives in the Prescribing and Administration
     of Medicinal Products* (Dublin: An Bord Altranais and the National Council for the
     Professional Development of Nursing and Midwifery, 2005), pp. 27–8.

16   'Power to Prescribe – Pushing an Open Door', *WIN*, 13, 11 (December 2005), pp. 20–1.

17   'The Final Push For Prescribing Powers', *WIN*, 14, 8 (September 2006), pp. 22–3.

18   'Future Proof', *WIN*, 20, 9 (November 2012), p. 28.

19   Ibid.

20   Barring some stipulations regarding controlled drugs such as morphine.

21   'Empty Promises', *WIN*, 17, 6 (June 2009), p. 27.

22   Oral history interview conducted with Annette Kennedy, 29 July 2016.

23   'The R.N. – Real Nurse', *WIN*, 1, 5 (September/October 1993), p. 14.

24   Oral history interview conducted with Annette Kennedy, 29 July 2016.

25   Ibid.

26   Ibid.

27   Ibid.

28   Ibid.

29   'Distance Learning: Moving Closer to Nurses' Needs', *WIN*, 3, 2 (May/June 1995), p. 14.

30   Minutes of meeting of INO Executive, 24 October 1944 (INMO Archives, Dublin,
     Archives Box).

31   'University Education in Nursing', *WIN*, 8, 1/2 (January/February 1979), p. 9.

32   Irish Nurses' Organisation, *INO Annual Report and Accounts, 1978/79* (Dublin: Irish
     Nurses' Organisation, 1979), p. 11.

33   Department of Health, *Report of the Working Party on General Nursing*, pp. 103–4, 111–
     12, 127.

34   McGowan, *Attitude Survey of Irish Nurses*, p. 94.

35   'Industrial Relations News, Nurse Tutors/Clinical Teachers Boycott Forthcoming Student
     Intake', *WIN*, 20, 4 (July/August 1991), p. 18.

36   'Industrial Relations News, E.C. Directives, 85/595', *WIN*, 21, 1 (January/February 1992),
     pp. 12–13.

37   'Are We Ready for University Education for Irish Nurses?', *WIN*, 20, 4 (July/August 1991),
     p. 22.

38   J. McFarlane, 'The Role of Nurse Graduates in the Health Service in the Year 2000', *Nurse
     Education Today*, 7, 1 (1987), pp. 38–41.

39   'Letters', *WIN*, 2, 2 (March/April 1994), p. 27.

40   An Bord Altranais, *The Future of Nurse Education and Training in Ireland* (Dublin: An
     Bord Altranais, 1994).

41   'Pay Rise of 4.6% Agreed For New Style Nurse Tutors', *WIN*, 3, 5 (November/December
     1995), p. 9.

42 'Employers to Foot Bill for Nursing Degree Fees', *WIN*, 8, 5 (June 2000), p. 8.

43 'Where to Now?' *WIN*, 4, 3 (May/June 1996), pp. 19–21.

44 'A Student Nurse's Account of the First Day on the Ward', *WIN*, 9, 7 (September 2001), p. 15.

45 Independent External Evaluation Team, *Nurse Education and Training Evaluation in Ireland* (Southampton: University of Southampton, 1998), p. 15.

46 Government of Ireland, *Report of the Commission on Nursing*, pp. 79–82.

47 'At Last the Status Nursing Deserves', *WIN*, 9, 10 (December 2001), p. 5.

48 Oral history interview conducted with Liam Doran, 24 February 2014.

49 Oral history interview conducted with Annette Kennedy, 29 July 2016.

50 For a moving tribute to Clare Spillane, see 'A Fearless Advocate for the Carers', *WIN*, 11, 8 (September 2003), p. 5.

51 'News', *WIN*, 14, 6 (November/December 1985), p. 12.

52 Oral history interview conducted with Annette Kennedy, 29 July 2016.

53 Oral history interview conducted with Liam Doran, 28 July 2016.

54 B. Girvin, 'The Republicanisation of Irish Society, 1932–48', in Hill (ed.), *A New History of Ireland vol. VII, 1921–84*, p. 145.

55 Remarks by T.J. O'Connell T.D., Dáil Éireann Debate, vol. 31 No. 3, 5 July 1929.

56 Remarks by T.J. O'Connell T.D., Dáil Éireann Debate, vol. 30 No. 4, 29 May 1929.

57 *Electoral (Amendment) (Political Funding) Act (2012)* Section 42.

58 Personal correspondence with the Nursing and Midwifery Board of Ireland in relation to the 2015 elections to the board.

59 Personal correspondence with the Irish Medical Council in relation to the 2013 elections to the council.

60 Personal correspondence with the Teaching Council in relation to the 2016 elections to the council.

61 *WIN*, 10, 5 (May 2002), p. 9.

62 See 'Misleading Political Message', *WIN*, 10, 6 (June 2002), p. 42; 'Upset at Political Message', *WIN*, 10, 7 (July/August 2002), p. 17.

63 Oral history interview conducted with Liam Doran, 28 July 2016.

64 'European Delivery', *WIN*, 13, 11 (December 2005), pp. 25–6.

65 'Our Voice in Europe', *WIN*, 13, 10 (November 2005), p. 21.

66 A. Kennedy, 'The Role of Irish Healthcare Representatives in Shaping the EU Debate: Past, Present and Future', in Irish Nurses' Organisation, *Forming EU Healthcare Policy, A Showcase of Irish Involvement* (Dublin: Irish Nurses' Organisation, 2007), p. 20.

67 'EFN/INMO Lobby Successfully for Better Sharps Injury Protection', *WIN*, 18, 5 (May 2010), p. 14.

68 Council Directive 2010/32/EU, 10 May 2010.

69 'Landmark Victory in EC Pay Case', *WIN*, 23, 1 (February 2015), p. 18.

70 'Soaring Living Costs Hit Nursing', *WIN*, 8, 10 (December 2000/January 2001), p. 6.

71 'Three Rs Remain a Mystery to Management', *WIN*, 10, 10 (November 2002), p. 5.

72 'No Place Like Home', *WIN*, 9, 4 (May 2001), pp. 16–17.

73 The Nursing Alliance, *Submission to the Benchmarking Body* (Dublin: Nursing Alliance, 2001).

74 'Benchmarking Fails to Address Conditions of Employment', *WIN*, 10, 8 (September 2002), p. 6.

75   This debate was to rumble on for years.
76   'Because You're Worth It', *WIN*, 10, 10 (November 2002), p. 21.
77   Oral history interview conducted with Liam Doran, 28 July 2016.
78   'Rejection of National Deal Speaks Volumes About Health Services', *WIN*, 12, 8 (September 2004), p. 6.
79   Labour Court Recommendation 18763 (9 November 2006).
80   'Action Plan Underway Following Endorsement by 96% of Members', *WIN*, 15, 3 (March 2007), p. 7.
81   70 per cent of INO members voted on the proposal with 54 per cent voting in favour and 46 per cent voting against; see 'NIB Proposals Accepted', *WIN*, 15, 6 (June 2007), p. 5.
82   Oral history interview conducted with Liam Doran, 28 July 2016.
83   Ibid.
84   K. Browne, 'Schooling, Capitalism and the Mental/Manual Division of Labour', *Sociological Review*, 29, 3 (July 1981), pp. 445–73.

CHAPTER 12

1   'Are We A Society Or Just An Economy?', *WIN*, 16, 10 (November 2008), p. 5.
2   *Financial Emergency Measures in the Public Interest Act (2009)* Section 2.
3   'Get Up – Stand Up', *WIN*, 17, 10 (November 2009), p. 5.
4   'HSE Confirms Education Cutbacks for 2009', *WIN*, 16, 11 (December 2008), p. 8.
5   Public Service Agreement (2010–14).
6   'INMO No Vote Highlights Challenges Ahead', *WIN*, 18, 7 (July/August 2010), p. 6.
7   'INMO to Challenge New Entrants' Pay Scale', *WIN*, 19, 1 (February 2011), p. 7.
8   'BCC Hears INO Complaint on RTÉ Broadcasts', *WIN*, 17, 5 (May 2009), p. 9.
9   'Croke Park Extension – Why the INMO Urges Members To Vote No in the Upcoming Ballot', *WIN*, 21, 3 (April 2013), pp. 6–7.
10   Oral history interview conducted with Dave Hughes, 10 November 2016.
11   Oral history interview conducted with Liam Doran, 28 July 2016.
12   Oral history interview conducted with Noreen Muldoon, 23 August 2013.
13   'Delegates Condemn 80% Graduate Pay Plan', *WIN*, 21, 5 (June 2013), p. 24.
14   Seventy-one per cent of members who voted chose to endorse the Haddington Road Proposals; see 'Haddington Road – The Final Ask', *WIN*, 21, 6 (July/August 2013), p. 5.
15   'Grad Boycott Hits Headlines', *WIN*, 21, 1 (February 2013), p. 51.
16   Oral history interview conducted with Phil Ní Sheaghdha, 27 October 2017.
17   'African Odyssey', *WIN*, 17, 2 (February 2009), p. 41.
18   'Ethiopia Update', *WIN*, 17, 9 (October 2009), p. 23.
19   '€6,000 Donation to ICN Relief Fund for Haiti', *WIN*, 18, 8 (September 2010), p. 10.
20   'Rising from the Ruins: Life in Tacloban After Typhoon Haiyan', *WIN*, 22, 8 (October 2014), p. 44.
21   'Turning Off The Red Light', *WIN*, 19, 5 (June 2011), pp. 22–3.
22   Oral history interview conducted with Clare Treacy, 22 November 2017.
23   *Criminal Law (Sexual Offences) Act (2017)* Section 25.
24   'Vote Yes for Equality', *WIN*, 23, 3 (April 2015), pp. 42–3.

25   Oral history interview conducted with Clare Treacy, 22 November 2017.

26   *Nurses Act (1950)* Section 45–6.

27   *Nurses Act (1985)* Section 38–47.

28   Oral history interview conducted with Clare Treacy, 22 November 2017.

29   Ibid.

30   Nursing and Midwifery Board of Ireland, *Annual Report 2014* (Dublin: Nursing and Midwifery Board of Ireland, 2015), p. 40.

31   Nursing and Midwifery Board of Ireland, *Annual Report 2015* (Dublin: Nursing and Midwifery Board of Ireland, 2016), p. 47.

32   'When Disaster Is Just A Heartbeat Away', *WIN*, 7, 6 (July/August 1999), p. 12.

33   Ibid., p. 13.

34   G. Marie, 'Women in union' (Dublin: University College Dublin, 1995), p. 57.

35   D.P. O'Donovan, *The Commission of Investigation into Leas Cross Nursing Home, Final Report* (Dublin: Department of Health, 2009), pp. 287, 290.

36   Irish Nurses' and Midwives' Organisation, *Annual Report 2015* (Dublin: Irish Nurses' and Midwives' Organisation, 2016), p. 51.

37   Oral history interview conducted with Clare Treacy, 22 November 2017.

38   'It's Time For Real Pay Restoration', *WIN*, 23, 5 (June 2015), pp. 22–3.

39   'Members Accept Lansdowne Road Deal', *WIN*, 23, 7 (September 2015), p. 9.

40   Irish Nurses' and Midwives' Organisation, *Submission to the Public Service Pay Commission* (Dublin: Irish Nurses' and Midwives' Organisation, 2017), p. 4.

41   Public Service Pay Commission, *Report of the Public Service Pay Commission* (Dublin: Public Service Pay Commission, 2017), p. 75.

42   Cunningham, *Unlikely Radicals*, p. 249.

43   Wren, *Unhealthy State*, p. 229.

44   'Cutbacks Deepen in Health Service', *WIN*, 17, 9 (October 2009), p. 12.

45   'Stop Health Cuts', *WIN*, 17, 5 (May 2009), p. 17.

46   R. Francis, *Report of the Mid Staffordshire NHS Foundation Trust Public Inquiry, Executive Summary* (London: The Stationery Office, 2013).

47   'Warning: Safe Care Must Always Come First', *WIN*, 19, 10 (December 2011/January 2012), pp. 18–20.

48   'INMO Asks HIQA To Inspect All Hospitals', *WIN*, 19, 8 (October 2011), p. 6.

49   Oral history interview conducted with Dave Hughes, 10 November 2016.

50   'The Pathway to an Equitable, Fair and Quality Assured Health Service', *WIN*, 24, 7 (September 2016), supplement.

51   Committee on the Future of Healthcare, *Sláintecare Report* (Dublin: Houses of the Oireachtas, 2017).

52   'Depth Of Crisis Spelled Out Repeatedly', *WIN*, 22, 8 (October 2014), p. 8.

53   Oral history interview conducted with Liam Doran, 28 July 2016.

54   'Public Health Service Faces Worst Crisis Yet', *WIN*, 17, 5 (May 2009), p. 7.

55   Ibid.

56   'Email from a "Broken" Member', *WIN*, 22, 8 (October 2014), p. 16.

57   'Proud and Passionate', *WIN*, 16, 7 (July/August 2008), p. 19.

58   Oral history interview conducted with Annette Kennedy, 29 July 2016.

59   'Future Proof', *WIN*, 20, 9 (November 2012), p. 29.

60   L.H. Aiken, D.M Sloane, L. Bruyneel, K. Van den Heede et al., 'Nurse Staffing and Education and Hospital Mortality in Nine European Countries: A Retrospective Observational Study', *The Lancet*, 383, 9931 (24 May 2014), pp. 1824–30.

61   'INMO Supports Nurse Forecasting Study', *WIN*, 18, 2 (February 2010), p. 18.

62   'HR Planning: Nurses and Nursing in Ireland', *WIN*, 19, 2 (March 2011), p. 12.

63   'Midwifery Survey Confirms Staffing Crisis', *WIN*, 22, 3 (April 2014), p. 6.

64   'If We Could Do It So Can You', *WIN*, 22, 5 (June 2014), pp. 27–8.

65   'Update on Major Current Issues, Taskforce on Staffing and Skill Mix in Nursing', *WIN*, 23, 10 (December 2015/January 2016), p. 10.

66   'Have Your Say On New Bill', *WIN*, 16, 1 (January 2008), p. 20.

67   'Talks With DOH On New Legislation Ongoing', *WIN*, 17, 7 (July/August 2009), p. 13.

68   Oral history interview conducted with Liam Doran, 28 July 2016.

69   *Nurses Act (2011)* Section 22.

70   E. Hanrahan, *A Social Study of the Training and Career Aspirations of Final Year Student Nurses*, pp. 154–5.

71   Oral history interview conducted with Anne Cody, 12 August 2013.

72   'Clarity and Quality Key to INO Submission on New Nurses and Midwives Bill', *WIN*, 16, 3 (March 2008), pp. 20–1.

73   'INO Seeks Guidance from An Bord Altranais', *WIN*, 177, 7 (July/August 2009), p. 7.

74   Robins, *Nursing and Midwifery in Ireland in the Twentieth Century*, p. 62.

75   Irish Nurses' Organisation, *Annual Report and Accounts, 1988–9* (Dublin: Irish Nurses' Organisation, 1989), p. 5.

76   'A Board in Crisis', *WIN*, 19, 2 (March/April 1989), p. 3.

77   'Breakthrough Likely in Nurses' Row', *Irish Independent*, 23 February 1989.

78   Irish Nurses' Organisation, *INO Annual Report and Accounts, 1988–9*, p. 5.

79   'Letters from the INO', *WIN*, 17, 6 (November/December 1988), p. 9.

80   'One-Day Nurses' Strike Disrupts St James's', *Irish Times*, 19 July 1989.

81   'The Nurses Bill, 1949', p. 7.

82   An Bord Altranais, *Submission to the Commission on Nursing* (Dublin: An Bord Altranais, 1997).

83   'INMO Agrees New Arrangements with An Bord', *WIN*, 19, 5 (June 2011), p. 6.

84   'Breaking News', *WIN*, 19, 4 (May 2011), p. 20.

85   Government of Ireland, *Report of the Commission on Nursing*, p. 57.

86   Letter from Paul Gallagher to each nurse and midwife, 3 November 2014.

87   'The Nurses Bill, 1949', p. 6.

88   NMBI Welcomes Large Numbers Paying Full Annual Retention Fee (ARF) 2015, 12 January 2015 (Nursing and Midwifery Board of Ireland).

89   Nursing and Midwifery Board of Ireland, *Annual Report 2015*, p. 41.

90   'Minister Calls on NMBI to Enter Direct Talks with Unions Over Fee Dispute', *WIN*, 23, 1 (February 2015), p. 6.

91   'Nursing Body Spent €96,000 on Executive Travel Abroad', *Sunday Business Post*, 14 June 2015.

92   Remarks by Senator John Crown, Joint Committee on Health and Children Debate, 16 July 2015.

93   Nursing and Midwifery Board of Ireland, *Annual Report 2014*, p. 29.

94 Crowe Horwath, *Final Report to Nursing and Midwifery Board of Ireland, Organisation Review* (Dublin: Crowe Horwath, 2015), pp. 2, 4.

95 Personal correspondence with Madeline Spiers.

96 Nursing and Midwifery Board of Ireland, *Annual Report 2015*, p. 41.

97 Oral history interview conducted with Liam Doran, 24 February 2014.

CONCLUSION, EPILOGUE … AND OVER TO YOU

1 'Plan to Ban Strikes in "Essential Services" Sparks Unions' Anger', *Irish Independent*, 23 May 2017.

2 Personal correspondence with Madeline Spiers.

3 Oral history interview conducted with Phil Ní Sheaghdha, 27 October 2017.

4 Ibid.

5 Ibid.

6 See European Court of Human Rights, Enerji Yapi-Yol Sen v. Turkey (Application no: 68959/01).

7 Oral history interview conducted with Phil Ní Sheaghdha, 27 October 2017.

8 Oral history interview conducted with Anne Cody, 12 August 2013.

9 Report of the Provisional Committee to the First Annual Conference of the INU, 1920.

Bibliography and Sources

Secondary Sources

Abel-Smith, B., *A History of the Nursing Profession* (London: Heinemann Educational Books, 1960).

Abrams, L., *Oral History Theory* (Abingdon: Routledge, 2010).

Adams, J., M. Carney and T. Kearns, *RCSI, Faculty of Nursing and Midwifery, 40th Anniversary History: 1974–2014* (Dublin: Royal College of Surgeons in Ireland, 2014).

Baly, M.E., *Nursing and Social Change* (3rd edn, London: Routledge, 1995).

Barrington, R., *Health, Medicine and Politics in Ireland, 1900–70* (Dublin: Institute of Public Administration, 1987).

Bew, P. and H. Patterson, *Seán Lemass and the Making of Modern Ireland, 1945–66* (Dublin: Gill and Macmillan, 1982).

Black, C., *King's Nurse – Beggar's Nurse* (London: Hurst and Blackett, 1939).

Blackburn, R.M., *Union Character and Social Class: A Study of White Collar Unionism* (London: Batsford, 1967).

Bostridge, M., *Florence Nightingale, The Woman and Her Legend* (London: Viking, 2008).

Boyd, A., *The Rise of the Irish Trade Unions* (Tralee: Anvil Books, 1972).

Boyle, J.W., *The Irish Labor Movement in the Nineteenth Century* (Washington: The Catholic University of America, 1988).

Brown, T., *Ireland: A Social and Cultural History, 1922–2002* (2nd edn, London: Harper Perennial, 2004).

Browne, N., *Against the Tide* (Dublin: Gill and Macmillan, 1986).

Brownmiller, S., *In Our Time, Memoir of a Revolution* (New York: Dell Publishing, 1999).

Brush, B.L. and J.E. Lynaugh (eds), *Nurses of all Nations: A History of the International Council of Nurses, 1899–1999* (Philadelphia: Lippincott, Williams and Wilkins, 1999).

Burke, H., *The People and the Poor Law in 19th Century Ireland* (Littlehampton: The Women's Education Bureau, 1987).

Byrne, S., *The Final Journey, An Autobiography* (Kiltimagh: Evelyn and Phil Byrne, 2005).

Callan, C., *The Irish National Painters' and Decorators' Trade Union and its Forerunners* (Dublin: Watchword, 2008).

Campbell, J., *'A Loosely Shackled Fellowship'*, *The History of Comhaltas Cána* (Dublin: The Public Service Executive Union, 1988).

—, *An Association to Declare: A History of the Preventive Staff Association* (Dublin: The Public Service Executive Union, 1996).

Carr, E.H., *What is History?* (2nd edn, London: Penguin, 1987).

Chaison, G. and B. Bigelow, *Unions and Legitimacy* (Ithaca: Cornell University Press, 2002).

Chuinneagáin, S., *Catherine Mahon: First Woman President of the INTO* (Dublin: Irish National Teachers' Organisation, 1998).

Clear, C., *Nuns in Nineteenth-Century Ireland* (Dublin: Gill and Macmillan, 1987).

Coakley, D., *Baggot Street: A Short History of the Royal City of Dublin Hospital* (Dublin: Royal City of Dublin Hospital, 1995).

Coleman, M., *IFUT: A History – the Irish Federation of University Teachers, 1963–99* (Dublin: Irish Federation of University Teachers, 2000).

Coleman, M., *The Irish Sweep: A History of the Irish Hospitals Sweepstake, 1930–87* (Dublin: University College Dublin Press, 2009).

Colson, I., *More Than Just The Money: 100 Years of the Victorian Nurses' Union* (Northcote: Prowling Tiger Press, 2001).

Connolly, J., *Socialism Made Easy* (Dublin: The Plough Book Service, 1971).

Connolly, L., *The Irish Women's Movement from Revolution to Devolution* (Dublin: The Lilliput Press, 2003).

Corlett, C. and M. Weaver (eds), *The Price Notebooks, Vol. I* (Dublin: Dúchas, 2002).

Cox, B. and J. Hughes, 'Industrial Relations in the Public Sector', in *Industrial Relations in Ireland, Contemporary Issues and Developments* (Dublin: Department of Industrial Relations, University College Dublin, 1987).

Crowley, M., *A Century of Service, 1880–1980: The Story of the Development of Nursing in Ireland* (Dublin: Faculty of Nursing, Royal College of Surgeons in Ireland, 1980).

Cullen Owens, R., *Smashing Times: A History of the Irish Women's Suffrage Movement, 1889–1922* (Dublin: Attic Press, 1984).

—, *Louie Bennett* (Cork: Cork University Press, 2001).

—, *A Social History of Women in Ireland, 1870–1970* (Dublin: Gill and Macmillan, 2005).

Cunningham, J., *Unlikely Radicals: Irish Post-Primary Teachers and the ASTI, 1909–2009* (Cork: Cork University Press, 2009).

Curran, O.A., *Two Hundred Years of Trade Unionism, 1809–2009* (Dublin: Irish Print Group, SIPTU, 2009).

Devine, F., *Organising History: A Centenary of SIPTU* (Dublin: Gill and Macmillan, 2009).

—, *A Unique Association: A History of the Medical Laboratory Scientists' Association, 1961–2011* (Dublin: Medical Laboratory Scientists' Association, 2012).

Dickenson, M., *An Unsentimental Union: The New South Wales Nurses' Association, 1931–92* (Sydney: Hale and Iremonger, 1993).

Dingwall, R., A.M. Rafferty and C. Webster, *An Introduction to the Social History of Nursing* (London: Routledge, 1988).

Dirrane, B., R. O'Connor and J. Mahon, *A Woman of Aran* (Dublin: Blackwater Press, 1997).

Dunsmore Clarkson, J., *Labour and Nationalism in Ireland* (New York: AMS Press, 1970).

Earner-Byrne, L., *Mother and Child: Maternity and Child Welfare in Dublin, 1922–60* (Manchester: Manchester University Press, 2007).

English, R., *Radicals and the Republic: Socialist Republicanism in the Irish Free State, 1925–37* (Oxford: Oxford University Press, 1994).

Farmar, T., *Patients, Potions and Physicians: A Social History of Medicine in Ireland* (Dublin: A. & A. Farmar and The Royal College of Physicians of Ireland, 2004).

Fealy, G.M. (ed.), *Care to Remember: Nursing and Midwifery in Ireland* (Cork: Mercier Press, 2005).

—, *A History of Apprenticeship Nurse Training in Ireland* (Abingdon: Routledge, 2006).

Ferriter, D., *Mothers, Maidens and Myths: A History of the Irish Countrywomen's Association* (Dublin: FÁS Training and Employment Authority, 1995).

—, *The Transformation of Ireland, 1900–2000* (London: Profile Books, 2005).

—, *Ambiguous Republic: Ireland in the 1970s* (London: Profile Books, 2012).

Finnegan, R.B. and J.L. Wiles, *Women and Public Policy in Ireland, A Documentary History: 1922–97* (Dublin: Irish Academic Press, 2005).

Flannery, T., *The Death of Religious Life* (Dublin: The Columba Press, 1997).

Foley, C., *The Last Irish Plague: The Great Flu Epidemic in Ireland, 1918–19* (Dublin: Irish Academic Press, 2011).

Forster, P.G., *The Esperanto Movement* (The Hague: Mouton Publishers, 1982).

Foster, R.F., *Luck and the Irish: A Brief History of Change, c. 1970–2000* (London: Penguin, 2007).

Fox, R.M., *Louie Bennett: Her Life and Times* (Dublin: The Talbot Press, 1958).

Frazier, A., *Hollywood Irish: John Ford, Abbey Actors and the Irish Revival in Hollywood* (Dublin: The Lilliput Press, 2011).

Gilligan, C., *In a Different Voice: Psychological Theory and Women's Development* (Cambridge: Harvard University Press, 1982).

Girvin, B., *The Emergency: Neutral Ireland, 1939–45* (London: Macmillan, 2006).

Gunnigle, P. and P. Flood, *Personnel Management in Ireland: Practice, Trends and Developments* (Dublin: Gill and Macmillan, 1990).

Hallam, J., *Nursing the Image: Media, Culture and Professional Identity* (London: Routledge, 2000).

Hart, C., *Behind the Mask: Nurses, their Unions and Nursing Policy* (London: Baillière Tindall, 1994).

—, *Nurses and Politics: The Impact of Power and Practice* (Basingstoke: Palgrave Macmillan, 2004).

Hawkins, S., *Nursing and Women's Labour in the Nineteenth Century: The Quest for Independence* (Abingdon: Routledge, 2010).

Hazard, M., *Sixty Years A Nurse* (London: HarperElement, 2015).

Hegarty, P., *Peadar O'Donnell* (Cork: Mercier Press, 1999).

Henry, H., *A History of the Irish Guild of Catholic Nurses: Seventy-Five Years of Service, 1922–97* (Dublin: Irish Guild of Catholic Nurses, 1998).

Hensey, B., *The Health Services of Ireland* (4th edn, Dublin: Institute of Public Administration, 1988).

Hill, J.R. (ed.), *A New History of Ireland, Vol. VII, 1921–84* (Oxford: Oxford University Press, 2003).

Hirsch, S. and L. van der Walt (eds), *Anarchism and Syndicalism in the Colonial and Post-Colonial World, 1870–1940* (Leiden: Brill, 2010).

Hyman, R., *Strikes* (2nd edn, Glasgow: Fontana/Collins, 1977).

Inglis, T., *Moral Monopoly, The Rise and Fall of the Catholic Church in Modern Ireland* (2nd edn, Dublin: University College Dublin Press, 1998).

Johnstone, M.J., *Bioethics: A Nursing Perspective* (5th edn, Chatswood: Elsevier, 2009).

Jones, M., *These Obstreperous Lassies: A History of the Irish Women Workers' Union* (Dublin: Gill and Macmillan, 1988).

Kearns, K.C., *Ireland's Arctic Siege: The Big Freeze of 1947* (Dublin: Gill and Macmillan, 2011).

Kiely, E. and M. Leane, *Irish Women at Work, 1930–60: An Oral History* (Sallins: Irish Academic Press, 2012).

Kimmel, M.S., *The Gendered Society* (2nd edn, New York: Oxford University Press, 2004).

Kostick, C., *Revolution in Ireland: Popular Militancy, 1917–23* (London: Pluto Press, 1996).

Leap, N. and B. Hunter, *The Midwife's Tale* (London: Scarlet Press, 1993).

Lee, J.J., *Ireland, 1912–85: Politics and Society* (Cambridge: Cambridge University Press, 1989).

Lewenhak, S., *Women and Trade Unions: An Outline History of Women in the British Trade Union Movement* (London: Ernest Benn, 1977).

Little, W., H.W. Fowler and J. Coulson, *The Shorter Oxford English Dictionary on Historical Principles* (London: Oxford University Press, 1944).

Logan, J. (ed.), *Teachers' Union: The TUI and its Forerunners in Irish Education, 1899–1994* (Dublin: A. and A. Farmar, 1999).

Mac Lellan, A., *Dorothy Stopford Price: Rebel Doctor* (Sallins: Irish Academic Press, 2014).

Maguire, M., *Servants to the Public: A History of the Local Government and Public Services Union, 1901–90* (Dublin: Institute of Public Administration for IMPACT, 1998).

—, *The Civil Service and the Revolution in Ireland, 1912–38: 'Shaking the Blood-Stained Hand of Mr Collins'* (Manchester: Manchester University Press, 2008).

—, *Scientific Service: A History of the Union of Professional and Technical Civil Servants, 1920–90* (Dublin: Institute of Public Administration for IMPACT, 2010).

Malcolm, E. and G. Jones (eds), *Medicine, Disease and the State in Ireland, 1650–1940* (Cork, Cork University Press, 1999).

McCarthy, C., *Trade Unions in Ireland, 1894–1960* (Dublin: Institute of Public Administration, 1977).

—, *Elements in a Theory of Industrial Relations* (Dublin: Irish Academic Press, 1984).

—, *Cumann na mBan and the Irish Revolution* (Cork: The Collins Press, 2007).

McCormick, E., *The INTO and the 1946 Teachers' Strike* (Dublin: The Irish National Teachers' Organisation, 1996).

McGann, S., *The Battle of the Nurses* (London: Scutari Press, 1992).

—, A. Crowther and R. Dougall, *A History of the Royal College of Nursing, 1916–90: A Voice for Nurses* (Manchester: Manchester University Press, 2009).

McGarry, F., *The Abbey Rebels of 1916* (Dublin: Gill and Macmillan, 2015).

Merrigan, M., *Eagle or Cuckoo? The Story of the ATGWU in Ireland* (Dublin: Matmer Publications, 1989).

Millerson, G., *The Qualifying Associations: A Study in Professionalization* (London: Routledge and Kegan Paul, 1964).

Molony, J., *The Worker Question: A New Historical Perspective on Rerum Novarum* (Dublin: Gill and Macmillan, 1991).

Moriarty, T., *Work in Progress: Episodes from the History of Irish Women's Trade Unionism* (Dublin and Belfast: The Irish Labour History Society and UNISON, 1994).

Morrissey, J., B. Keogh and L. Doyle (eds), *Psychiatric/Mental Health Nursing: An Irish Perspective* (Dublin: Gill and Macmillan, 2008).

Munro, A., *Women, Work and Trade Unions* (London: Mansell Publishing, 1999).

Murphy, J., *Bartenders' Association of Ireland: A History* (Dublin: Bartenders' Association of Ireland, 1997).

Nevin, D. (ed.), *Trade Unions and Change in Irish Society* (Dublin: Mercier Press, 1980).

— (ed.), *Trade Union Century* (Cork: Mercier Press, 1994).

Nolan, P., *A History of Mental Health Nursing* (Cheltenham: Stanley Thornes, 1993).

Ó Céirín, K. and C. Ó Céirín, *Women of Ireland* (Kinvara: Tir Eolas, 1996).

O'Connell, T.J., *A History of the Irish National Teachers Organisation, 1868–1968* (Dublin: Irish National Teachers' Organisation, 1970).

O'Connor, E., *Syndicalism in Ireland: 1917–23* (Cork: Cork University Press, 1988).

—, *A Labour History of Ireland: 1824–2000* (Dublin: University College Dublin Press, 2011).

O'Connor, M.E., *Freed to Care, Proud to Nurse: 100 Years of the New Zealand Nurses' Organisation* (Wellington: Steele Roberts Publishers, 2010).

O'Connor, P., *Emerging Voices: Women in Contemporary Irish Society* (Dublin: Institute of Public Administration, 1998).

Ó Drisceoil, D., *Peadar O'Donnell* (Cork: Cork University Press, 2001).

Ó Duigneáin, P., *Linda Kearns: A Revolutionary Irish Woman* (Manorhamilton: Drumlin, 2002).

Ogle, B., *Off the Rails: The Story of ILDA* (Dublin: Currach Press, 2003).

Ó Gráda, C., *A Rocky Road, The Irish Economy Since the 1920s* (Manchester: Manchester University Press, 1997).

Ó Loingsigh, P., *Gobnait Ní Bhruadair* (Baile Átha Cliath: Coiscéim, 1997).

O'Morain, P., *The Irish Association of Directors of Nursing and Midwifery, 1904–2004: A History* (Dublin: The Irish Association of Directors of Nursing and Midwifery, 2004).

—, *The Health of the Nation: The Irish Healthcare System, 1957–2007* (Dublin: Gill and Macmillan, 2007).

Parkes, S.M. (ed.), *A Danger to the Men? A History of Women in Trinity College Dublin: 1904–2004* (Dublin: The Lilliput Press, 2004).

Pavri, J.M., *Honoring Our Past, Building Our Future: A History of the New York State Nurses' Association* (Franklin: Q Publishing, 2000).

Pelling, H., *A History of British Trade Unionism* (3rd edn, Harmondsworth: Penguin, 1976).

Prendergast, E. and H. Sheridan, *Jubilee Nurse: Voluntary District Nursing in Ireland, 1890–1974* (Dublin: Wolfhound Press, 2012).

Price, L., *Dr Dorothy Price: An Account of Twenty Years' Fight Against Tuberculosis in Ireland* (For private circulation only, 1957).

Raw, L., *Striking a Light: the Bryant and May Matchwomen and their Place in Labour History* (London: Continuum Books, 2009).

Redmond, S., *The Irish Municipal Employees Trade Union: 1883–1983* (Dublin: The Irish Municipal Employees' Trade Union, 1983).

Reverby, S.M., *Ordered to Care: The Dilemma of American Nursing, 1850–1945* (Cambridge: Cambridge University Press, 1987).

Richardson, J.E., *Analysing Newspapers: An Approach from Critical Discourse Analysis* (Basingstoke: Palgrave Macmillan, 2007).

Ritchie, D.A., *Doing Oral History* (3rd edn, Oxford: Oxford University Press, 2015).

Robins, J., *Nursing and Midwifery in Ireland in the Twentieth Century: 50 Years of An Bord Altranais (The Nursing Board), 1950–2000* (Dublin: An Bord Altranais, 2000).

Rouse, P. and M. Duncan, *Handling Change: A History of the Irish Bank Officials' Association* (Cork: The Collins Press, 2012).

Ryan, L., *Irish Feminism and the Vote: An Anthology of the* Irish Citizen *Newspaper, 1912–20* (Dublin: Folens, 1996).

Scanlan, P., *The Irish Nurse, A Study of Nursing in Ireland: History and Education, 1718–1981* (Manorhamilton: Drumlin Publications, 1991).

Smithson, A. (ed.), *In Times of Peril: Leaves from the Diary of Nurse Linda Kearns from Easter Week 1916 to Mountjoy 1921* (Dublin: The Talbot Press, 1922).

—, *Myself – and Others* (Dublin: The Talbot Press, 1944).

Steele, K., *Women, Press, and Politics During the Irish Revival* (New York: Syracuse University Press, 2007).

Strachan, G., *Labour of Love: The History of the Nurses' Association in Queensland, 1860–1950* (St Leonards: Allen and Unwin, 1996).

Sweeney, G., *In Public Service: A History of the Public Service Executive Union, 1890–1990* (Dublin: Institute of Public Administration, 1990).

Swift, J., *History of the Dublin Bakers and Others* (Dublin: Irish Bakers', Confectionery and Allied Workers' Union, 1948).

Thompson, P., *The Voice of the Past, Oral History* (Oxford: Oxford University Press, 1978).

Tweedy, H., *A Link in the Chain: the Story of the Irish Housewives' Association, 1942–92* (Dublin: Attic Press, 1992).

Vicinus, M., *Independent Women: Work and Community for Single Women, 1850–1920* (London: Virago Press, 1985).

Von Prondzynski, F. and W. Richards, *European Employment and Industrial Relations Glossary: Ireland* (London: Sweet and Maxwell, 1994).

Wallace, J., P. Gunnigle, G. McMahon and M. O'Sullivan, *Industrial Relations in Ireland* (4th edn, Dublin: Gill and Macmillan, 2013).

Walsh, O., *Anglican Women in Dublin: Philanthropy, Politics and Education in the Early Twentieth Century* (Dublin: University College Dublin Press, 2005).

Ward, M., *Unmanageable Revolutionaries, Women and Irish Nationalism* (London: Pluto Press, 1983).

Webb, S. and B. Webb, *The History of Trade Unionism* (New edn, London: Longmans, Green and Company, 1911).

Whelan, B. (ed.), *Women and Paid Work in Ireland, 1500–1930* (Dublin: Four Courts Press, 2000).

Whyte, J.H., *Church and State in Modern Ireland, 1923–79* (2nd edn, Dublin: Gill and Macmillan, 1980).

Wren, M.A., *Unhealthy State: Anatomy of a Sick Society* (Dublin: New Island, 2003).

Yeates, P., *Lockout, Dublin 1913* (Dublin: Gill and Macmillan, 2000).

—, *A City in Wartime: Dublin, 1914–18* (Dublin: Gill and Macmillan, 2011).

Newspapers

Anglo-Celt
Bean na h-Éireann
Clare Champion
Connacht Tribune
Connaught Telegraph
Evening Herald

Evening Telegraph
Freeman's Journal
Irish Citizen
Irish Daily Mail
Irish Independent
Irish Press
Irish Times
Kerryman
Kildare Observer
Leitrim Observer
Limerick Leader
Munster Express
Nenagh Guardian
Northern Standard
Sunday Business Post
Sunday Independent
Sunday Tribune
Weekly Irish Times

Journals, Periodicals and Circulars

American Journal of Nursing
American Journal of Sociology
Archivium Hibernicum
British Journal of Nursing
European Journal of Women's Studies
Industrial and Labor Relations Review
International Journal of Nursing Studies
Irish Nurse
Irish Nurses' and Midwives' Union Members' Circular
Irish Nurses' Journal
Irish Nurses' Magazine
Irish Nurses' Union Gazette
Irish Nursing and Hospital World
Irish Nursing News
Journal of Advanced Nursing
Journal of the Statistical and Social Inquiry Society of Ireland
Journal of Women's History
Labour History

Labour/Le Travail
The Lancet
Nurse Education Today
Nursing Ethics
Nursing History Review
Nursing Inquiry
Nursing Research
Political Studies
Saothar
Sociological Review
Studies
Translocations: Migration and Social Change
Women's History Review
World of Irish Nursing

Unpublished Sources

Bashford-Synnott, M., 'Annie M.P. Smithson: romantic novelist/revolutionary nurse, a literary biography' (Dublin: University College Dublin, 2000).

Bates, D., 'Keepers to nurses? A history of the Irish Asylum Workers' Trade Union, 1917–24' (Dublin: University College Dublin, 2010).

Buckley, A., 'Delia Larkin and the founding of the Irish Women Workers' Union' (Dublin: Trinity College, 1996).

Fealy, G.M., 'A history of the provision and reform of general nurse education and training in Ireland, 1879–1994' (Dublin: University College Dublin, 2002).

Ferriter, D., '"A peculiar people in their own land" Catholic social theory and the plight of rural Ireland, 1930–55' (Dublin, University College Dublin, 1996).

Horgan Ryan, S., 'The development of nursing in Ireland, 1898–1920' (Cork: University College Cork, 2004).

Loughrey, M., 'A history of the Irish Nurses' Organisation, 1919–99' (Dublin: University College Dublin, 2015).

Madden, P.J., 'The unionateness of the Irish Nurses' Organisation: The formation of a working trade union for nurses, 1978–90' (Keele: University of Keele, 1991).

Marie, G., 'Women in union' (Dublin: University College Dublin, 1995).

McMahon, E.A., 'The regulation of midwives with special reference to aspects of the regulation of midwives in Ireland, 1918–50' (Dublin, University College Dublin, 2000).

Legislation, European Union Directives and Labour Court Recommendations

Midwives (Ireland) Act (1918)
Nurses Registration (Ireland) Act (1919)
Garda Síochána Act (1924)
Local Government Act (1925)
Midwives Act (1931)
Local Government Act (1941)
Trade Union Act (1941)
Industrial Relations Act (1946)
Health Act (1947)
Nurses Act (1950)
Health Act (1953)
Health Act (1970)
Anti-Discrimination (Pay) Act (1974)
Council Directive 77/453/EEC of 27 June 1977
Health (Family Planning) Act (1979)
Nurses Act (1985)
Labour Court Recommendation 15450 (7 March 1997)
Labour Court Recommendation 16083 (9 February 1999)
Labour Court Recommendation 16084 (9 February 1999)
Labour Court Recommendation 16261 (31 August 1999)
Labour Court Recommendation 16330 (27 October 1999)
Labour Court Recommendation 18763 (9 November 2006)
Financial Emergency Measures in the Public Interest Act (2009)
European Court of Human Rights, *Enerji Yapi-Yol Sen v. Turkey* (Application no: 68959/01)
Council Directive 2010/32/EU of 10 May 2010
Nurses Act (2011)
Electoral (Amendment) (Political Funding) Act (2012)
Criminal Law (Sexual Offences) Act (2017)

Reports, Government/Official Publications and Corporate Authorships

An Bord Altranais, *Code for Nurses* (Dublin: An Bord Altranais, 1985).
An Bord Altranais, *The Code of Professional Conduct for Each Nurse and Midwife* (Dublin: An Bord Altranais, 1988).

An Bord Altranais, *The Future of Nurse Education and Training in Ireland* (Dublin: An Bord Altranais, 1994).

An Bord Altranais, *Submission to the Commission on Nursing* (Dublin: An Bord Altranais, 1997).

An Bord Altranais, *Review of Scope of Practice for Nursing and Midwifery* (Dublin: An Bord Altranais, 2000).

An Bord Altranais and the National Council for the Professional Development of Nursing and Midwifery, *Review of Nurses and Midwives in the Prescribing and Administration of Medicinal Products* (Dublin: An Bord Altranais and the National Council for the Professional Development of Nursing and Midwifery, 2005).

An Bord Altranais/Nursing and Midwifery Board of Ireland, *Annual Reports.*

W. Beveridge, *Social Insurance and Allied Services* (London: His Majesty's Stationery Office, 1942).

Committee on the Future of Healthcare, *Sláintecare Report* (Dublin: Houses of the Oireachtas, 2017).

Crowe Horwath, *Final Report to Nursing and Midwifery Board of Ireland, Organisation Review* (Dublin: Crowe Horwath, 2015).

Deloitte and Touche, *Value for Money Audit of the Irish Health System, Main Report* (Dublin: The Department of Health and Children, 2001).

Department of Health, *Report of the Working Party on General Nursing* (Dublin: The Stationery Office, 1980).

Department of Industry and Commerce/Central Statistics Office, Census of Population: 1926; 1936; 1946; 1951; 1961; 1966; 1971; 1981; 1986.

Dublin Trades Union and Labour Council, *Report of Irish Labour Delegation to Union of Socialist Soviet Republics* (Dublin: Dublin Trades Union and Labour Council, 1929).

R. Francis, *Report of the Mid Staffordshire NHS Foundation Trust Public Inquiry, Executive Summary* (London: The Stationery Office, 2013).

Government of Ireland, *The Health Services and their Further Development* (Dublin: The Stationery Office, 1966).

Government of Ireland, *Outline of the Future Hospital System: Report of the Consultative Council on the General Hospital Services* (Dublin: The Stationery Office, 1968).

Government of Ireland, *Report of the Commission on the Status of Women* (Dublin: Stationery Office, 1972).

Government of Ireland, *Programme for Competitiveness and Work* (Dublin: The Stationery Office, 1994).

Government of Ireland, *Report of the Commission on Nursing* (Dublin: The Stationery Office, 1998).

E. Hanrahan, *A Social Study of the Training and Career Aspirations of Final Year Student Nurses* (Dublin: Irish Matrons' Association, 1971).

Independent External Evaluation Team, *Nurse Education and Training Evaluation in Ireland* (Southampton: University of Southampton, 1998).

The Independent Labour Party and Labour Research Department, *Trade Unions in Soviet Russia* (London: The Independent Labour Party and Labour Research Department, 1920).

International Labour Office, *Employment and Conditions of Work of Nurses* (Geneva: International Labour Office, 1960).

Irish Housewives' Association, *The Irish Housewife: The Irish Housewives' Association Yearbook* (Dublin: Irish Housewives' Association, 1948).

Irish Nurses' Organisation, *Irish Nurses' Organisation Souvenir Book* (Dublin: Irish Nurses' Organisation, 1947).

Irish Nurses' Organisation, *50th Anniversary Souvenir Book* (Dublin: Irish Nurses' Organisation, 1969).

Irish Nurses' Organisation, *Submission to the Commission on Nursing* (Dublin: Irish Nurses' Organisation, 1997).

Irish Nurses' Organisation, *Forming EU Healthcare Policy, A Showcase of Irish Involvement* (Dublin: Irish Nurses' Organisation, 2007).

Irish Nurses' Organisation, *Celebrating 90 Years of Growth: 1919–2009* (Dublin: Irish Nurses' Organisation, 2009).

Irish Nurses' and Midwives' Organisation, *Submission to the Public Service Pay Commission* (Dublin: Irish Nurses' and Midwives' Organisation, 2017).

Irish Nurses' Organisation/Irish Nurses' and Midwives' Organisation, *Annual Reports*.

P.R. Kaim-Caudle and J.G. Byrne, *Irish Pension Schemes, 1969* (Dublin: Economic and Social Research Institute, 1971).

J. McGowan, *Attitude Survey of Irish Nurses* (Dublin: Institute of Public Administration, 1979).

Ministry of Health, *First Report of Nurses' Salaries Committee, Salaries and Emoluments of Female Nurses in Hospitals* (London: HMSO, 1943).

Ministry of Health, *Report of the Committee on Senior Nursing Staff Structure* (London: HMSO, 1966).

The Nursing Alliance, *Submission to the Benchmarking Body* (Dublin: Nursing Alliance, 2001).

D.P. O'Donovan, *The Commission of Investigation into Leas Cross Nursing Home, Final Report* (Dublin: Department of Health, 2009).

Paul VI, *Humanae Vitae* (Rome: 1968).

Pius XI, *Quadragesimo Anno* (Rome: 1931).

Public Service Pay Commission, *Report of the Public Service Pay Commission* (Dublin: Public Service Pay Commission, 2017).

South Eastern Health Board, *The History of the South Eastern Health Board, 1971– 2004* (Kilkenny: The Health Service Executive, 2005).

B. Tierney, *Stress in Irish Nursing* (Dublin: An Bord Altranais, 1988).

Archives

Cork City and County Archives, Cork.

Dublin Diocesan Archives, Dublin.

Irish Nurses' and Midwives' Organisation Archives and Library, Dublin.

Irish Labour History Society Archives, Dublin.

James Hardiman Library Archives, Galway.

Military Archives, Dublin.

The National Archives, Kew, England.

The National Archives of Ireland, Dublin.

Nursing and Midwifery Board of Ireland Archives, Dublin.

Miscellaneous

Dáil Éireann Debate transcripts.

Seanad Éireann Debate transcripts.

Joint Committee on Health and Children Debate transcripts.

Abbreviations

DCU:	Dublin City University
EEC:	European Economic Community
ICN:	International Council of Nurses
ICPSA:	Irish Conference of Professional and Service Associations
ICTU:	Irish Congress of Trade Unions
ICU:	Intensive Care Unit
IHA:	Irish Housewives' Association
ILO:	International Labour Office
IMPACT:	Irish Municipal, Public and Civil Trade Union
INMO:	Irish Nurses' and Midwives' Organisation
INO:	Irish Nurses' Organisation
INU:	Irish Nurses' Union
ITGWU:	Irish Transport and General Workers' Union
ITUC:	Irish Trade Union Congress
IWWU:	Irish Women Workers' Union
MEP:	Member of the European Parliament
NHS:	National Health Service (United Kingdom)
NMBI:	Nursing and Midwifery Board of Ireland
NUIG:	National University of Ireland, Galway
NUIM:	National University of Ireland, Maynooth
PLAC:	Pro-Life Amendment Campaign
PNA:	Psychiatric Nurses' Association
RCSI:	Royal College of Surgeons, Ireland
SEN:	State Enrolled Nurse
SIPTU:	Services, Industrial, Professional and Technical Union
TCD:	Trinity College, Dublin
UCD:	University College, Dublin
WUI:	Workers' Union of Ireland

Index

Note: Page locators in italics refer to pictures and illustrations.

and a 40-hour week in 1970, 179–82,
181–2
Prunty, Mary, *123*
psycho-prophylactic method of childbirth,
the, 113, *114*
Public Health Bill (1945), 97–8
public health nurses, 87, *126*, 126–8, 138, 154,
160, 214, 238, *251*
public health provision, 131, 132
Public Hospitals Bill (1933), 61–4
Public Sector Pay Commission, the, 291–2
public sector pay freeze, the, 282
puerperal sepsis, 36–7

Quadregesimo Anno (Papal Encyclical), 101–3
Quinn, Sheila, 141, 159, 162

rationing, 74
RCN (Royal College of Nursing), 140, 147,
196, 200
RCSI (Royal College of Surgeons, Ireland),
26, 190
recruitment ads, *173–4*
recruitment embargo on the health service,
xxi, 213, 283, 285, 291
recruitment to the INU, 19–21
Reeves, Alice, 25–6
refresher courses, 77, *78*, *98*, 98–9, 149, 156,
162, *188*
Reidy, Margaret, 101, *102*
Report of the Commission on Nursing (1997),
228, 299
*Report of the Commission on the Status of
Women*, 175, 211
*Report of the Irish Free State Hospitals'
Commission*, 68, 73, 89
*Report of the Working Party on General
Nursing*, 214, 269
Rerum Novarum (Papal Encyclical), 125, 132
Retired Members' Section, INO, *156*
reversal of health services cuts, xxv, 291
*Review of Scope of Practice for Nursing and
Midwifery*, 252
Richmond Hospital, the, xi, *39*, 189, 219, 258,
299–300, *301*

RN4CAST project, the, 298
Rogers, Kelvin, 79
Royal City of Dublin Hospital, Baggot Street,
10, 16, *253*
*Rushcliffe Report (First Report of Nurses'
Salaries Committee)*, the, 85
Russell, George, 2
Ryan, Dr James, 90, 93, 98, 103–5

salary scales and increments, 87, 105, 135,
138–9, 176–7, 182, 225–6, 227, 229, 243,
251, 291; and standardised scales, 29, 74,
85, 86–7, 95
*Salmon Report (Report of the Committee on
Senior Nursing Staff Structures)*, the, 157
scientific method of nursing work, the, 162,
191–2, 214–15, 217
Second World War, the, 73, 95
secondments for student nurses, 189
sections (INO member subgroups), 125–8,
128, 129, *129*, 131, *148*, 149, *156*, 157,
160, 287–8
SEN (State Enrolled Nurse) grade, 160, 161
senior nurse staffing in Britain, 157
service-obligations to patients and strike
action, 125, 235–6, 239, 278, 308, 311;
and Annie Smithson on, 57–8; and
impact on negotiating leverage, 46,
138, 245; and incompatibility with their
professional status, 23, 24, 56, 185, 241
Shelly, J., 22
Sheridan, Jean, 74–6
Shields, Adolphus, 16
Shields, Arthur, 18
shift work, 193
Sinn Féin, 33
SIPTU (Services, Industrial, Professional and
Technical Union), 224, 225, 232
Sister Lauras Food, *30*
Sláintecare Report, the, 295
Sligo General Hospital, 246–7
Smithson, Annie, 48, *57*, 57–8, *64*, 81, 83,
109–10, 124–5, 245; as INO Secretary,
70–3, *71*; and sweepstakes fundraising,
59, 60; writing talents of, 48, 66, 86, 92